Contents

Rehabilitation in adult nursing practice

Edited by

Mike Smith MSc RGN

Senior Lecturer, Faculty of Health, South Bank University, London

Foreword by

Fred Middleton FRCP

Consultant in Rehabilitation Medicine, Clinical Director,
Spinal Injuries Unit, Royal National Orthopaedic Hospital Trust,
Stanmore, Middlesex

CHURCHILL
LIVINGSTONE

EDINBURGH LONDON NEW YORK PHILADELPHIA SYDNEY TORONTO 1999

CHURCHILL LIVINGSTONE
An imprint of Harcourt Brace and Company Limited

© Harcourt Brace and Company Limited 1999

⚓ is a registered trademark of Harcourt Brace and Company Limited

First published 1999

ISBN 0443 06012 6

British Library Cataloguing in Publication Data
A catalogue record for this book is available from the British Library.

Library of Congress Cataloging in Publication Data
A catalog record for this book is available from the Library of Congress

Note
Medical knowledge is constantly changing. As new information becomes available, changes in treatment, procedures, equipment and the use of drugs become necessary. The editors, contributors and the publishers have, as far as it is possible, taken care to ensure that the information given in this text is accurate and up-to-date. However readers are strongly advised to confirm that the information, especially with regard to drug usage, complies with the latest legislation and standards of practice.

C2126563

The
publisher's
policy is to use
**paper manufactured
from sustainable forests**

Printed in China
NPCC/01

Contributors

Deborah Barnett BSc(Hons) RNT
Lecturer in Health Studies,
Edge Hill University College, Ormskirk, Lancashire

Peter Davis MA BEd(Hons) CertEd RN DN(Lond) ONC
Principal Lecturer,
South Bank University, London

Kathleen P Dean BA RGN DipN(Lond) CertEd
Senior Lecturer (Orthopaedic, trauma and spinal lesions nursing),
South Bank University, London

Amanda Pearson RGN
Rehabilitation Process Coordinator, Trauma and Rehabilitation
Directorate, Leicester Royal Infirmary NHS Trust, Leicester

Anne Seaman RN DRSN BSc(Hons)
Lecturer Practitioner in Spinal Cord Injury,
The Duke of Cornwall Spinal Treatment Centre,
Salisbury District Hospital, Salisbury, and
Institute of Health and Community Studies,
Bournemouth University, Bournemouth

Jo Seymour MSc RGN
Ward Manager, Hume Unit,
Ryehope General Hospital,
City Hospitals, Sunderland

Mike Smith MSc RGN
Senior Lecturer, South Bank University,
Nurse Education Department,
Royal National Orthopaedic Hospital,
Stanmore, Middlesex

Paul Street MSc BSc(Hons) DipN(Lond) RGN EN
Practice Development Nurse,
Greenwich Healthcare Trust and
The University of Greenwich, London

David Thomas MSc RGN
Rehabilitation Nurse Specialist,
formerly Spinal Unit,
Royal National Orthopaedic Hospital,
Stanmore, Middlesex

Sylvie Thorn RGN DipN BSc(Hons)
Nurse Research and Development Coordinator,
Rivermead Rehabilitation Centre, Oxford

Susan Tripp EN RGN MSc CertPCAT
Clinical Nurse Specialist,
Rehabilitation Unit,
Royal National Orthopaedic Hospital,
Stanmore, Middlesex

Greg Wain BSc RGN RMN
Clinical Nurse Manager (Tissue Viability),
Royal National Orthopaedic Hospital,
Stanmore, Middlesex

Foreword

Historically in the UK, rehabilitation has been perceived as something carried out by other people, usually somewhere else. The location of the rehabilitation centres, most of them away from general hospitals or indeed even urban areas, promoted this view. For most professionals, rehabilitation was a rather remote and poorly understood process.

In the early 1970s, Royal Commissions under Tonbridge and Mayer attempted to raise the profile of rehabilitation, both by emphasising the physical, psychological and social parameters of the process and by attempting to promote the subject within district general hospitals. They emphased that the majority of patients have need of rehabilitation following illness or injury and that all specialties and disciplines should be involved. As a result, during the later 1970s and the 1980's there was considerable development of services for the management of people with disabilities, particularly in the community, and enthusiasm for multi-disciplinary teams. In most instances, however, within the district general hospital the only tangible change was the alteration of the signs over the physiotherapy unit from 'Physiotherapy' to 'Rehabilitation', supporting the ward medical and nursing view that rehabilitation was still something which went on somewhere else, carried out by other people, albeit more locally.

More recently the profile of rehabilitation has been raised through greater recognition of the extent of disability throughout society, its massive cost and the suspicion that much of it is unnecessary.

This increasing interest is also driven by other factors, not least of which are the expectations of patients. Even those with the most serious disability quite rightly retain expectations of returning to the community, or returning to work, indeed of regaining a significant place in society, not fundamentally different from their pre-injury or illness aspirations. Support for these expectations is given by information disseminated through newspapers, television and increasingly via the internet. The understanding of many within society of the potential of micro-processor technology, genetic manipulation or rehabilitation engineering is far beyond what is provided in reality. The realisation that rehabilitation is primarily a learning experience is gradually spreading.

The traditional perceived role of nursing providing care for those who are sick or injured seems to be at odds with the basic concept of rehabilitation promoting independence. Indeed, it is suggested that medical and nursing aspects of health care lead to dependency and a culture of helplessness, and that the recovery process involves procedures being done to patients rather than patients becoming involved in an active process which requires considerable work on their part. The idea that nurses cannot assist people through this process is not supportable. In practical terms, it should be noted that most of the discharge planning which has been developed within general hospitals over the last decade has been carried out by nurses.

More difficult may be the patient's perception of the nurse as someone in the health care system who is on the patient's side, somehow collaborating against the doctors, therapists and others who are making interventions to try to cure the illness or injury. This nurse's roles of both carer and advocate/supporter may be seen by other members of the rehabilitation team as incompatible with being a primary member of that team.

To confine the nurse to the caring role is to diminish the nursing profession. In addition to care, there is no doubt that many nurses have enormous skills in providing education, psychological support and indeed medical expertise and knowledge which are the essential components of rehabilitation. The skills and roles required within the interdisciplinary rehabilitation team may be apparent, but argument and uncertainty remain as to the allocation of these roles among the different disciplines. The reality is that the vast majority of the roles can be fulfilled by the vast majority of the team members and it is only in areas of specific techniques (e.g. intravenous therapy, low bath techniques for spasticity, wheelchair prescription) that the individual skills of particular disciplines become involved.

There is a tendency for nurses to become the natural leaders within the rehabilitation team where they are fully involved and hence their predominance in the roles of key worker or case manager. If nurses are to play these roles to their full potential it is essential that their understanding of the rehabilitation process, the conceptual approaches, the technical issues and the potential interventions must be fully developed.

Many believe that the key worker or case manager concept will further develop and become increasingly important within many specialties, such as cardiology, oncology, neurology. This book, which sets out so comprehensively the concepts of rehabilitation and the roles that nursing could and should play within it, is very timely and it is hoped that it will be read not only by those already working within designated rehabilitation services, but also by those who work in district general hospitals, in the community and in health care generally.

1999   FRI Middleton

Preface

Rehabilitation nursing occurs in any specialty or clinical environment where the aim is to minimise disability and handicap in clients with particular impairments. There are, therefore, few adult nursing practice environments in which rehabilitation is not taking place – this book is designed to be applicable to the majority of these practice areas.

Traditionally, nurses in rehabilitation environments, unlike their colleagues in other areas, have found it difficult to define their roles and to actively influence practice. This text presents six key roles for nurses, illustrating that nursing has practice roles that should be clearly defined and valued. Unless nurses perform these roles, optimal outcomes for clients will not be achieved. The clear definition of these roles will enable nurses to contribute and respond to changes in health care systems, client needs and the socio-political climate.

In a format and language appropriate for qualified rehabilitation nurses, this text aims to provide the reader with information that can be applied to practice, including:

- assessment of client needs
- frameworks to enable development of nursing programmes and systems to meet client needs
- clear rationale and explanations for such systems
- criteria against which programmes and systems can be evaluated
- information relating to other resources available to provide additional knowledge.

In those sections that deal with theory, a link is made to the practice of the rehabilitation nurse.

The lack of a clear general rehabilitation nursing text has been detrimental not only to nurses in this area but also to the clients for whom they provide services. I hope that this text will, in some way, address this problem.

MS, 1999

The nature of rehabilitation

Mike Smith

1

INTRODUCTION

In starting this exploration into rehabilitation in adult nursing practice we must begin with an examination of the very nature of the term rehabilitation. It is only then we can investigate the roles of nursing, and the specific elements of those roles, within rehabilitation.

This chapter will aim to shed light on the basic underpinning concept of rehabilitation through identifying the common threads and principles that run through rehabilitation in whichever speciality it is deemed to take place.

The premise on which this book is based is that rehabilitation occurs across many specialities. It is rather unfortunate that the majority of the literature on rehabilitation appears to be related to neurological, spinal cord injury and elderly care, which may have influenced the thinking that other specialities would not benefit from the approaches used. Within this text I would wish to challenge this presumption. Although practical application in each clinical nursing practice area will obviously be different, as indeed it is within the rehabilitation 'specialities' above, it is worth emphasising that these principles *are* transferable to all specialities. Examples of specialities that have more recently embraced a greater use of rehabilitation principles, particularly in the USA and increasingly within the UK, are the areas of cardiac rehabilitation following myocardial infarction, and pulmonary rehabilitation following respiratory disease. It must be equally valid to classify as rehabilitation the process of an individual coming to terms with and learning to manage diabetes mellitus, or ongoing renal dialysis. One could surely also describe as rehabilitation the interventions required by a woman following mastectomy, which may include education, psychological support during adjustment, and an exercise programme to prevent limitation of physical functioning in the arm on the affected side.

This chapter is designed to take the reader through a step-by-step examination of the principles involved in rehabilitation, and is split into four distinct sections. The first section explores the aims and characteristics of rehabilitation. These characteristics will be defined and examined, thus enabling the reader to examine his own practice area against these characteristics. The place of rehabilitation within health care generally is described. In the second section models or frameworks which could be used in a rehabilitation environment are critically analysed. As a result of this analysis a new model is proposed. The third section examines processes perceived as useful within rehabilitation, again encouraging the reader to assess their suitability for use with patients or clients within their clinical area. In the fourth section, the resources required for rehabilitation are briefly discussed, exploring basic concepts of team-working, the location of rehabilitation and financial implications. Finally, in the summary, key points are highlighted to reinforce these concepts.

This approach and order has been chosen because, without a clear description of the aims and expectations relating to outcome of a service, one cannot develop an effective framework or model for rehabilitation services. It is the principles, philosophies and frameworks proposed within this model which will facilitate the development of processes to meet the aims and outcomes of rehabilitation. Once such processes have been defined, the resources required to deliver the processes can be ascertained.

Finally, it is worth emphasising at this point that examination of the service against proposed outcomes and delivery of processes using formal evaluation methods should take place. This will facilitate the refining of aims and processes and demonstrate deficits in resources in order to improve service delivery. Although evaluation of rehabilitation is covered in detail in Chapter 7, I hope that the reader will use the information within this chapter to begin to look at their own practice area.

AIMS AND CHARACTERISTICS OF REHABILITATION

WHAT IS REHABILITATION?

In an attempt to identify both aim and purpose, definitions of rehabilitation have been proposed by numerous authors. There appear to be common identifiable threads that exist across these definitions. Commonly quoted definitions include 'an educational, problem-solving process aimed at reducing disability and handicap' (McGrath & Davies 1992). Whiteneck et al (1992) proposed that the aim of rehabilitation should be the successful return to the life and social activities which society and the client himself expect, through reintegration into the community as independent and productive members of society. The idea of education being fundamental to rehabilitation was also discussed by Anderson (1988), who concluded that use of an educational model is consistent with the components of the rehabilitation process. Such components include relearning of lost skills, the acquisition of new skills and adjustment to the imposed alterations in previous lifestyle. In building upon this idea and discussing the interaction between rehabilitation team members and clients, Schofield (1993) suggested that an educational model also corresponds to the characteristics of the rehabilitation relationship. Such central characteristics should encompass a philosophy and practice of guidance, cooperation and mutual participation between the rehabilitation team and client.

In view of the above, it appears there are key characteristics involved in the aims and expectations of rehabilitation. These are outlined in Box 1.1 and discussed further below.

■ BOX 1.1 Characteristics of rehabilitation

• Reduction of disability and handicap
• Independence
• Empowerment
• Problem-solving
• Client centred
• 'Holistic' approach
• Educational process

Reduction of disability and handicap

The World Health Organisation (WHO) (1980) proposed the international classification of impairment, disability and handicap. This classification is now commonly used in the context of rehabilitation.

Impairment

Impairment can be defined as: 'Loss or abnormality of psychological, physiological or anatomical function or structure'. Disturbance to the person can therefore be thought of as being at organ level. Examples of impairment include blindness, traumatic brain injury, fractured neck of femur and myocardial infarction.

Disability

Disability has been defined as 'a restriction or lack of ability to perform an activity in the manner considered normal for a human being.' Disturbance of function is therefore at the person level (e.g. reduced ability to communicate, walk or dress). It is the focus on reduction of the impairment and its effects on the physical and mental function that appears to be the basis of the so-called 'medical model' of rehabilitation, which has received criticism from many recent authors (Finklestein 1993, French 1993, Oliver, 1987). Such a focus does not reflect the limitations imposed by the society within which an individual lives, and as a result the psychological and social aspects of disability are often only briefly and somewhat inadequately covered within rehabilitation.

Handicap

Handicap has been defined as 'a disadvantage resulting from impairment or disability that limits or prevents the fulfilment of a role which is normal (depending on age, sex and social and cultural factors) for that individual' (WHO 1980), and can be thought of in terms of how an individual is able to function within society. Examples include being able to move around one's own environment and maintaining social activities and relationships.

The classification of handicap, despite the often negative connotations of the actual word, has in recent years become an increasingly popular topic of discussion within rehabilitation. Some would propose that rehabilitation programmes should be based on examination of the effects on the individual's societal functioning of injury or illness, within the six dimensions proposed by the WHO (see Fig. 1.2) (Whiteneck et al 1992). This is discussed in more detail later when rehabilitation models are explored.

Although a significant proportion of handicap is as a result of societal attitudes, an idea commonly expressed by some authors (Finklestein 1993, Oliver 1987, Robinson 1988), entering into this topic more fully is not within the remit of this chapter. However, I would suggest that neither an entirely physical nor an entirely social focus should form the basis of rehabilitation. Instead, the emphasis should be away from the hospital-based rehabilitation programme, which often appears impairment and disability focused (following either a 'medical' or therapy-type 'functional' model), to community living. This may be through positively affecting the ability of an individual to interface as satisfactorily as possible with the environment he chooses to be part of. It is this that is the basis of reducing handicap. This clearly does not, and is not intended to, exempt the political system or society in general from the responsibility for effecting the major changes in attitude, policy and environment that are indisputably required.

Empowerment

Empowerment is the process of an individual becoming more in control of himself and his health and life through mobilisation of appropriate resources to enable his needs to be met. Key characteristics inherent in this process include:

- becoming self-directed, thus taking control
- learning assertiveness, so that control can be facilitated
- a recognition that making mistakes is part of the learning process
- being open to change and proactive in changing one's life.

If rehabilitation professionals are actually going to embrace empowerment fully as an essential underpinning principle for practice and process delivery, a change in perspective incorporating the following four points must be taken on board.

1. Health belongs to the individual. Rehabilitation professionals have a responsibility to promote health in the individual, and as part of this must acknowledge the social influences on health, which should be incorporated within and addressed through any programme of rehabilitation.

2. Individuals have the ability to make decisions for themselves, and should be enabled to do so through the provision of information and assisted where appropriate (as defined by that individual). Provision of such information and assistance must be a key role of rehabilitation professionals.

3. Individuals empower themselves; it cannot be done by rehabilitation professionals. It may be encouraged through promoting a sense of internal control and self-reliance in the individual, and by using and developing

available resources, including an environment and working practices that facilitate this.

4. Rehabilitation professionals should foster an environment of co-operation and partnership with the individual, relinquishing control and the attitude that they know what is best for that individual. This involves the ability to accept as valid the rejection by an individual of their suggestion or assistance. Therefore, relationships between rehabilitation professionals and clients should be seen by both parties as collaborative, neither party being viewed as superior or inferior. Essential to this is the presence of trust, mutual respect and effective negotiation.

It is questionable whether these principles are actually fully applied by rehabilitation team members, if at all, looking at the evidence from their apparent working practices. Applying them most certainly requires a major shift from the traditional beliefs and processes involved in health care to date. The reader is encouraged to examine the above points in relation to his own practice environment, and to examine how many are reflected beyond the lip-service which is often given to empowerment within rehabilitation.

It would be unfair to be over critical, however, as progress seems to have been made. Attitudes are changing, professionals are listening to the voices of those they are there to serve, and the very fact that the concept of empowerment is a topic of discussion is a positive step forward. There does, however, appear to be a significant way to go at this stage before we can state unequivocally that we are enabling empowerment through rehabilitation.

Independence

Independence has been described in broad terms as an individual having the choice of how to live his life within his capacity and means, which takes into account the individual's own values and preferences. There is a clear, direct relationship with the concept of empowerment as discussed above. 'Independence' has been part of healthcare vocabulary for many years, but the author would suggest that a word that so easily seems to slip off the tongue may not be completely addressed either in health care generally or, more specifically, within rehabilitation.

Several dimensions of independence can be discussed, including:

- social independence, i.e. having the power to demand rights of society
- economic independence, i.e. having the ability to provide for oneself and meaningful others
- physical independence, i.e. related to mobility and other daily living activities
- mental independence, i.e. the ability to problem-solve.

There are identifiable similarities between the above dimensions and the dimensions of societal function proposed by the WHO (1980), which are discussed later.

The process of attaining independence is often an arduous one, not only because of the limitations resulting from the interface of the individual (with the effects of an illness or injury) with his community, as previously mentioned, but also because of the further limitations imposed through a rehabilitation environment which does not facilitate concepts of empowerment. Often, a system which is based on medical or allied professional working practices may be imposed. This may have the effect of decreasing the personal decision-making of an individual and removing self-esteem and motivation; and may, in turn, ultimately result in reinforcing an individual's belief that independence is undesirable or even impossible.

Problem-solving

The art of problem-solving is a skill learnt from childhood and developed through life as new experiences and knowledge are taken on by an individual. One could argue that problem-solving is a component of being a person within society (reference has already been made above to the component of mental independence). One must be able to apply one's skills and previous knowledge to new situations. Clearly, coping with an illness or injury often requires a major change in the lifestyle for the individual. Rehabilitation should aim to facilitate and develop further such an individual's problem-solving skills, providing new knowledge and 'training for life' to enable effective decision-making (McGrath & Davies 1992). This is the reason for involving the client in the decision-making processes of his rehabilitation, thereby encouraging the development of problem-solving skills. Additionally, this highlights the role of the rehabilitation professional as facilitator rather than 'dictator'.

Client-centred rehabilitation

Both within healthcare environments and in the literature (Schofield 1993), much has been afforded, in the way of lip-service, to the notion of client-centred or focused care. But true client-centred care involves an environment that enables the individual, facilitating his empowerment and so promoting independence. It cannot be achieved through the work of one or even a group of healthcare professionals, but is a shared responsibility and is only possible through the collaboration and vision of a whole organisation. All services must be geared towards management of individuals as individuals. The focus of attention in philosophical thinking must be shifted from addressing professionally perceived patient problems to meeting client need. Professional and bureaucratic barriers must be removed. In other words, management at local and organisational level, research, audit, team-working, processes, job titles and roles, education, contracting and all affiliated services must be focused on meeting clients' needs resulting from injury or illness. Having experienced the workings of the worlds of rehabilitation practice, management and education, I admittedly find it hard to imagine the existence of such a utopian situation. However, there is surely much that can be achieved by striving to attain such an elusive vision.

The 'holistic' approach

The concept of holism suggests total well-being, which has been defined as 'that state of harmony between mind, body, emotions and spirit in an ever changing environment' (American Holistic Nurses Association 1992). In the literature the term 'holism' is commonly used in the spheres of complementary therapies and nursing and paramedical professions, and this may have contributed to the confusion regarding use of the term (Owen & Holmes 1993). Owen and Holmes have criticised the nursing profession as having a poor understanding of the complexity and meaning of holistic principles and their resulting implications. Although I would agree to an extent with these concerns, it is surely still important that these concepts are promoted. Rehabilitation professionals must, as a whole team, attempt to integrate more fully the ideology of viewing the person as a whole into both rehabilitation theory and practice, rather than adhering to a predominantly systems approach, which these authors imply is currently in existence. It may be unreasonable to expect the junior prastising rehabilitation professional to understand completely the concept of holism, and indeed all of the ever-changing theoretical concepts that underpin health care within the various disciplines. However, it is surely the role of rehabilitation education to contribute to the development of understanding, rather than potentially to alienate developing junior practice-based rehabilitation workers through such criticism, which appears to ignore progress made to date.

It is clear that a truly holistic profession does not and will not exist despite the apparent claims of some rehabilitation authors, particularly those from paramedical and nursing disciplines (Barnitt & Pomeroy 1995, Johnson 1995). Additionally, such authors may inadvertently be promoting the idea of generic rehabilitation therapists or workers. It is right to promote the idea that rehabilitation requires the skills of many disciplines, all of which should contribute to the concept of a holistic approach, but these are provided by a team of professionals. This approach will contribute to synergistic team-working (i.e. produce more than each individual discipline could accomplish on its own). Indeed, it could be suggested that the similarities that exist between the concepts of 'client-focused' rehabilitation and 'holism', and the apparent lack of consensus which surrounds the use of the term holism, perhaps merit scrapping the term entirely from the rehabilitation vocabulary, in order to end once and for all what seems a meaningless debate.

An educational process

Reference has already been made to the suggestion that the principles of rehabilitation and education possess similar characteristics. These similarities may not only be pertinent, but indeed it could be suggested that they are vital in guiding the processes of rehabilitation. Through examination of theories of adult learning one could perhaps positively influence the engagement of a client in a rehabilitation programme. Rogers (1969) proposed key principles of learning, which emphasised the importance of relevance to an individual, participation and involvement by the individual in learning, self-evaluation by the individual, and the absence or minimisation of threat during learning. Knowles (1990) promoted the concept of andragogy (an approach to adult learning), suggesting a contrast with methods used in the teaching of children (pedagogy). Again although written in an educational context the following underlying assumptions seem relevant to rehabilitation.

1. The individual must know why they need to learn something.
2. The concept of self-directed learning, where the individual takes the responsibility for their own learning, is central.
3. Adults have experiences that can serve as a rich resource for learning.
4. Adults' readiness to learn is related to the need to know and do things in real life.
5. This life-centred orientation to learning involves problem-solving and task-centred approaches.
6. Adult motivation to participate in learning is largely internal, being focused, for example, on self-perceived quality of life and self-esteem. Therefore, by ensuring that any rehabilitation programme has at the centre what is important to the individual (this being achieved by transfer of 'power' from the professional), motivation will be increased.

Again, Knowles (1990) and other authors have suggested that certain practices of such facilitators of learning are relevant across any learning situation. Such practices put into a rehabilitation context would suggest that the rehabilitation professional should be involved in:

- developing an environment conducive to adult learning, or rehabilitation in this case
- involving individuals in the mutual planning of rehabilitation programmes
- assisting individuals to diagnose their needs for rehabilitation
- encouraging individuals to form their own rehabilitation objectives
- assisting individuals in identifying resources and strategies for achieving such objectives, so forming a plan
- assisting in the carrying out of such plans
- involving individuals in the evaluation of their rehabilitation.

THE 'EXPERT' PERSPECTIVE

It is somewhat perturbing that there is little evidence of users of rehabilitation services having input into defining the aims, purposes and processes involved in rehabilitation. In recent years the voice of the 'consumers' of health care has undoubtedly become louder. Obvious examples are the introduction of the patients' charter and the plethora of patient satisfaction surveys that seem to be used in significant numbers of National Health Service (NHS) services in an effort to demonstrate quality. However, the author would suggest that these are, at best, frequently methodologically unsound, and often appear to contribute very little to the development of client-focused services.

■ **BOX 1.2 Key factors in rehabilitation**

- Individual differences and needs must be taken into account.
- Rehabilitation, in its broadest context, may take a minimum of 2 years following SCI, depending on the individual.
- Rehabilitation involves the emotional, physical and practical skills needed for living.
- A major, if not dominant, need is emotional rehabilitation.
- Peer support can be invaluable in emotional rehabilitation.
- Goal planning is a useful process.
- It is essential that patients regain control of their lives.
- Individuals must be allowed to take risks.
- Individual needs should dominate over the hospital programme.

Surely the people who have actually been subjected to some of the rehabilitation methods currently employed are in a prime position to make a valid and valuable contribution, and indeed they should actually be perceived as the 'experts' (as they have lived the situation), rather than the professionals. This leads to the question of how we may best find out what the aims of rehabilitation should be from this 'expert' perspective. Such issues are covered in detail in Chapter 7, which discusses the rehabilitation nurse as auditor and how we measure the effectiveness of our care, but it is worth mentioning at this stage a project undertaken at the London Spinal Cord Injury Unit (Smith 1996). Part of the project was to identify what users of that particular service believed were the fundamentals of rehabilitation. The key points are outlined in Box 1.2.

THE PLACE OF REHABILITATION WITHIN HEALTH CARE

It is worth briefly exploring where the concept and principles of rehabilitation fit into the scheme and process of healthcare provision generally. As previously stated, the concepts involved in the term rehabilitation may be perceived as the underlying background in the majority of healthcare situations. As rehabilitation occurs within both hospital and community settings, clearly the exact nature of the process will depend on the individual circumstances, and therefore various entry points to the process must exist. Figure 1.1 illustrates this, indicating three potential entry points depending on what predisposes to the need for rehabilitation, whether a period of hospitalisation is required or whether the individual can remain within their community.

Entry point A may be appropriate should an individual require an elective period of hospitalisation, for example for corrective surgery (e.g. hip replacement) or to engage in a formal rehabilitation programme (e.g. for chronic back pain). Involved in this stage would be optimising the

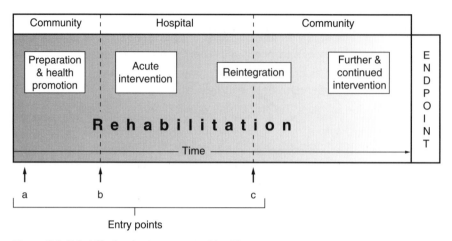

Figure 1.1 Rehabilitation in the context of health care.

health status of the individual, education, clarification and, perhaps, formal planning of what will occur during the following hospitalisation period, and psychological preparation and support related to the imminent intervention. Examples of this in practice include the use of pre-admission clinics, which facilitate this process. Additional social preparation involving arrangements related to work and home circumstances may be made during this period.

Entry point B would be relevant for those who have sustained an acute injury or have acute illness. During the following period, as with those individuals who have entered at point A, the appropriate acute intervention will be actioned and may incorporate so-called 'life-saving' or 'life-improving' procedures. Aspects of rehabilitation will continue to run throughout, as well as after, this period of acute intervention. Examples include preservation of existing function through maintenance exercise, commencement of education relating to living with the consequences of the injury or illness, psychological support of both the individual and meaningful others, and gathering information about the individual's social circumstances to enable an assessment of need to be made. This highlights the requirement for either acute interventions to occur within areas that can subsequently rehabilitate an individual, or clear effective working links to be maintained between areas deemed as acute units and rehabilitation units.

The process of reintegration involves ensuring an effective, successful return of the individual to his community. Although it is perhaps slightly artificial to separate this aspect from rehabilitation generally, it does help to emphasise essential key elements in the interface between hospital and community. These include early, effective discharge planning and involvement and co-working of hospital and community professionals with the patient, thus facilitating a smooth transition between stages and smooth transfer of care. Planning for further interventions and follow-up, if appropriate, should also occur as part of this stage.

Entry point C will be for those for whom rehabilitation is to occur entirely within their own community. As for those clients who have entered at points A and B, the clear advantage of this period is the fact that the environment in which rehabilitation is taking place is entirely realistic. Much of this stage is self-directed, the individual adjusting to a new set of life circumstances and the processes involved in regaining control and independence. Further interventions may be required and may be actioned on a hospital outpatient basis or entirely through community healthcare services.

The time-scale for reaching the endpoint will clearly depend on the specific social, psychological and physical circumstances of the individual. Additionally, it is worth pointing out that, for individuals with chronic conditions, reaching a formal endpoint may take a significant amount of time, and it may not be reached at all, with the necessity of continually using different entry points throughout life.

REHABILITATION MODELS

McFarlane (1986) suggested that a model for nursing 'identifies and defines the factors or phenomena at work in a [nursing] situation'. A model for rehabilitation as a whole should reflect rehabilitation as it occurs in reality, because it has a primary function in assisting all rehabilitation team members and clients to understand their situation and guide practice. Additionally, such a model should be the basis on which rehabilitation processes are devised and delivered, resources determined and utilised, and developments in rehabilitation practices undertaken.

Before exploring models currently utilised in rehabilitation, it seems logical to begin by outlining criteria by which a model should be judged. A model should encompass all aspects of an individual's lifestyle, thus enabling comprehensive services to be developed that meet all aspects of need.

The move to reject impairment and functional models in favour of a more society-focused model not only seems more relevant to the individual, but also ensures that the focus is on the needs of the client rather than on the problems as perceived by professionals. Through this focus a model will match the situation of the individual in the reality of their own life.

In accepting the principles raised previously relating to facilitating empowerment and independence, through decision-making and responsibility being with the individual rather than with the professional, it is essential that any model is 'client-friendly'. Too often, models seem complex and scattered with professional language. Therefore, to allow understanding of, and thus participation in, rehabilitation, models need to be written in the language of the client and have a framework that is simple yet comprehensive.

A related point is that a model should be capable of being understood and used by all members of the rehabilitation team at all levels. It would seem reasonable to assume that if frameworks for rehabilitation are in the language of the client, then they should be understood by professionals.

■ **BOX 1.3 Criteria for developing or appraising a model of rehabilitation**

- Comprehensive
- Relevant to and focused on the needs of the client
- Client-friendly
- Rehabilitation team friendly
- Provides a framework for practice and service development

Finally, a model should provide a framework for practice and clearly guide practice developments by adhering to the principles inherent the model. The key criteria for appraising or developing an appropriate model for rehabilitation are summarised in Box 1.3.

If it is accepted that rehabilitation is a team task and that the practices and processes involved should all be focused on the client, the relevance and usefulness of different models for different disciplines within such a team must be questioned. A model that achieves the goal of usability across all disciplines not only seems to be desirable, but surely would also reduce interdisciplinary misunderstanding, facilitate communication and focus, and provide a clear basis for rehabilitation developments. Although development of such a model may be arduous initially, the potential end result would appear worth the effort. Concerns regarding threat to individual disciplines have no basis in rationale and indeed the clarity which such a model would provide should strengthen the roles of the variety of disciplines and bury the concept of the generic therapist.

Model frameworks which may be used in the rehabilitation context will be outlined and evaluated using the criteria proposed above.

DISABILITY MEASURE BASED MODELS

Methods commonly used in measuring the extent of disability include the Functional Independence Measure (FIM) (Hamilton et al 1987) and the Barthel index (Mahoney & Barthel 1965). These methods include the rating of various self-care activities, which may be used as a basis for rehabilitation. As an example, the self-care activities incorporated in the FIM are listed in Box 1.4.

These reinforce the approach that disability and rehabilitation may often be thought of in terms of the individual being able or unable to successfully perform various physical or mental activities.

A HANDICAP BASED MODEL

As stated previously, assessment of handicap is based on dimensions of societal functioning. The WHO (1980) proposed six such dimensions, as illustrated in Figure 1.2 and described below.

■ **BOX 1.4 The items in the Functional Independence Measure (FIM)**

Self-care
Eating
Grooming
Bathing
Dressing: upper body
Dressing: lower body
Toileting

Sphincter control
Bladder management
Bowel management

Mobility
Transfers:
   Bed, chair, wheelchair
   Toilet
   Bath, shower

Locomotion
Walking or wheelchair
Stairs

Communication
Comprehension
Expression

Social cognition
Social interaction
Problem-solving
Memory

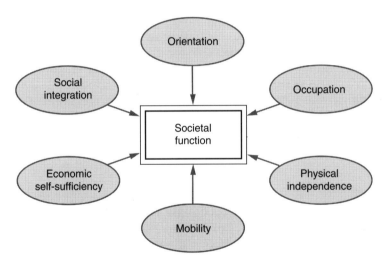

Figure 1.2 The six dimensions of societal functioning.

Physical independence

Physical independence is the ability of an individual to sustain accepted effective existence, and involves the performance of self-care activities and responsibility in directing care effectively to others in order to overcome any physical disability. Clearly, any existing physical consequences of injury may have a pronounced impact on this dimension, but psychological and social factors resulting from these consequences may have just as much effect on whether the client fulfils his potential. Education related to the maintenance of health, and the provision of support in developing assertiveness and problem-solving skills (part of which is the promotion of a rehabilitation environment that facilitates empowerment) are key factors in achieving physical independence. If personal assistance is required, support through the employment of an appropriate person and methods to assist in the maintenance of that relationship seem obvious issues within rehabilitation which may reduce handicap in this dimension.

Mobility

The dimension of mobility concerns the ability of an individual to move about effectively within his environment. It focuses on two main potential handicapping factors in relation to the effects on the individual following illness or injury. First is the amount of time that the client is able to spend outside the immediate environment of his home. Psychological issues following injury, for example altered body image or depression, may be a major factor in an individual's desire to venture out. Clearly, this desire may be influenced by and formed through perceptions of other people's attitudes, and through experiences of interaction with other people in society. Second are the potential limitations on independence caused by limited accessibility of transport. By removing such barriers through the provision of information (e.g. on the possibility of driving, albeit in cars that have adapted controls, and advice relating to travelling abroad), handicap may be reduced. Access to or provision of a personal assistant, who as part of his role is responsible for driving the individual at a time that the individual wishes, would also reduce handicap. In addition, there currently remain major barriers within society itself, such as poor access to buildings and public transport systems. Sensory impairments due to cognitive problems associated with head injury, or a lack of appropriate signs may make successful and safe negotiation of even short journeys difficult, although for obviously different reasons.

Occupation

The ability of an individual to occupy his time in a manner related to his age, gender and culture relates to the dimension of occupation. As well as formal employment, aspects of this dimension may include schooling, home-making, home maintenance, volunteer work, recreation and sports activities, and self-improvement activities. Problems with employment following major physical disability have been well documented in the literature, which consistently seems to emphasise poor statistics relating to return to work. Rehabilitation within this dimension may include effective formal employment rehabilitation, the use of 'buddies' through the voluntary sector or the employment of a paid personal assistant. Although these measures may prove to be successful to some degree, the attitudinal barriers from potential employers towards people with physical disabilities may well be part of, or indeed the major handicapping factor in this dimension. The impact of formal employer training may help to reduce these barriers, and may be an important part of such employment rehabilitation programmes.

Social integration

The dimension of social integration is commonly heavily impacted upon by the effects of chronic illness or disability. It encompasses the participation in and maintenance of accepted social activities and relationships. As well as romantic and sexual relationships, relationships with family, friends, and business or work colleagues may be affected. In the case of traumatic brain injury (TBI), for example, there are many reports in the literature that focus on the effects on the relatives of the characteristics which their spouse, partner or family member who has sustained TBI may exhibit. Any such situation may be exacerbated, creating further strain on the existing relationship, if a relative or partner is the main carer of the person with a physical disability. The person rehabilitating following myocardial infarction (MI) may exhibit a dramatic change in social behaviour due to the fear of recurrent MI in the home situation, and may have major concerns regarding re-engaging in sexual activity with his or her partner. Social interaction with work and business colleagues depends to some degree on the individual's ability and opportunity to return to work, as discussed above. Closely related to all the above factors and also included within this dimension is initiation of conversations, and communication with others by telephone or writing. The general attitude of society to people with disabilities does not facilitate social integration, as evidenced by the constant barrage of the apparent unacceptability of physical differences in the media. Involvement of meaningful others within rehabilitation through education and formal support systems may assist reduction of handicap within this dimension, as may input with the individuals themselves. Such input could include formal goal setting in a general life context and psychological support, through the provision of counselling and peer support provided by other people in similar situations.

Economic self-sufficiency

Economic self-sufficiency, a dimension described as the ability of the individual to sustain socio-economic activity and independence (WHO 1980), has a clear link to the occupational dimension, as included within this is the generation of income. Other activities encompass management of personal finances, including purchasing and budgeting. Characteristics such as immaturity, decreased initiative and decreased learning may all have an influence on an individual's performance in the practical aspects of handling money.

Orientation

The dimension of orientation, defined as the ability of the individual to orientate himself to his surroundings, is more difficult to objectify and therefore its measurement is more complex (Whiteneck et al 1992). This dimension may be particularly relevant in those with degrees of sensory handicap and those with cognitive impairments resulting in memory problems. Again, substantial improvements could be made within society itself, for example in the provision of signs that can be read by those with less severe visual impairments. Overall performance and handicap in the other dimensions seems to have been accepted as guidance. If one accepts this as a premise, the interventions designed to minimise handicap in other areas will be of positive influence on this area.

AN AREAS OF NEED MODEL

A programme of rehabilitation based on an 11 areas of need model is used in some spinal cord injury units in the UK. The underpinning principle is one of ensuring that the rehabilitation team addresses all relevant aspects within the life of an individual, so that goals planned within these areas are comprehensive and relevant to the individual.

Physical well-being

Physical well-being refers to aspects of the maintenance of general health relating to the effects of illness or injury on relevant systems of the body. Examples would be management of nutrition, eliminatory functions, joint and muscle function, respiratory function and general fitness.

Accommodation

This dimension addresses the suitability of the individual's home following any physical limitations resulting from injury or illness. With the advent of major disability, a full formal home assessment may be required, adaptions and aids prescribed and their usage taught. Some individuals with more severe disability or complicated social circumstances may require re-housing, and the arrangement of this would be part of this dimension.

Mobility

This incorporates all aspects of the ability of the individual to move around his environment. In addition to aids for walking, wheelchairs and cushions, and exercise programmes that may be needed to use such equipment, aspects of driving and use of public transport would be relevant to this area.

Psychological well-being

Recognising the often major psychological impact on an individual of illness and injury, this area focuses on adaption to living with such effects. This often involves providing the individual with information about where help is available, and arranging such if required.

Finance

Particularly when a change of employment status is necessary or during long periods of sickness, an individual may need assistance in managing the resulting financial implications. Again, often this involves referral to the relevant person for advice, particularly relating to entitlement to state benefits, sick pay and legal advice concerning compensation if required.

Functional independence

This area encompasses the ability to perform daily life activities, which may be made more difficult through the effects of the injury or illness. The focus is on training the individual in new techniques and providing relevant aids to enable them to undertake activities such as washing, dressing, cooking and writing.

Sexuality

The area of sexuality incorporates management of changes in sexual functioning, aspects of fertility and, possibly, relationship counselling. It is rather unfortunate that the area of sexual health seems to have developed a predominant focus on HIV and AIDS, which is clearly a less than comprehensive approach towards this topic. Aspects of sexual health are explored in detail in Chapter 4.

Social reintegration

This area relates to the individual re-establishing his previous lifestyle in terms of previous social roles. Involved in this dimension are roles at home, at work and with friends. This is again particularly relevant in major illness or injury, where a long period of hospitalisation and an inability to return to previous employment may have an impact. A programme of re-establishing contacts during the period of hospital rehabilitation may be used to facilitate reintegration. In addition, a resettlement officer or adult education department may be involved in providing assistance with obtaining alternative employment or retraining, as appropriate.

Family support

Social support networks may be particularly important in some individuals' adaption to illness and injury. Such networks may only be actioned fully if there is a level of understanding regarding the individual's circumstances. In addition, there is a requirement for psychological support for close family in their adjustment.

Self-care and independence

This area relates to the individual regaining responsibility and full control of his life during rehabilitation. Enabling the individual to achieve this may involve the teaching of problem-solving skills, and could involve a stay in a halfway house or a self-care unit as part of the rehabilitation process.

Communication

Obviously, communication may become a major issue with those who have sensory or speech impairments. However, probably more common is the effect of communication problems on social reintegration and psychological well-being, in that an individual may feel inhibited due to a poor self-image. Those with major physical disability may have problems communicating with their environment. Environmental control systems or other aids may be useful in circumventing this.

EVALUATION OF FOUR MODEL FRAMEWORKS

Four potential model frameworks are evaluated here. The elements of the first three of these have been described above.

- Disability based model. As described above, a framework can be developed on the basis of the elements incorporated in an outcome measure (e.g. FIM) (Hamilton et al 1987).
- Handicap based model. As described above, this is based on six dimensions of societal function (WHO 1980).
- Eleven areas of need model. As described above.
- Existing healthcare model. An existing model framework currently used in health care and familiar to nursing, for example Activities of Living (Roper et al 1985), could be used.

The features and usability of these four types of model are compared in Table 1.1.

A NEW FRAMEWORK FOR REHABILITATION

In reviewing the above models the author proposes a framework based on the adaptions suggested to the second and third model frameworks. The new framework consists of five dimensions, as illustrated in Figure 1.3. The key elements are described below. The influence and input of nursing within this model framework are discussed in Chapter 2.

Physical health and independence

This could include, for example:

- provision of information and education which facilitates client choice relating to potential methods to promote and maintain health
- demonstration and supervision of practical skills to manage physical aspects of the above
- enabling and assisting the individual in developing the ability to direct others in assisting with care needs

Table 1.1 Comparison of four potential model frameworks

	Model framework basis			
	Disability	Societal function	11 areas of need	Activities of living
Comprehensive	No. Psychological aspects limited, social aspects absent. Focus therefore predominantly on physical ability	Yes, but dimension of orientation appears irrelevant as covered within other elements. Assumed psychological aspects are a common thread	Yes, although perhaps repetitious (e.g. functional independence and mobility, sexuality and psychological well-being)	No. The focus is predominantly on the physical, with no obvious direct link to aspects of living in society
Relevant to and focused on client needs	No, due to limitations. Professional orientation	Yes. Societal living focus	Yes. Needs focused	No, due to limitations
Client-friendly	No, due to professional language and emphasis	No, due to professional language	No, due to possible confusion related to repetition and language. Elements may be difficult to recall	No, due to professional language and emphasis
Rehabilitation team friendly	Yes, language appropriate	Yes, but requires a change in team thinking generally	Possible confusion related to repetition and language. Elements may be difficult to recall	Commonly used in nursing. Although adapted, not whole-team friendly due to limitations
Could provide framework for practice	No, limited	Yes	Yes	No, limited
Usability	No	Adaptions required in language, and inclusion of psychological health	Adaptions required in language and reduction of number of elements to remove potential confusion	No

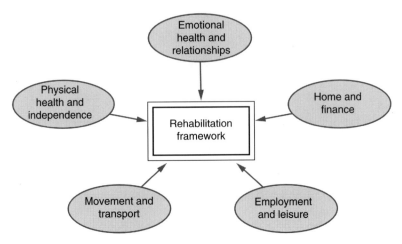

Figure 1.3 A new rehabilitation framework.

- providing training, both to the individual and to personal assistants, in managing the client/assistant relationship.

Emotional health and relationships

This could include, for example:

- supporting and promoting the individual, through all aspects of a rehabilitation programme, in taking responsibility and control for living with his new situation
- offering training in problem-solving, reflection, personal goal setting and assertiveness if desired by the individual
- providing support for the family under the guidance and instruction of the individual
- providing education and support relating to physical aspects of sexual function
- offering support for the psychological aspects of sexuality through provision of counselling, both with and without the partner present
- utilising other individuals in offering 'peer support' and positive role models in the reality of living with the consequences of their illness and disability in today's society.

Movement and transport

This could include, for example:

- Enabling the individual, through physical training and exercise, to safely utilise appropriate (deemed by the client) forms of mobility which are suitable for their lifestyle and environment.
- Offering training in practical skills and, where possible, adapting the individual's social environment in order to minimise the physical limitations imposed by that environment. This should

include training the individual in offering advice and giving information to others to minimise the effects of their environment.

- Providing information and relevant training regarding options related to driving (assisted or non-assisted) and travel, with reference to the identified needs and desired lifestyle of that individual.

Employment and leisure

This could include, for example:

- providing the information required for the individual to make choices regarding employment
- enabling the individual to take up such choices through provision of formal vocational rehabilitation, which may include:
  - setting up appropriate training or re-training programmes through suitable educational establishments
  - working with potential employees to minimise the limitations imposed by the working environment
- providing information and opportunity to enable access to desired sports and recreational activities.

Home and finances

This could include, for example:

- assisting the individual in obtaining accommodation which can either be used immediately or can be adapted to meet their needs
- providing information and advice relating to available benefits and financial management training if desired.

REHABILITATION PROCESSES

GOAL PLANNING IN REHABILITATION

Setting goals is commonplace within education and rehabilitation. Educational psychologists suggest that learning goals should possess particular characteristics in order to facilitate achievement. That is, goals should be 'specific, reasonable, moderately challenging and attainable within a short space of time' (Schunk 1991). These short-term goals should be seen in the context of long-term achievement. It is the ongoing process of identification of, and interventions related to meeting, individualised, need-focused goals, that now commonly forms the basis of established rehabilitation programmes. Such a programme often includes formal 'goal-planning meetings', during which the client will be present along with relevant rehabilitation team members. Measurable goals will be set and broken down into targets, with indications given of who is responsible for meeting aspects of the goal, under what conditions the goal will be met and what constitutes success. There is nothing particularly health exclusive about this approach; similar processes are used in appraisal systems within many spheres of business and employment and, as stated previously, within education, often in the form of learning contracts.

Davies et al (1992) described a set of conditions considered necessary for a rehabilitation goal-setting process to be effective. It was suggested that goals should be client centred and prioritised, be coordinated (with specific personnel assigned to specific tasks) and give a prediction of the client's immediate future.

Clearly, the ideal is to have the patient central to the goal-setting process, involving him in the decision-making and evaluation relating to the goals set. Indeed, the primary member of the team is the client himself; it is his needs and expectations relating to societal function that should dictate the activities, interactions and processes of the rehabilitation team, with the obvious inclusion of relatives or meaningful others, as appropriate. Davies et al (1992) stated that the aim of an interdisciplinary approach to rehabilitation was 'to be able to form objectives across disciplines involving clients and significant others, thus moving towards a client centred approach as opposed to a professional approach.'

Key to the success of this principle is the language that is used within the process. As with any professional discipline, medicine and its allied professions has its own particular language and jargon, which may not be entirely comprehensible to a lay person. If the individual client is as much an integral part of the rehabilitation team as any other member, it is imperative that the language used is appropriate.

Based on previous work by Houts & Scott (1985) and evidence from a behavioural mapping study in a rehabilitation environment, Kennedy (1988) suggested a method of goal planning utilising a key worker system. Such a system has been used successfully in some rehabilitation units for a number a years, and an evaluative study on the efficacy of this approach (Kennedy et al 1991) concluded 'that the goal planning system used is an effective way of maximising the therapeutic potential of the rehabilitation environment.' A survey by Walker & Alden (1993), relating to patient satisfaction with, and participation in, the goal-planning system showed positive attitudes.

There seems to be agreement that some degree of coordination is required to run a goal-planning system effectively. A key worker (any suitably trained member of that client's team) is allocated to the coordination role. Other rehabilitation teams have felt that the term 'coordinator' is preferable, the rationale being that the term 'key worker' implies a greater responsibility and input than could be reasonably expected from individual team members (Davies et al 1992). However, it could be strongly argued that, although the input required as a key worker is substantial, this level of personal responsibility for one client is of benefit both to the client, in having a key worker as advocate, and to the rehabilitation process, by ensuring that responsibility is taken by someone for coordinating the system effectively. An alternative term, which in the past was predominantly used in America but is now also used in the UK, is 'case manager'. Such roles are often not confined to the hospital environment. While ideally commencing involvement during the acute stage following injury or illness, the role also extends into the community after discharge from a hospital-based rehabilitation programme, continuing the input in collaboration with community healthcare professionals. It is a logical progression from this to consider the possibility of the client himself functioning as the key worker, with the benefit of regaining earlier control of his life though greater participation in the process, which is congruent with the principles of independence and empowerment discussed earlier. Obviously, this may not be possible for those clients who have cognitive difficulties or have a reduced psychological capacity initially (Swanson et al 1989), but as reintegration becomes more imminent and coping and adaptive mechanisms are increasingly established, there may be a possibility of the client taking over the role of key worker to some degree at a later stage.

Such a system utilised on a continuous basis is probably most beneficial to those individuals whose disability is perceived as complex. However, one can certainly envisage the goal-planning process being useful for all individuals requiring rehabilitation, particularly as nursing and paramedical disciplines across all areas currently report the use of goals within their systems.

The key components of goal planning are summarised in Box 1.5.

THE USE OF REFLECTION IN REHABILITATION

Now commonly used in education, including that of healthcare professionals, the concept of reflection has achieved widespread acceptance as a valid and valuable technique in the education of adults. Obvious similarities exist with experiential learning models, and reflection provides the basis for effective development of the individual by facilitating continuous improvement in competence when dealing with similar situations. In view of this it may be worth considering the process of reflection as used with clients in a rehabilitation context. Such a process is cyclical (Fig. 1.4).

A concrete practical experience that the individual may perceive as being problematic or of interest forms the topic for reflection. The experience is

---

■ BOX 1.5 Key components of a goal-planning system

- Client-centred (ideally client led)
- Relevant
- Needs broken down into goals and targets, including timescales
- Language of the patient
- Realistic goals
- All relevant professionals contribute to process
- Documented within framework of chosen rehabilitation model
- Progress evaluated

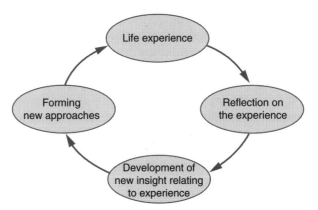

Figure 1.4 The reflective process.

evaluated, with the individual gathering any relevant observations and information. This analysis of the experience may result in the individual developing new insight related to the circumstances that contributed to the result of the experience. These insights and theories can then be utilised to generate new practical approaches when the individual is faced with similar situations or circumstances in the future (Box 1.6).

■ **BOX 1.6 Reflection – a practical checklist**

(a) Write a description of the experience and highlight the key issues which merit attention.

(b) Reflect on:
   – the aim of the activity
   – the results of the activity
   – the implications of the experience on you and others
   – how you felt during the experience.

(c) What factors both from previous experience and previous knowledge influenced your actions?

(d) What experiences and knowledge which you did not possess prior to the event would have helped your decision-making?

(e) What alternative choices could have been made and what may have been the result?

(f) What learning has taken place? Consider:
   – how this experience has increased your personal knowledge and will change your practice in the future when faced with similar events
   – how you feel now about the event and what support is available to assist in dealing with those feelings
   – should this learning be shared with others to add to their knowledge?

To my knowledge this process has not been formally used in the rehabilitation of individual clients. However, it does seem possible that this process could help in encouraging the individual client to problem-solve, and come to terms with his new situation. It is certainly congruous with suggestions made previously of using the individual's own experiences, and the need for relevance of learning to an individual's life.

If reflection is to be a benefit within a rehabilitation environment, then the emphasis of the role of the rehabilitation professional is again on the need to act as a facilitator of learning rather than as a traditional dictatorial teacher or instructor.

RESOURCES FOR REHABILITATION

The resources required for rehabilitation include the environment in which rehabilitation will take place, the personnel needed to provide a comprehensive rehabilitation service, and financial resources.

TEAM-WORKING IN REHABILITATION

It is commonly accepted that a team approach to rehabilitation, utilising the skills of various disciplines, is the method by which rehabilitation is best delivered and the client's needs met (Davies et al 1992, Whiteneck et al 1992). This is the case with rehabilitation in any healthcare setting, whether following back surgery or the more complex disabilities resulting from spinal cord injury. It is this philosophical importance of a team approach which indicates the need to measure team-working itself when the concern is with outcome, process and practice. A study that examined what a rehabilitation team thought rehabilitation actually consisted of, found different perceptions in different disciplines (Davies et al 1992). This is surely an undesirable situation, as any organisation must possess a clear, united vision in order to remain motivated and work effectively (Buchholz & Roth 1982). Focusing on the role of the rehabilitation nurse within elderly care rehabilitation, Waters & Luker (1996) suggested that team perceptions were not clear either within nursing itself or in other disciplines. Further work in relation to rehabilitation team-working suggested that there may often be a conflict in interprofessional relations, and staff may perceive an encroachment on professional territory despite the acknowledgment of the value of a team approach in rehabilitation (Strasser et al 1994). It would not be surprising that such a conflict, if it exists, would itself lead to disharmony and demotivation within the team and in individuals; but, in addition, there would be a perceived absence of recognition by other team members of the contributions made in attempts to provide what is considered beneficial for the client. Herzberg et al (1959) suggested that recognition is one of the major motivating factors for an individual at work, and that demotivation is likely to occur if recognition is withheld. He also considered that achievement, responsibility, progress and personal growth, and satisfaction in the nature of the work are other major individual motivation factors, and if these are not available in the workplace then demotivation may ensue. The team members themselves, and their peers, are as responsible as the managers of the team for ensuring that these motivational needs are met, and they may have either a positive or a negative influence in this.

Various team approaches have been adopted in health care, namely multidisciplinary, interdisciplinary and, less frequently used to date, transdisciplinary. Such approaches are discussed in detail in Chapter 6.

LOCATION OF REHABILITATION SERVICES

The question of where rehabilitation should take place should be explored. As previously stated, an underpinning principle of this book is that rehabilitation should occur across specialities. It is, however, too simplistic to state that rehabilitation can or should occur anywhere, even though rehabilitation principles may be transferable. There are clear issues relating to the suitability of an environment for the rehabilitation of any individual. At a basic level, it would be an inappropriate use of resources for a specialised neurorehabilitation unit to house a patient following myocardial infarction, or a long-term ventilated high-level quadriplegic to be treated within a chronic back pain programme. In addition, the appropriate allocation of resources must be extended outside the hospital environment. Community rehabilitation, either total or as a continuation of a hospital programme, is a reality, and the possibilities of expanding this further are already being realised through various 'hospital at home' schemes (Clarke 1997), for example, following hip replacement.

However, if suitable services are going to be developed, one must be able to define what constitutes an appropriate environment for an individual undergoing rehabilitation. In an attempt to do this, one could propose the dimensions of what constitutes quality. The dimensions of quality suggested by Maxwell (1984) may be adequate indicators of appropriate location.

Appropriateness

This relates to the relevance of the service to the needs of the client. The locations mentioned above could be deemed prime examples of inappropriateness. Indeed, a strong rationale for the increase in community programmes is that they provide the most realistic environment for the rehabilitation of an individual (i.e. his own society).

Availability of expertise is paramount within this area. The effects of a lack of this expertise seem obvious, with at best there being a lack of fulfilment of the potential of the individual, and at worst actual harm to him. The aggregation of expertise, in particular within specialised units, or indeed on a more general scale with the development of specialities within health care, suggests additional advantages such as the opportunity of undertaking meaningful research. Primarily, one would suggest that this facilitates new developments designed to improve available services and techniques to minimise the impact of illness and injury.

Equity

This is the duty to provide equal services for all. On a broad level this may mean the opportunity for all patients to have equal access to a specialised programme of rehabilitation relevant to their needs (e.g. all patients with spinal cord injury having access to spinal injury units or all individuals following myocardial infarction being able to be part of a formalised cardiac rehabilitation programme). Equally, one can focus on more specific aspects of rehabilitation; for example, the client should have the opportunity to attend a formal patient education programme or have access to appropriate support from community rehabilitation nurses.

Accessibility

Accessibility is defined as the ease with which services are available. This may encompass limitations in mobility capability, waiting times and knowledge that services exist. Examples related to this include ensuring that a service is able to provide information about appropriate support groups within a local area, or receipt of accurate information relating to recent developments that may impact positively on a person's level of disability. At a basic level it may mean that the environment empowers the individual (e.g. that toilets or washing facilities are accessible, or that equipment is available to facilitate such activities).

Acceptability

This focuses on the degree to which the reasonable expectations of the client are satisfied. It is clear that to achieve this we must actually know what expectations the client has of rehabilitation. This should be achieved to some degree if rehabilitation teams are employing a truly client-focused service. Although infrequently examined experimentally, available peer support, from other individuals 'in the same boat', appears beneficial to significant numbers of people with chronic illness or disability. For evidence of this one need look no further than the plethora of support groups that exist.

FINANCIAL ASPECTS OF REHABILITATION PROVISION

It is clear to all who work within health services, both nationally and internationally, that resources available for health care are continuously under scrutiny. In addition, the costs of health care are rising globally, as advances in technology, although improving health, are often expensive. Increased life expectancy and, therefore, an increase in the elderly population, and higher public expectations are all key factors contributing to the current situation.

In view of this, it would be folly to ignore the financial aspects of the provision of rehabilitation, and somewhat naive not to strive for cost-effectiveness (i.e. quality provision at the lowest cost). Although concern about finance often does not appear to sit well with the role of healthcare professionals, from the ward orderly to the senior professional, it is a fact of life and cannot be ignored. Anecdotally, resources for rehabilitation appear to have been hit in recent years, possibly due to the appeal of the quick-fix mentality of having 'as many bums in beds' as possible, which seems to be so popular in today's political climate. It is clear, however, that it is only through demonstrating that formal rehabilitation does make a difference that we can validly fight for additional resources; and we must look for new ways of working that maximise the resources available. This will ultimately result in the provision of quality rehabilitation to as many clients as possible. Surely the clarification of the role of nursing within a rehabilitation context, ensuring better working practices and correctly focused and meaningful educational input to enable nurses to rehabilitate effectively, can go some way to facilitating good use of resources. This is one of the aims of this book.

Finally, on a broader point, the barriers created by separate health and social service remits and funding must be resolved. This could be achieved through joint purchasing and collaborative planning via an effective case-management system. Clearly this is something we may not be able to influence as individuals, but as a body of professionals rehabilitation workers should be shouting about it from the rooftops.

EVALUATION OF REHABILITATION

This issue is addressed in detail in Chapter 7, and therefore just a brief outline of the major points is given here. Reference has already been made to the benefits of demonstrating effectiveness in rehabilitation for the provision of financial resources. However, in addition, and one could suggest more importantly, when providing health care it is ethically correct to strive for the optimum from the patient's or client's perspective. All rehabilitation professionals are bound through the relevant codes of conduct to aim for this. It is essential that we do not lose sight of this, despite the cynicism that healthcare professionals may have about government motives for promoting evidence-based health care.

SUMMARY

The aim of this chapter was to offer guidance to the reader regarding the principles of rehabilitation, not only in order to increase understanding, but also to facilitate and promote appraisal of current rehabilitation practice within the reader's own area. To summarise, it may be useful to reiterate some of the key principles discussed.

1. Definition of the key aims, expectations and characteristics of rehabilitation is the vital first stage in developing effective and meaningful rehabilitation services. Without this, inappropriate models, processes and practices may be developed. Key characteristics include empowerment, independence, reduction of disability and handicap, and a client centred approach. The involvement of individuals who have used rehabilitation

services is invaluable. It is clear that the focus of rehabilitation should be on the interface of the individual with his community within society, rather than on impairment or physical functioning.

2. The criteria for the development and utilisation of a model include that it is comprehensive, relevant, focused on the needs of the individual, and user-friendly (both to the client and the professional). Such a model should be serviceable across all disciplines, utilising an interdisciplinary team approach. In addition, the model should form the basis of practice evaluation and development.

3. Formal goal planning is an established and useful process within rehabilitation and health care generally. The individual should be central to this process and goals should be set to meet his perceived need. An additional process that may be of benefit within goal setting is that of reflection, whereby the individual uses his own experience to facilitate learning to live with his new situation.

4. Rehabilitation requires coordination through a named key worker or case manager. Ideally, this role should be transferred to the patient or client at an appropriate stage.

5. Following the principles of adult learning, rehabilitation professionals should be facilitators within the process, rather than dictators. Control should be transferred to the individual, enabling him to become empowered.

6. As rehabilitation occurs across all spheres of health care, these principles should be transferable. The ideal location for rehabilitation depends on the specific circumstances and needs of the individual.

7. It is folly to ignore the current financial constraints on rehabilitation. To ensure the viability of rehabilitation services, evidence must be produced that demonstrates the effectiveness of rehabilitation in achieving positive outcomes. This is not only vital from a financial perspective, but we are ethically bound through our professional duty to provide this evidence.

REFERENCES

American Holistic Nurses Association 1992 Description statement. AHNA, Flagstaff, Arizona
Anderson T P 1988 Rehab treatment (versus training) for recovery. Archives of Physical Medicine and Rehabilitation 69:312–317
Barnitt R, Pomeroy V 1995 An holistic approach to rehabilitation. British Journal of Therapy and Rehabilitation 2(2):87–92
Buchholz S, Roth T 1982 Aligned on a purpose – sharing a vision. In: Creating the high-performance team. Wilson Learning Corporation/Wiley, New York, ch 4, pp 53–67
Clarke A M 1997 Benefits and drawbacks of hospital at home schemes. Professional Nurse 12(10):734–736
Davies A, Davis S, Moss N et al 1992 First steps towards an interdisciplinary approach to rehabilitation. Clinical Rehabilitation 6:237–244
Finklestein V 1993 The commonality of disability. In: Swain J, Finklestein V, French S, Oliver M (eds) Disabling barriers – enabling environments. Sage, London
French S 1993 Disability, impairment or something in between? In: Swain J et al (eds) Disabling barriers – enabling environments. Sage, London
Hamilton B, Granger C V, Sherwin F S, Zielezny M, Tashman T S 1987 A uniform national data system for medical rehabilitation. In: Fuhrer M J (ed) Rehabilitation outcomes analysis and measurement. Brooks, Baltimore

Herzberg F, Maisner B, Snyderman B 1959 The motivation to work. Wiley, New York

Houts P, Scott R A 1985 Goal planning with developmentally disabled persons: procedures for developing. In: Individualised client plan. Milton Hershey Center, Pennsylvannia

Johnson J 1995 Achieving effective rehabilitation outcomes: does the nurse have a role? British Journal of Therapy and Rehabilitation 2(3):113–118

Kennedy P, Fisher K, Pearson E 1988 Ecological evaluation of a rehabilitative environment for SCI people – behavioural mapping and feedback. British Journal of Clinical Psychology 27: 239–246

Kennedy P, Walker L, White D 1991 Ecological evaluation of goal planning and advocacy in a rehabilitation environment for spinal cord injured people. Paraplegia 29: 197–202

Knowles M 1990 The adult learner: a neglected species, 4th edn. Gulf, Houston

McFarlane J 1986 The value of models for care. In: Kershaw B, Savage J (eds) Models for nursing. John Wiley and Sons, Chichester

McGrath J R, Davies A M 1992 Rehabilitation – where are we going and how do we get there? Clinical Rehabilitation 6:225–235

Mahoney F, Barthel D W 1965 Functional evaluation – the Barthel index. MD State Medical Journal 14:342–346

Maxwell R J 1984 Quality assessment in health. British Medical Journal 288:1470–1471

NHS Executive 1994 Priorities and planning guidance for the NHS 1995/96, NHS Executive, Leeds, EL(94) 55

Oliver M 1987 Redefining disability: a challenge to research. Research, Policy and Planning 5(1):9–13

Owen M J, Holmes C A 1993 'Holism' in the discourse of nursing. Journal of Advanced Nursing 18:1688–1695

Robinson I 1988 Rehabilitation of long term physical impairments: the social context of roles. Clinical Rehabilitation 2:339–347

Rogers C 1969 Freedom to learn. Merill, Columbus, Ohio

Roper N, Logan W, Tierney A 1985 The elements of nursing, 2nd edn. Churchill Livingstone, Edinburgh

Schofield G 1993 Ethical considerations in rehabilitation medicine. Archives of Physical Medicine and Rehabilitation 74:341–346

Schunk D H 1991 Learning theories: an educational perspective. Merrill, New York

Smith M J 1996 Expectations of rehabilitation – a focus group project. Paper presented at the American Association of SCI Nurses Conference, Las Vegas

Strasser C, Falconer J A, Saltzmann D 1994 The rehabilitation team: staff perceptions of the hospital environment, the interdisciplinary team environment, and interprofessional relations. Archives of Physical Medicine and Rehabilitation 75:177–182

Swanson B, Cronin-Stubbs D, Sheldon J 1989 The impact of psychological factors on adapting to physical disability: a review of the research literature. Rehabilitation Nursing 14(2): 64–68

Walker L, Alden P 1993 The key worker system – a comparison of staff and patient perceptions. Presented at the International Medical Society of Paraplegia Conference, Ghent, Belgium

Waters K R, Luker K A 1996 Staff perceptions on the role of the nurse in rehabilitation wards for elderly people. Journal of Clinical Nursing 5:105–114

Whiteneck G, Charlifue S, Gerhart K, Overholser J, Richardson G 1992 Quantifying handicap. A new measure of long term outcomes. Archives of Physical and Medical Rehabilitation 73:519–526

World Health Organisation 1980 World Health Organisation international classification of impairments, disabilities and handicaps. A manual of classifications relating to the consequences of disease. WHO, Geneva

Nursing and rehabilitation

Mike Smith

2

INTRODUCTION

This chapter provides an overview of nursing and rehabilitation of the adult following injury or illness, thereby setting the scene for subsequent chapters. The functions and roles of nursing in the rehabilitation setting, using the previously described rehabilitation framework, are briefly explored. The central concept of empowerment to rehabilitation is discussed further, exploring how nursing may need to change to overcome any potential barriers.

The types and sources of knowledge required to undertake these roles are given, with examples from clinical practice.

Finally, the ideas discussed in the chapter are summarised through examples of how the rehabilitation framework, client goals and nursing roles and interventions interrelate.

REHABILITATION AND THE CORE ELEMENTS OF NURSING

Fawcett (1984) explored what nursing should actually be concerned with in order to identify the beliefs and values that form the discipline of nursing. She proposed the existence of four core elements:

- person
- environment
- health
- nursing.

However, some authors argue that nursing *is* the discipline, i.e. it is the whole rather than a specific part (Melesis 1991, Parse 1992), and therefore cannot be described as a core element. Newman et al (1991) suggest that a fundamental element of nursing is the concept of caring. This is reflected in the work of many others (Benner & Wrubel 1989, Leininger 1986, Watson 1988). In addition, Roach (1985) describes nursing as the 'professionalisation of the human capacity to care', and states that this may be achieved through the acquisition and use of the knowledge and skill required for prescribed nursing roles. Kirby & Slevin (1992), in describing the essential nature of nursing practice, discuss nursing as an activity involving three elements: caring, relationships and health.

In view of the above, I would suggest the following as the core elements of nursing.

1. *Person* (the patient or client). This encompasses the relevant fundamental beliefs regarding clients, which were discussed in Chapter 1 in the context of rehabilitation (e.g. empowerment and independence). In addition, a key concept is that of developing services which are client centred and focused on the needs of the whole individual, rather than on a particular impairment. These needs of the whole individual form the basis of the rehabilitation framework.

2. *Environment* (physical and social environment in which nursing takes place). This means the specific location in which rehabilitation takes place, and it includes the issues of the realism of the environment and also the availability of relevant social support, including that of others with similar health problems.

3. *Health* (aspects of both illness and well-being). Quite simply this is the potential deficits in health (in its broadest context) specific to that individual and his circumstances, which will determine the particular rehabilitation programme required. This will also determine the types of intervention required (e.g. health education, which will enable the individual to minimise development of future health problems).

4. *Caring* (helping and being with others at time of need). As previously mentioned, the concept of caring in nursing has been perceived as a key element by many authors. True caring in rehabilitation involves the gradual transfer of responsibility and control to the individual, and the provision of support in this process.

It is this combination of core elements and a discrete body of underpinning knowledge which nursing practice should reflect, and this should form the basis of the development of a nursing philosophy (Box 2.1).

NURSING AND REHABILITATION MODELS

If one accepts that there is a need for a general model or framework

---

■ BOX 2.1 Developing a philosophy for rehabilitation nursing

- Using the core elements described in the text and the principles of rehabilitation, identify the key values and beliefs involved in nursing from a rehabilitation perspective.

- A philosophy should be owned by the whole team. To enable this, all team members should be involved in identifying these values and beliefs. This can be achieved through a number of means (e.g. in-ward questionnaire, ward meeting). It may also be of benefit to include representatives from other disciplines, to not only to aid in development, but also to facilitate cross-discipline understanding of what nursing is all about.

- A draft philosophy consisting of key statements relating to the elements should be made available for final comment by the ward team.

- Final amendments should be made and a date for review of the philosophy set.

for rehabilitation which should be used by all disciplines, then it is the rehabilitation framework introduced in Chapter 1 (see Fig. 1.3) which should be used to guide and reflect nursing in rehabilitation of the adult. Here, potential nursing practice within the dimensions of the framework are outlined, as a means of defining the role of the nurse in rehabilitation, and as a preliminary scene-setting for the forthcoming chapters.

PHYSICAL HEALTH AND INDEPENDENCE

Key to this dimension is the provision of information and education, which enables promotion and maintenance of the client's health. Adaption to a new health status will include, as a first stage, assessment of what the potential health risks may be. To make this assessment the nurse must possess a degree of technical expertise within the relevant speciality, and have the ability to perform aspects of related care, initially to maintain the safety and well-being of the individual until he is in a position to be able to take responsibility for himself. This is the role nurses have traditionally aspired to and, one could suggest, possibly feel most comfortable with. Indeed, issues surrounding bowel and bladder function, nutrition and assistance with hygiene needs have been commonly described as primary nursing areas within rehabilitation (Johnson 1995, Waters & Luker 1996). It is the transfer of responsibility that some may find more difficult, particularly when the individual is being encouraged to choose particular interventions or forms of managing a particular health problem for himself. It is the recognition of this process and the ability to effectively support an individual through it that define the particular skills of the rehabilitation nurse.

Inherent within this process is the education of an individual which comprises two components:

- A theoretical component, which will enable the individual to make informed decisions.
- The practical skills which an individual must learn in order to promote and maintain health. Incorporated within this is the ability to problem-solve should the need arise.

A degree of technical expertise will be required by the nurse to be able to determine both the key areas in which the individual may need to problem-solve and potential solutions to such problems, as the nurse must be able to give appropriate information to the client.

There may be a need for diagnostic tests before or during the rehabilitation stage, and these may contribute to the assessment of potential health problems or determine the success, or otherwise, of prescribed medical interventions. The nurse often acts as coordinator, ensuring that such tests are organised and undertaken. Increasingly nurses are performing some of these diagnostic tests themselves, as part of nurse-led or nurse-assisted clinics. Obvious examples would be in the areas of phlebotomy, diabetic investigations and, more recently, urodynamic studies to assess bladder and sphincter function and objective pressure measurement as part of tissue viability clinics. Once again this highlights the role of the nurse as a technical expert within rehabilitation, and it is often these expanded skills, along with the other attributes which nursing can bring to health care, that have formed the basis of the development of specialist nursing roles within rehabilitation.

Finally within this dimension, if an individual is unable to perform many activities without assistance on a long-term basis, it is vital for that individual's independence that he is enabled to direct others to provide this assistance. This is often termed 'verbal independence'. One way of supporting this may be to carry out the training programmes of such personal assistants under the direction of the individual client. It may seem obvious to the reader, but it is worth reiterating, that the technical expertise required will depend on the particular speciality involved and on the individual capabilities and desires of the client.

EMOTIONAL HEALTH AND RELATIONSHIPS

The major change in health status that may result from illness or injury, which may be of a chronic nature, will often have significant effects on the lifestyle of that individual. Such lifestyle changes will often result in a period of adaption to a new way of living and be emotionally traumatic. For example, the individual may experience a change in his body image, role changes within his life, or a self-perceived change in or loss of sexuality. Additionally, anxieties may exist related to the health condition itself, with the potential recurrence of the initial condition or the development of related complications (e.g. following myocardial infarction).

The nurse is at the frontline of these issues due to the unique 24 hour nature of nursing work and the 'intimacy' of the nurse – patient relationship which often exists. Clearly, therefore, the nurse can be perceived as having a primary role in the emotional support of both the client and his meaningful others.

The concepts of empowerment and independence were discussed in Chapter 1 as key elements within rehabilitation. The first stage within these is to enable the individual, through providing emotional support in all aspects of a rehabilitation programme, to begin to take responsibility and control for living with his new situation.

MOVEMENT AND TRANSPORT

Traditionally, movement or mobility has been perceived as a primary concern of physiotherapy and, occasionally, occupational therapy. It is quite clear, however, that nursing too has a vital role. This may often be to reinforce the programmes prescribed by therapy colleagues who cannot work with individuals on a continuing basis as the nurse does. What has often been described as 'carrying on the work of others' has received endorsement in the rehabilitation nursing literature (Johnson 1995, Waters & Luker 1996). In addition, authors on orthopaedic nursing have stressed mobility as a central theme within that speciality (Davis 1994, Footner 1992), often in terms of nursing being central in minimising potential problems and promoting health in the individual relating to the causes and effects of reduced mobility. Examples of these include the management of pain, pressure sore prevention and management, preventive measures to minimise the risk of deep vein thrombosis, and preventing problems associated with wearing a plaster cast or orthosis.

Again it is clear that the nurse, whatever the speciality, must have the relevant technical expertise, not only to carry out these prescribed interventions, but also to provide emotional support and to encourage the client through this period of physical learning. In addition, this continual nature of nursing highlights another key role as rehabilitation team worker, i.e. in reporting client progress. Not only is it essential for therapists to be aware of the performance of the individual outside a therapy gym, but also reports are required of any actual or potential problems that the client is having with the prescribed programme. The key to this is to be able to provide accurate information. This highlights the need to measure the input and impact of nursing in rehabilitation.

EMPLOYMENT AND LEISURE

Employment is not generally perceived as falling within the remit of the nurse. However, in this field, the ability of the nurse to offer advice at a basic level and refer appropriately is crucial.

From a recreational perspective, the necessity for the individual to be independent in relation to physical needs may be a goal, in order that he can participate in social activities. Again the nurse requires information relating to referral to suitable organisations that offer appropriate opportunities. It is also important that recreation should be perceived as broader than sporting activities. I remember one individual clearly stating 'I didn't spend years bunking off games at school, to be forced to do sport just because I've had a spinal injury.' This surely reinforces that recreation should be perceived as any social activity that the individual enjoys. This may indeed be a sporting activity, or it may quite simply be sharing the company of others in a pub or enjoying a meal at a favourite restaurant.

HOME AND FINANCES

Once again the role of the nurse as team worker is fundamental. Gathering appropriate information and appropriate referral are essential elements within this role. The information can highlight the need for referral, enabling a more detailed assessment by other professional disciplines. Discharge from hospital may be complicated and may involve the cooperation of many agencies and departments, and good coordination is essential in order to facilitate a smooth transition from hospital to home, particularly for those individuals with complex disability. Nurses are often the key players in this process, undertaking this coordination role. Indeed, nursing case management, which is described in detail in Chapter 6, emphasises this as a vital role, and one which nursing is in a prime position to provide successfully.

NURSING ROLES IN REHABILITATION OF THE ADULT

As the reader may have recognised, throughout the proposed rehabilitation framework there are identifiable common threads, which seem to indicate the fundamental nursing roles within rehabilitation. In view of this I suggest the existence of six key nursing roles within the rehabilitation of an adult. These are given in Figure 2.1, which indicates their relationship to the dimensions of the rehabilitation framework. The six roles are described below, reiterating the points made previously.

TECHNICAL EXPERT AND PROVIDER OF CARE

This incorporates the technical expertise required to perform prescribed nursing interventions, and those nursing actions prescribed by other professionals. In addition, it involves the provision of 'care', not only in times of dependence and illness, but also in terms of the transfer of decision-making and independence to the client.

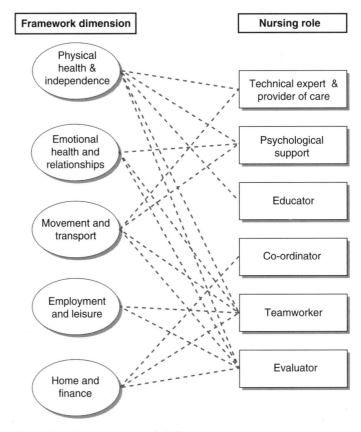

Figure 2.1 Nursing roles in rehabilitation.

PSYCHOLOGICAL SUPPORT

As discussed previously, due to her 24 hour involvement and regular intimate contact with the client, it is the nurse who provides first-line psychological support. This not only involves general issues relating to adaption to a new set of life circumstances imposed by the client's condition and by society, but will often also encompass the individual's concerns regarding his relationships with others (e.g. as a partner or parent). The nature of rehabilitation and health care generally is that during daytime hours individuals are often occupied, and their thoughts and efforts relate to the more functional aspects of their condition. It is during the evening and at night or at weekends when the individual may more fully contemplate the impact of what has happened. No other discipline retains the 24-hour contact as does nursing. It is therefore the nurse who initially must deal with these expressed feelings and concerns. There are obvious limits on how much support a nurse can provide, depending on the particular issue and the knowledge the nurse has. These limits must be acknowledged and acted upon through referral to particular specialists (e.g. clinical psychologist or counsellor). These issues are the detailed focus of Chapter 4.

EDUCATOR

Previous reference has been made to education as a key component within rehabilitation. Nurses are in a prime position to provide the theoretical and practical education needed to enable the individual to regain responsibility for his physical independence and prevention of further health problems. Education is required, not only for the client himself, but also for carers and relatives/meaningful others, particularly as social support appears to play such a key role within rehabilitation. These issues are discussed in more depth in Chapter 3.

COORDINATOR

More than any other professional, the nurse is central to the coordination of patients' activities during the day. It is the nurse who works over the whole day within the social environment of the rehabilitation area, and to a degree manages the interaction in the 'community' of the rehabilitation environment. Likewise, it is the community nurse who will often co-ordinate rehabilitation activities in the individual's home environment, ensuring that the appropriate professionals are mobilised. Such issues are discussed in Chapter 6.

TEAM WORKER

This incorporates two essential elements: first, all those nursing activities that involve carrying out care prescribed by other rehabilitation team members over the 24 hour period; secondly, the need to report the result of nursing interventions that may impact on the client meeting required goals. Aspects of the role of team worker are covered in more depth in Chapter 6.

EVALUATOR

The nursing role of evaluator relates to all rehabilitation dimensions. The role is quite simply based on the need to demonstrate effectiveness and identify the outcome of interventions in whatever we do as nurses. This area is the focus of Chapter 7, which explores measurement of nursing in rehabilitation.

PERFORMING NURSING ROLES WITHIN REHABILITATION

Having offered the theoretical basis for nursing and rehabilitation, it is time to focus on the practical aspects of delivering these nursing roles. This section will concentrate on three key areas. The rationales for focusing on these three elements are as follows.

1. If the principle of empowerment is fundamental to nursing and rehabilitation, and so is based on collaboration and cooperation, then one needs to explore the nature of this relationship and offer practical solutions to potential problems. One could describe this as 'a partnership in care'.

2. To perform these roles effectively and comprehensively, nurses must possess certain types of knowledge. Through defining these types and their content, effective programmes of rehabilitation education can be identified.

3. A process by which the concepts and philosophies can be translated into the prescription of practical nursing interventions must be outlined. Through providing this, one should be able to offer both a comprehensive system which ensures assessment of all client needs, and a comprehensive plan to meet these needs. In addition, this may point to possible ways in which to document the rehabilitation process and the nursing contribution within it.

A PARTNERSHIP IN CARE

As outlined in Chapter 1, a key principle relating to empowerment is that of establishing an environment of collaboration. This should result in the nurse relinquishing control, and so enabling the individual to regain control following a period of relative dependence.

As this complex relationship or partnership between the client and nurse is fundamental to the rehabilitation of adults, it is worthy of brief exploration.

This will be approached from a problem-solving approach, identifying potential barriers to such a partnership, and proposing possible solutions. It is worth stressing that such barriers will be specific both to the particular environment and to the client, and they may encompass some or all of the factors discussed below. The approach suggested in Box 2.2 could

■ BOX 2.2 A seven-stage problem-solving approach

1. Identification of the particular problem area to be examined.
2. Definition of the ideal situation.
3. Critical analysis of the existing situation, resulting in identification of current deficits.
4. Development of an action plan to address the identified deficits, including responsibilities, time-scales and indicators of success.
5. Implementation of action plans.
6. Evaluation of the effect of the intervention.
7. Return to step 3 and repeat until a satisfactory outcome is obtained.

be used in collaboration with other professionals, or perhaps ideally with a group of nurses and clients.

Barriers to an effective partnership

There are many potential barriers to the development of an effective partnership between client and nurse which could affect the final aim of an empowered individual.

Common broad sources are illustrated in Figure 2.2 and are briefly discussed below, together with some possible solutions.

Locus of control

Much of the initial work relating to locus of control originates from social learning theory. A key proponent of this concept, often still quoted in

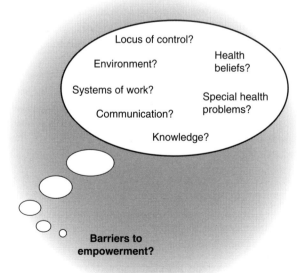

Figure 2.2 Potential barriers to empowerment.

related literature, was Rotter (1966), who proposed that an individual may have either a perceived external or internal locus of control. There is a suggestion that, not only is an internal locus of control consistent with the principle of empowerment, but it is likely to result in an individual becoming compliant in rehabilitation processes and with central advice (Rheiner 1995). This is, of course, key in ensuring that aspects of health education are taken on board by the individual. In addition, it seems to reinforce the principles of adult learning that were discussed in the context of rehabilitation in Chapter 1.

Therefore if there is a rehabilitation environment where the individual's decision-making capabilities are limited and nursing and other disciplines take the responsibility for decisions relating to that individual, not only does this go against the basic principles outlined earlier, but it may also result in the individual inadvertently not taking advice on board and developing complications. It is essential, therefore, to develop a perceived internal locus of control in the client. The individual must be part of any decision-making, not only in being able to express his particular goals relating to rehabilitation, but also in the planning of how to meet these goals. Interventions must be supported through the provision of comprehensive information and must be acceptable to the individual. Consequently, the nurse must be able to accept the decision of the client after pointing out potential health problems and consequences; the client must be allowed to make mistakes, and the consequences must be managed in a supportive manner by the nurse. The reflective analysis technique outlined in Chapter 1 may be a useful and appropriate approach in such circumstances.

One must acknowledge the difficulty that this may cause, particularly if the safety of the individual is compromised, and such actions often result in the 'problem-patient' label. However, bearing in mind the issues discussed previously, I suggest that, unless the result of an individual's perceived non-compliance would be severe immediate danger, it is very difficult to endorse any alternative approach. This is clearly a move away from what has traditionally been the case in nursing and health care generally.

Health beliefs

Health beliefs are those things which it is believed will influence health either for the good or the bad. There are three components relating to health beliefs which may result in a change in behaviour. The individual client must believe:

- that there may be a susceptibility to a particular health problem
- that the particular health issue will impact on quality of life in some way
- that a particular course of action may actually result in the health problem being prevented.

Such health beliefs may be present in both the client and the nurse. From the nurse's perspective, health beliefs should be based on evidence, highlighting once again the need for measuring the effectiveness of rehabilitation nursing interventions. Without this evidence the position of the nurse is severely weakened, and indeed it is not beyond the realms of possibility that the intervention itself may even be flawed. One needs to look no further than some interventions that have been delivered by nursing in times past which have since been abandoned (e.g. the use of Eusol for dressings, or 'ring cushions' as a prophylactic measure for pressure sore development) for evidence that this may be the case.

From the client's point of view, health beliefs are often created throughout the life of the individual as a result of his particular life experiences and the experiences of others he has come into contact with. This may be by direct contact or through a third party, such as the media. Clearly, such sources are often far from reliable and may promote beliefs that are to the detriment of the individual's safety.

In exploring potential solutions, the following points are proposed.

1. Examine the evidence for existing health beliefs about nursing and rehabilitation, ensuring that practical nursing interventions and advice are based on the best available evidence, and examining those areas for which sufficient evidence is not available.

2. Identify the areas in which the individual client's health beliefs do not seem to be congruent with the evidence-based information that underpins the health beliefs of the nurse. An effective method of highlighting a potentially flawed opinion of the client is to point out previous consequences of his actions. Alternatively, one could consider actually presenting relevant documented evidence to the individual.

3. In discussing the potential effects of a behaviour, highlight not only the physical effects on that individual but also other effects (e.g. effects on social activity, on meaningful others or on employment/leisure).

Lack of knowledge

It is clear that the process of education involves more than just the provision of information; it actually results in a potential change in behaviour or attitude. Therefore, we cannot promote the use of information sheets alone as a means of educating patients in terms of self-care. You need only look at the number of individuals that require re-application of plasters or dressings, after having received of a set of 'instructions'. One would again encourage the reader to look back at the principles relating to the education of adults raised in Chapter 1 and examine whether these match how nurses attempt to provide education for patients. Once again it is worth emphasising the knowledge needed by the nurse to enable her to provide not only the physical but also the psychological aspects of a rehabilitation programme. Certainly my own experience and anecdotal evidence from many others would seem to suggest that education for nurses often falls short of what may be required.

Communication barriers

Communication barriers may exist and these may impact on the ability of the individual to participate fully in the care partnership. Such barriers may be physical, attitudinal or language related.

Physical barriers may often be due to previous or resulting health circumstances of the client. Obvious examples include the presence of visual and hearing impairments. It is vital that methods for overcoming such barriers are addressed as part of any rehabilitation programme. Use of external agencies with the relevant expertise and assistance is a worthwhile step (e.g. Royal National Institute for the Blind (RNIB) and Royal National Institute for the Deaf (RNID). However, the more common-sense techniques (e.g. positioning oneself in front of the individual while talking, and providing written materials in large print) are often sufficient. It is obvious, but nevertheless worthwhile stating, that such methods must be adopted by and communicated to the whole of that client's team.

The last point leads into the next category of communication barriers, that of attitudinal barriers. Such barriers may result from any existing prejudice which either the client or the nurse may hold. The outcome of such a situation may be that communication is limited to a basic level only. The exchange of incomplete information may detract from what is gained from the partnership.

It is essential that the nurse recognises and acknowledges his own attitudes that result in barriers to communication. From a professional ethics viewpoint, such feelings must not be allowed to get in the way of rehabilitation. Therefore these attitudes must be addressed, perhaps through supporting the nurse in assessing his feelings towards the client. If they are not resolvable, other nurses must take on the primary care of that client.

Problems that arise due to the attitudes of the client must again be recognised and acknowledged, usually with the assistance of a professional as a first stage. Again, if the problem is unresolvable through appropriate support, it is worth considering reassigning that individual to another nurse or, in extreme cases, to another rehabilitation area.

Special health problems

Special health problems which are a barrier to participation, and so empowerment, may often be cognitive in nature. Obvious examples include the individual with brain injury, an existing mental health problem (e.g. schizophrenia) or the confused elderly client. The first stage must be the identification and management of any underlying condition that may be creating or exacerbating the situation. An example of this would be the treatment of an acute confusional state in an elderly patient due to dehydration and electrolyte imbalance. Once this has been treated it is essential that prompt referral is made to those professionals who are able to maximise or stabilise that individual's abilities to participate (e.g. a clinical psychologist or psychiatrist). Such programmes may be lengthy in nature, and cannot be covered in detail here. However, some of the relevant issues are addressed Chapter 4.

Environment

The environment may play a large part in the client's ability to participate in rehabilitation and barriers to empowerment may simply be a result of the fact that the person is in hospital. Some authors have suggested that individuals may automatically take on the role of passive, receiving 'patient' as soon as they enter a hospital environment. Consequently, one of the first tasks for the nurse immediately following admission, is to outline the nature of any rehabilitation programme, with a description of what the aims, expectations and responsibilities of both the team and the client are. Consistency and reinforcement of this approach must be adopted not only by all the nursing staff, but also by other team members. The provision of written information containing the above principles may well be beneficial to reinforce this further.

The second major environmental barrier may be the layout of the rehabilitation area itself. It is impractical to suggest that nurses must start to knock down walls in order to make the environment more client-friendly. However, it is worth endorsing the involvement of nurses in planning new clinical areas. In addition, there are some fairly simple and practical things that can be done to improve the ward environment in order to facilitate participation. The following are some fairly simple and, importantly in the current economic climate, low cost ideas gleaned from clinical environments in which I have worked.

1. If a client is expected to perform a particular practical intervention for himself (e.g. placing a self-intermittent catheter, changing a dressing, injecting insulin, or caring for his own personal hygiene and grooming), then all the necessary equipment should be accessible to that individual. The client needs to be able to set up any equipment for himself (and dispose of any rubbish safely).

2. Areas within the clinical environment should be clearly marked with appropriate signs and even markings on the floor (these are frequently employed in elderly care environments). Signing should extend beyond just toilets and bathrooms, and should include rooms that will be used for other purposes (e.g. goal-planning meetings, case conferences, meetings with other professionals).

3. The rehabilitation environment should not resemble an obstacle course. Although there are certainly valid concerns that rehabilitation areas are usually not particularly realistic in terms of what the individual may have to overcome within the community, it is reasonable to have a specific area that is set up appropriately as the client is learning new skills.

Systems of work

Barriers to partnership can be attributed to more than one systems factor. First, there may be programme barriers in that the rehabilitation may be too complex for either the client or the professional to participate in fully, leading to difficulties in developing a good care partnership. This was discussed in Chapter 1 with reference to criteria for rehabilitation models.

In addition, there may be constraints imposed by the organisation due to internal or external factors. A key factor in enabling a partnership to develop is being able to invest sufficient time. Readers will probably readily identify with this. Time seems ever more precious as nurses are expected to do more and more in less time. No one disputes that nurses are working harder, but it is possible to work smarter in order to create more time. It is difficult to offer standard suggestions that will be applicable to all working environments, but some ideas are given below.

1. Explore alternative shift times. Do they match what is needed in terms of the required level of nursing input?

2. Look at the demands of other professionals or agencies on nursing and rehabilitation. Are these truly patient focused or do they operate to the detriment of nursing provision for rehabilitation? For example, if a client is scheduled for a physiotherapy appointment at 09.30, does this give the allocated nurse the necessary time to promote independence, given the assistance and education that may be necessary? Or must the nurse curtail the client's potential independence for fear of missing an appointment which has been arranged simply because there is a slot in the rehabilitation colleague's diary?

3. Although there are concerns regarding the use of healthcare assistants, given appropriate training and supervision such assistants could relieve some of the workload of the qualified rehabilitation nurse. This issue is explored in greater depth in Chapter 8.

4. Examine the administration tasks that a nurse undertakes during a day (e.g. through a time analysis). Look at the analysis and question if any tasks could be made easier or quicker through the use of information technology, or even the employment of further administration support. Examples of such tasks include completion of forms, collection of specimens, off-duty rotas, completion of timesheets and telephone answering. Again the tasks will depend on the nature of the work.

It is clear from the above that a fundamental shift in nursing culture may be required. This shift must occur not only in nurses themselves, but also in the organisational structure, both on a micro-level, within the particular clinical environment, and at a macro-level, throughout the organisation, in order to minimise any barriers that may arise from external sources.

KNOWLEDGE OF NURSING

Founded in practice, nursing knowledge is the facts and information held to be true by the discipline of nursing on the basis of the best evidence available. It is this knowledge that enables relevant nursing roles to be fulfilled in the environment in which nursing is taking place.

Nursing knowledge may be divided into four dimensions (Carper 1978) (Fig. 2.3). These dimensions of nursing knowledge are discussed below in the context of adult rehabilitation in nursing, and examples are given as appropriate.

Empirics

Often described as 'the science of nursing', knowledge in this dimension can be gained from observation of the world and is positivist in nature. Primarily, empirical knowledge is perceived as being quantitative, and therefore is usually considered to be objective and scientific. Much of the

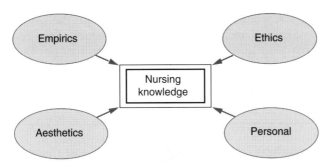

Figure 2.3 The knowledge of nursing.

technical expertise required by the nurse within rehabilitation will be based on empirical knowledge. Examples of this include:

1. Knowledge of the potential health complications relating to a particular condition (e.g. in the individual who is an insulin-dependent diabetic). This knowledge will enable the nurse to recognize such complications if they occur, and educate the individual in how to prevent them.
2. Practical skills (e.g. utilisation of an optimum pressure relieving device).
3. Acting as a client advocate by being able to provide a rationale in disputing suggested possible interventions which may compromise another aspect of the client's health. This situation may not be uncommon when dealing with new junior medical staff.

Ethics

This incorporates nursing knowledge based on moral values. It comprises decisions of a moral nature that nursing imposes on the individual, guiding what the discipline considers to be right or wrong, good or bad. Examples of such knowledge within rehabilitation are the principles of empowerment and independence, which would be perceived as good. Conversely, the development of exclusive nursing or other professional power to the detriment of client decision-making and self-reliance would not be perceived as ethically good within the rehabilitation context.

Aesthetics

Aesthetics implies a subjective comprehension. Commonly referred to as the 'art of nursing', knowledge within this dimension promotes the ability of the individual nurse to act appropriately to a situation without the need for deliberation on what needs to be done. It is aesthetic knowledge that is fundamental in defining the 'expert' practitioner, as described by Benner (1984). Increasingly, reference is made in the literature to the role of intuition in nursing. In addition, aesthetic knowledge could include the ability to manage the social environment and coordinate the ward area in rehabilitation. Providing this knowledge directly is often difficult, if not impossible, in a standard classroom setting. Perhaps the key is for nurses to develop skills and techniques which will enable this knowledge to develop in the practical clinical setting. Such techniques could include encouragement of the use of reflective skills or peer critical incident analysis.

Personal

Personal knowledge is developed from the individual nurse possessing a knowledge and awareness of self, and therefore promotes the ability for the nurse to acquire knowledge and awareness of others. This is at the heart of 'caring' and is related to empathy and being with others at a time of need. The old-school philosophy relating to the need to keep a distance is not congruous with this concept. It has been proposed that 'the nurse needs to get inside the skin of each of her patients in order to know what he needs' (Henderson 1964). It is difficult to assess competency of caring in the individual nurse as it 'goes beyond the identification of observable performance of skills alone but must also include related broader considerations such as intention, choices and judgments that underlie the performance' (Gaut 1986). In addition, it encompasses the ability to extend the potential of the client, thus facilitating the empowerment of that individual. Again direct teaching can provide a theoretical basis for caring, but real learning can only take place during clinical interaction with clients. Possibilities for developing personal knowledge may focus on using the life experiences of the individual to explore his own attitudes in role play and reflection.

Summary

It is nursing knowledge in these four dimensions that guides nursing activity in practice. Should one accept that these dimensions encompass all that is necessary for the client, one could logically suggest that the knowledge present in all four dimensions should produce nurses who are able to deliver truly client centred rehabilitation, thus meeting the needs of the whole client. The issues around ways in which such knowledge may be obtained is the focus of Chapter 9.

ASSESSMENT AND PLANNING WITHIN NURSING AND REHABILITATION

All readers will be familiar with the need to assess and develop plans based on the identification of goals. This section in essence attempts to bring together the previous theoretical framework and concepts. Table 2.1 gives examples that illustrate the relationship between the dimensions within the rehabilitation framework and possible goals that the client could identify. The framework is designed so that the relevant interventions within the nursing roles can then be identified. Detailed descriptions of relevant interventions are given in subsequent chapters. Without an actual

Table 2.1 Examples of the relationship between the dimensions of the rehabilitation framework, client-identified goals and the nursing role

Dimension	Identified individual goals	Nursing role and intervention	Target date
Physical health and independence	To be physically independent in performing intermittent catheterisation	Technical expert: knowledge of procedure and underpinning theory Psychological support: offer support relating to changes in bladder function Educator: teach the patient about the changes in bladder function, and supervise practical procedure Coordinator: arrange urodynamic studies; liaise with community professionals Team worker: report progress to urology team	
Emotional health and relationships	To be able to express potential concerns relating to changes in body image following lower limb amputation	Technical expert: knowledge of potential impact of illness or injury on body image, and use and types of limb prosthesis Psychological support: allow and encourage the client to express what he is feeling; stress the positive aspects of disability Educator: teach the client about the use of the prosthesis; demonstrate ways in which the aesthetic issues surrounding wearing the false limb can be minimised Coordinator: refer client to clinical psychologist if necessary Team worker: participate in setting staged goals that allow the client to adapt to wearing the prosthesis	
Home and finance	Have awareness of entitlement to state benefits	Technical expert: have basic knowledge relating to benefit entitlement; know about the system through which this can be facilitated Team worker: refer client to social worker/benefits entitlement officer	
Employment and leisure	To be able to attend Carlisle United football match	Technical expert: knowledge of what is required in the way of preparation Psychological support: encourage the individual to discuss the feelings associated with regaining this aspect of his social life, emphasising the positive nature Educator: discuss any potential problems that may impact on his experience, and ways to solve them; train carers as appropriate	

Table 2.1 (contd)

Dimension	Identified individual goals	Nursing role and intervention	Target date
Movement and transport	To be able to shop at supermarket	Technical expert: knowledge of what is required in the way of preparation Psychological support: encourage the individual to discuss the feelings associated with regaining this aspect of his social life, emphasising the positive nature Educator: discuss any potential problems that may impact on his experience, and ways to solve them; train carers as appropriate	
Physical health and independence	To be able to direct others when assisting with washing and dressing	Technical expert: knowledge of client's abilities and skills in maximising these; able to state these and use in practice (these should be specified in a care plan situation) Psychological support: provide support in coming to terms with being reliant on others for specific aspects of care Educator: enable the client to become verbally independent through teaching others what assistance is required. Coordinator: arrange a session where a health care assistant acts as a carer would; supervise the session Team worker: provide feedback to team regarding the ability of the client and potential readiness for discharge	
Emotional health and relationships	To have less anxiety regarding the possibility of recurrent myocardial infarction	Technical expert: demonstrate knowledge of myocardial infarction and ways in which potential recurrence can be minimised Psychological support: support the client through allowing him to express how he feels; provide meaningful practical techniques that may assist in controlling his anxiety (e.g. relaxation exercises) Educator: educate the client relating to minimising risk of recurrence; educate client's partner Coordinator: liaison with psychologist or counsellor if necessary; arrange support services within the community Team worker: report that anxieties exist to team after discussion with patient, so that their interaction and intervention do not exacerbate this	

Table 2.1 (contd)

Dimension	Identified individual goals	Nursing role and intervention	Target date
Employment and leisure	To be able to return to work	Technical expert: able to recognise the potential abilities rather than disabilities in the individual, and how these may translate into the work situation Psychological support: offer support and encourage positive thinking relating to potential change in employment Educator: assist the individual in maximising his physical abilities related to the form of employment which he wants to undertake Coordinator: liaison with occupational therapist relating to potential assistive devices, and disabled resettlement officer; liaison with current employer if appropriate Team worker: report progress in using prescribed aids	
Physical health and independence	To minimise the risk of unsafe blood sugar levels	Technical expert: ability to monitor blood sugar levels and take remedial action if adverse; able to titrate and administer insulin as prescribed Psychological support: assist the client in adapting to injecting himself; provide reassurance that blood sugar level is controllable Educator: assist the patient in learning to monitor his own blood sugar levels, eat a diet which is appropriate and inject insulin. This should be staged: (a) dependence on the nurse with explanation (b) supervised practice (c) independence for each of the three aspects Coordinator: organise education sessions and liaise with dietitian as appropriate Team worker: Report progress relating to success or otherwise of controlling blood sugar levels; highlight problems with insulin dosage as appropriate	

Table 2.1 (contd)

Dimension	Identified individual goals	Nursing role and intervention	Target date
Emotional health and relationships	To be able obtain erection through use of an 'erectaid' vacuum device	Technical expert: be able to operate the vacuum device; demonstrate awareness of potential complications Psychological support: be aware of limitations in providing support relating to sexual health; encourage the individual to discuss sex and sexuality; look for positive cues that may enable 'safe' initiation of such a conversation Educator: teach the use of the device, including prevention of potential complications Coordinator: organise obtained 'erectaid' Teamworker: report or refer to sexual health team as appropriate relating to progress	
Movement and transport	To be able to put on a spinal brace independently	Technical expert: able to apply the brace while minimising movement of affected area; able to demonstrate means by which limitations in function through wearing the brace can be overcome Psychological support: there may be issues regarding body image relating to wearing the brace; encourage the client to express how they feel about wearing the brace Educator: teach the individual to put on the brace; explanation of potential complications if they do not adhere to this is essential Coordinator: liaison with orthotics about allocating time for fitting, and regarding subsequent alterations to brace size and shape Team worker: report progress towards goal	
Home and finance	To identify potential issues in preparation for discharge through spending weekend at home	Technical expert: knowledge of current client abilities; able to advise on practical solutions to potential problems Psychological support: discuss before and arrange session after the weekend to discuss how it felt to be back home; offer practical solutions to any anxieties expressed; reassure that support is available via the telephone from the clinical area continually throughout the weekend Educator: educate regarding problem-solving techniques Coordinator: organise with the client any medication and equipment required Team worker: liaise with team to ensure everything is in place to facilitate going home; arrange for the district nurse to visit if appropriate	

client to use as an example the interventions suggested are broad in nature. These will obviously be more specific in the real situation.

SUMMARY

The prophets of doom may suggest that nursing is under threat, and indeed it is correct to suggest that this is indeed true for nursing as we know it *today*. However, nursing has been, is and will be subject to continual change, and it is axiomatic that this should be the case. The basis for change should be in response to meeting client need effectively, and it must be seen in the context of the overall provision of health care and, of course, rehabilitation. There will be a role for nursing in health care, and although this role may change, nursing services will remain rooted in the core elements and based in practice. The opportunities to develop nursing to meet client need effectively through expanding nursing practice have been increased through the 'scope of professional practice'. The knowledge base unique to nursing will not only enable this to occur, but will also ensure that all the elements required to provide client-centred rehabilitation nursing services remain intact. This necessitates a proactive approach, with nursing leading such changes rather than sitting back waiting for changes to be imposed.

Six key nursing roles within rehabilitation have been described within the rehabilitation framework. There needs to be a recognition, both within nursing itself and within other disciplines, that rehabilitation does not fall entirely within a traditional therapy remit. Conversely, the wide scope of nursing and the role it has within rehabilitation over the entire 24 hour period suggests that now, more than ever, rehabilitation nursing is valuable and should be valued.

REFERENCES

Benner P 1984 From novice to expert: excellence and power in clinical practice. Addison-Wesley, New York
Benner P, Wrubel J 1989 The primacy of caring. Addison-Wesley, New York
Carper B 1978 Fundamental patterns of knowing. Advanced Nursing Science 1(1):13–23
Davis P 1994 Nursing the orthopaedic patient. Churchill Livingstone, Edinburgh
Fawcett J 1984 The metaparadigm of nursing: present status and future requirements. IMAGE: Journal of Nursing Scholarship 16:84–87
Footner A 1992 Orthopaedic nursing, 2nd edn. Baillière Tindall, London
Gaut D A 1986 Evaluating caring competencies in nursing practice. Topics in Clinical Nursing 8(2):77–83
Henderson V 1964 The nature of nursing. American Journal of Nursing 64:62–68
Johnson J 1995 Achieving effective rehabilitation outcomes: does the nurse have a role. British Journal of Therapy and Rehabilitation 2(3):113–118
Kirby C, Slevin O 1992 A new curriculum for care. In: Slevin O, Buckenham (eds) Project 2000: the teachers speak. Campion Press, Edinburgh
Leininger M 1986 Care facilitation and resistance factors in the culture of nursing. Topics in Clinical Nursing 8(2):1–12
Melesis A I 1991 Theoretical nursing: development and progress, 2nd edn. Lippincott, New York
Newman M A, Sime A M, Corcoran-Perry S A 1991 The focus of the discipline of nursing. Advances in Nursing Science 14(1):1–6

Parse R R 1992 Human becoming: Parse's theory of nursing. Nursing Science Quarterly 5(1):35–42

Rheiner N W 1995 A theoretical framework for research on client compliance with a rehabilitation programme. Rehabilitation Nursing Research 4(3): 90–97

Roach S M 1985 A foundation for nursing ethics. In: Carmi A, Schnieder S (eds) Nursing law and ethics. Springer-Verlag, Berlin, pp 170–177

Rotter J B 1966 Generalized expectancies for internal versus external control of reinforcement. Psychological Monographs 80(1):1–28

Waters K R, Luker K A 1996 Staff perceptions on the role of the nurse in rehabilitation wards for elderly people. Journal of Clinical Nursing 5:105–114

Watson J 1988 Nursing: human science and human care – a theory of nursing. National League of Nursing, New York

The rehabilitation nurse as educator

3

The education of clients

Deborah Barnett

WHY EDUCATE CLIENTS?

In recent years there has been an increasing awareness surrounding the need for provision of patient education (Luker & Caress 1989, Noble 1991, Fleming 1992). Both nurses and their patients are now realising that issues surrounding health and health promotion should not be solely confined to the professionals, but that knowledge should be cascaded down through all levels from those who provide the care to those who receive the care.

As far back as 1966, classic nursing authors such as Henderson perceived part of the nurse's role as being to improve patients' levels of understanding, and therefore promote their health. According to the nurse's Code of Professional Conduct (United Kingdom Central Council of Nursing, Midwifery and Health Visiting (UKCC) 1992, Section 5) each registered nurse, midwife or health visitor must 'work in an open and cooperative manner with patients, clients and their families, foster their independence and recognise and respect their involvement in the planning and delivery of care.' Encompassed within the concept of fostering independence is the provision of education to enable this to be achieved. Patients should be facilitated to become empowered, encouraged to take a more active role, and ultimately lead in the decision-making process regarding their care. Therefore, as nurses it is unreasonable to consider that patients will have the ability to cooperate without having received adequate information about their condition and the care that accompanies it. This has been reemphasised in two major government led documents: *The Health of the Nation* and *The Patient's Charter* (Department of Health 1992, 1995). Both documents suggest that nurses should be encouraging people to lead healthier and safer lives, and promote the availability of healthy choices. It is also emphasised that patients have the right to have any proposed treatment, including the risks involved in that treatment and any other alternatives, clearly explained to them before they decide whether to agree to it.

Nurses must realise and appreciate that, whether they are in agreement or not, health education is no longer a desirable and optional element in patient care within the rehabilitation process following injury or illness, but is a compulsory and essential one. Therefore, nurses must appreciate that they have a legal, moral and professional responsibility to ensure that patients are kept informed and have their questions answered. This concept should be incorporated in daily practice, as it is undoubtedly one of the key components of everyday nursing practice. According to Antrobus (1997), 'The role of the nurse as health worker should be to assist individuals to attain equilibrium with both their internal and external environment as they strive to participate in the world.' To be able to meet the challenges that this role of educator brings to any rehabilitation environment, nurses must be familiar with why, how and who they should be educating. The aim of this chapter is therefore to provide the reader with the tools to develop patient education programmes that are effective and achieve the above aims.

WHY EDUCATE IN REHABILITATION?

The nature of illness or injury often results in a temporary if not permanent disability, requiring that individual to adapt to a new lifestyle, with many physical and social changes challenging their independence and well-being. According to Dean-Baar (1996), cited in Hoeman (1996), 'In the rehabilitation setting the process focuses on the individual's need to incorporate adaptive behaviour into his or her lifestyle.' The whole concept of rehabilitation is based around the process of maximising the potential of an individual, and using this to restore independence to an optimal level for all the major components of life.

Nurses play a vital role in the process of patient education in all clinical settings. In the rehabilitation setting education is focused on helping the patient to increase independence through the acquisition of new skills, knowledge, values, beliefs and behaviour. As outlined in earlier chapters, the main aim is to develop and encourage the patient towards a self-governing state, so that he feels empowered in knowing that he has a responsibility for his own well-being and still has the right to make informed choices regarding his life. It is a way of ensuring both physical and verbal independence (i.e. the ability of the patient to direct his care needs to others, such as personal assistants).

There may be a danger that there are those who perceive patient education as a way of ensuring compliance and making patients fit into a new way of life, a new way of thinking, and/or a new role. The patient is told what he needs to know and what the nurse feels he should know. This method allows no scope for the individual requirements of the patient. The patient adopts the 'sick role' and behaves in the way in which he is expected to. It is only too common for the patient who asks questions and expects answers to be labelled as a 'problem patient'. If we are actually providing education to enable empowerment and independence, this is surely desirable rather than a problem situation.

The more modernistic way of thinking, and the one promoted throughout this book, is one that includes involving patients within the educational process and helping them as individuals to identify what their needs are. This information is then used by patients to build upon their existing

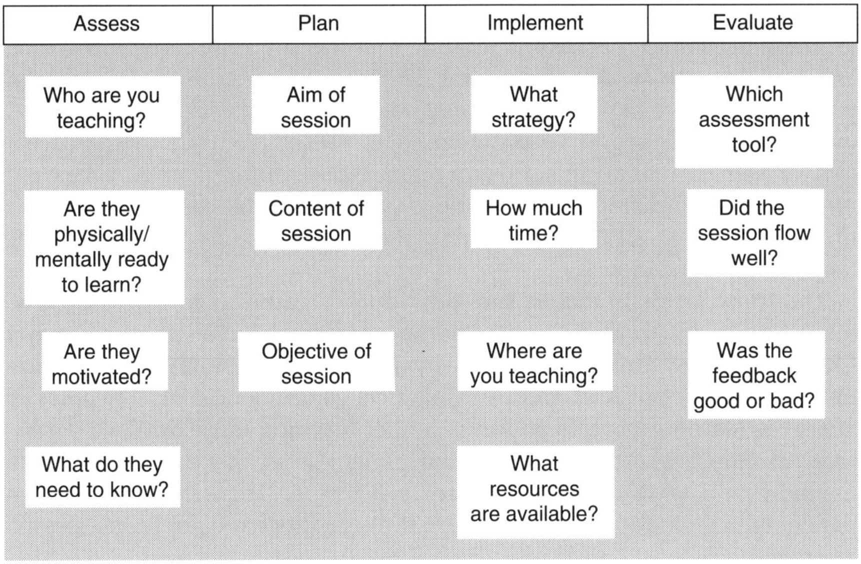

Assess	Plan	Implement	Evaluate
Who are you teaching?	Aim of session	What strategy?	Which assessment tool?
Are they physically/ mentally ready to learn?	Content of session	How much time?	Did the session flow well?
Are they motivated?	Objective of session	Where are you teaching?	Was the feedback good or bad?
What do they need to know?		What resources are available?	

Figure 3.1 The patient teaching and learning process.

knowledge and skills base, helping them towards self-directive behaviour and the ability to control their own destiny. According to Spicer (1982a), 'If the nurse is to be an effective teacher she must do more than just pass on facts; she must engage her patient in learning.' This is further supported by Wilson Barnett (1988) when she acknowledges that 'The shift of focus from the teacher to the client or patient as the main influence when deciding the content, style and pace of teaching is reflected in current thinking around education generally within the concept of adult learning.' Once the particular client group has been identified the process for development of a relevant and meaningful package can begin. This process is outlined in Figure 3.1 and forms the basis of this chapter.

ASSESSMENT OF NEEDS

Before any teaching programme or learning can take place, the nurse must recognise the need to assess three major factors that could influence this process. If the nurse lacks the ability to assess the patient, then effective teaching is not going to take place.

First, it must be identified what it is the patient needs to learn. This will obviously differ depending on the particular health situation of the individual and the individual needs and desires of that person with regard to returning to community living. Teaching a person something that they already know or something that is totally irrelevant to them and their life is a total waste of both the nurse's and the patient's time and can lead to much frustration (Spicer 1982b). The nurse must enter the process objectively and accept that patients are individuals and therefore have individual needs and individual ways of learning.

Second, the patient's ability to learn must be ascertained. This will determine the way in which any programme is delivered and, possibly, the eventual outcome. It is easy to assume that the key principles of teaching and learning can be adapted to any learning situation, including that of patient education. However, this may not always be the case. For example, individuals with cognitive problems (e.g. following head injury or the elderly with chronic confusion) will often require different approaches and may necessitate different expectations. It may be the case that they are unable to take on all that is required, and it is the family who will be the focus of the education.

The third factor is that of the individual's readiness to learn. Clearly, many patients who require education programmes have suffered a major life catastrophe. This is discussed by Luker & Caress (1989), who emphasise that the physical and psychological consequences of ill health can affect the learning process and thus render teaching more difficult. Therefore one must question whether the patient is at the right stage, both mentally and physically, to engage in learning. There are times when patient education fails simply because these factors have not been assessed accurately.

The key areas that the nurse must take into account when planning an education programme are described below.

IS THE PATIENT'S BIOLOGICAL/PHYSICAL STATUS CONDUCIVE TO LEARNING?

During the acute period of illness prior to entering the stage of rehabilitation, the patient may have experienced extensive homeostatic imbalance or been subject to certain neuromuscular disturbances. The nurse must be aware of these factors and ensure that the patient feels well enough to participate in any learning programme. It is of little use attempting to conduct a teaching session with a patient who is in severe pain or who is distracted because he is feeling anxious or restless due to breathlessness. As stated previously, each patient who has experienced cognitive impairments due to, for example, trauma or stroke requires a different approach.

HAS THE PATIENT ACCEPTED HIS CONDITION/PROGNOSIS?

It is important that the nurse appreciates the relationship between body image and self-concept, responses to changes in body image, and strategies for adjustment to changes in body image secondary to disease or injury (Drench 1994). Many patients entering the rehabilitation setting may have suffered changes in body image or have a chronic physical disability. Whether these changes are internally or externally visible has little significance. What matters more is whether the patient has reached the stage within the recovery process where he has begun to adjust to his new life situation. According to Dean-Baar (cited in Hoeman (1996)), clients who are anxious or in denial may state they have never been provided with information that the rehabilitation team are known to have given to the client. Another example of this is the individual who is unable to pass urine and requires an intermittent catheterisation programme. If he believes he will get better, there may be a reluctance to be 'educated', as it is of no relevance. Price (1986) suggested that education is the means by which the patient can re-own his own health care; the assessment of readiness is the first stage in reaching this aim.

IS THE PATIENT SUFFICIENTLY MOTIVATED TO LEARN?

It is envisaged that learning has taken place when there has been a noticeable change in a person's behaviour (Gagne 1970, Rogers 1983). According to Noble (1991), behaviour will only change if there is a need within the patient for the information. Therefore, motivation plays a major part in the learning process. Motivation patterns include both cognitive and affective processes that help direct the patient towards the initiation and the maintenance of achievement, which in turn help towards learning. The cognitive component helps the patient to recognise the importance and need for entering the learning process, and the affective part helps to enhance feelings of achievement and satisfaction when the patient has made the effort to learn. Both the cognitive and affective domains hold an influence over the patient's commitment to learn. Simplistically, it can be said that there are both intrinsic and extrinsic factors acting on the patient. The intrinsic factors come from the patient himself and the extrinsic factors are imposed upon the patient by the environment surrounding him. Intrinsic sources include the way the patient perceives that his illness/disability affects him, the symptoms he is experiencing, his personality and any other related factors that he may have previously experienced. Extrinsic factors may include other patients that he meets with similar or related conditions, information and facts received from the media, the healthcare team responsible for his care, and the response from his family and significant others. Strategies to encourage motivation are covered in Chapter 4.

WHAT DOES THE PATIENT NEED TO LEARN?

It is relatively easy for an experienced nurse, using his experience with other individuals with the same diagnosis, to assess a patient's medical condition and be comfortable in thinking that he knows what that patient needs to learn. Although this may be true to a certain extent, it is equally important that the nurse also includes in his assessment what the patient feels 'he needs to learn'. Every person has their own personal hierarchy of human needs (Fig. 3.2). Biological requirements, social pressures and individual interests all combine together to produce a particular response to a situation. Therefore, when assessing the patient's priorities, the nurse must take into account the type of person he is dealing with, including that person's individual past experiences and present circumstances.

Roper et al (1980) suggest that, after a serious accident, the fulfilment

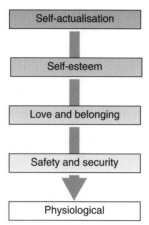

Figure 3.2 Hierarchy of human needs.
(From Roper et al 1980, with permission.)

of physiological and safety needs becomes of paramount importance and submerges all others. This has a significant influence on the order of learning; topics that seem to be of prime importance to the nurse seem irrelevant to the patient at that particular time in their rehabilitation. An example is teaching a patient who is confined to bed because of a sacral pressure sore the topic of 'how to maintain his wheelchair'. In this particular situation at that particular point in time, the patient is not even allowed to get up and sit in his wheelchair. This will not lend itself to the patient being able to see the relevance of learning about how to maintain it. Although obviously the patient will eventually need to know about this subject, at that point they would benefit more from the nurse teaching them about skin management and how to prevent future pressure sores from occurring. Therefore, although the nurse can produce a formal timetable for her teaching, it is important that there is also a patient-centred approach that incorporates a degree of flexibility to take account of changes in need according to the particular circumstances. Learning is significant when the person can relate it to their experiences, and this in turn leads to greater compliance with an education programme.

METHODS OF EDUCATION

Once a thorough assessment of learning needs has been made, the next stage is to decide on the methods through which these needs are to be met. There is a variety of methods that the rehabilitation nurse can employ to deliver a determined education programme. It would be folly to suggest that one method is the only one to be used, as individuals learn in different ways and, therefore, using a combination of methods will often achieve the desired result. Some of these potential methods are discussed in detail below, and potential approaches within these are examined.

A patient-centred programme that can utilise a contract-style, goal-setting approach to education has been advocated by Coles (1989). It was suggested that this approach should be used because people learn best when they are helped to define their own problems. In addition, it may also help to break down any hierarchical barriers that may exist between the patient and the nurse, and thus assist towards developing the 'partnership in care' discussed in Chapter 2. It could be suggested that this less threatening environment, as well as being conducive to the concepts of rehabilitation, will result in improved learning, and therefore a more positive outcome in terms of the promotion of health and prevention of complications. So, prior to discussing specific strategies, it is worth exploring the use of a goal-setting approach to meet the education needs of clients in rehabilitation.

USING A 'GOAL-SETTING' PROCESS FOR PATIENT EDUCATION

As discussed in Chapter 2, goal-setting is becoming a valued tool in areas of rehabilitation and can be a vital part of the assessment, planning, delivery, evaluation and documenting of education, which will achieve satisfactory learning outcomes.

Why have individual goal-setting for learning?

- It allows the patient to make productive use of a learning experience and provides a way of measuring its success.
- It allows the patient to focus on problems individual to their learning needs.
- It allows the patient to reflect upon progress and to self-assess.

How do you organise individual goal-setting?

- The patient and nurse ascertain the identity of specific learning goals, based around the expected learning outcomes of a subject area.
- The patient and the nurse identify the resources necessary to achieve the learning and the process around how to achieve them.
- Documentation is formulated in order to demonstrate progress made towards learning and how often re-evaluation will take place.
- It is identified how the achieved goals will be assessed and by whom.

To reinforce previous points, goals should always be relevant to the patient and motivating. If the patient cannot see the relevance of a particular goal then he will lack motivation in achieving it. When setting goals consider the acronym:

R   relevant
U   understandable
M   measurable
B   behavioural
A   achievable

IDENTIFYING LEARNING RESOURCES AND STRATEGIES

This incorporates a combination of human and material resources and activities required for the patient to achieve the identified goal. Strategies incorporate the actual nurse activity or approach (e.g. teaching and observation of psychomotor skills). Resources may include the nurse as a teacher, involvement of the stoma therapist, literature, models, etc. The patient may require a combination of resources and strategies to achieve one particular outcome.

A ONE-TO-ONE TEACHING APPROACH

Many theorists have compared the strategy of individual learning against that of group learning (Felton 1976, Linderman 1972). They have reached the conclusion that group teaching can be as effective and more efficient than individual teaching. Group teaching allows for peer support and discussion, something which is absent from a one-to-one approach, and is also more cost-effective in terms of teaching resources. Although this may be the case, there are many instances in rehabilitation where individual instruction is clearly beneficial, and where group teaching is not the optimum option in isolation. Indeed, in some situations group teaching can be counterproductive, either to an individual or to other group members. Examples of situations where group learning may not be the most suitable strategy and the nurse would be advised to educate the patient on an individual basis are when the patient:

- has concentration difficulties
- has special needs (e.g. learning disabilities or cognitive problems)
- is extremely apprehensive and anxious about learning new knowledge relating to their condition
- is very elderly or very young
- has language or cultural differences.

A patient with a condition unfamiliar to the environment he is being nursed in, has different educational needs from the other patients. It is true to say that by using a medical model approach, any condition has a set curriculum for an educational programme to follow. For example, a patient found to be suffering from diabetes will be required to know about the nature, complications and management of hypoglycaemia and hyperglycaemia. The beauty of individual teaching is that, in addition to the set curriculum, it allows for flexibility and the ability to negotiate the content between the nurse and the individual patient. For example, with a diabetic patient, particular dietary likes and dislikes, sport and fitness, relationships, and concerns regarding the education of family and others can be addressed which may be relevant just to that individual. It should not be forgotten that much education can and does occur when providing 'care' to individuals. This informal teaching could be deemed as equally important as formally planned sessions, as it provides the opportunity to ascertain progress on a continual basis. If formal sessions are planned, they should be 'timetabled' into the patient's day, as perhaps therapy sessions are. Not only does this approach facilitate the nurse being able to organise his time effectively, but it also helps to emphasise the importance of education to other team members, who may not perceive this rehabilitation nurse role as quite as important as their session. Ozbolt Goodwin (1979) was one of the first nurses to employ a contract learning approach to patient education. While working in a cardiac rehabilitation setting she devised a booklet giving a step-by-step approach to learning. Each patient was assessed and the way that they used the booklet was based on their recovery rate and their individual ability. Evaluation studies of this method proved extremely positive, and the patients had far fewer side-effects.

GROUP LEARNING

For subject areas that have a 'generic' content, a suitable strategy may be that of group learning. In the first instance, for group learning to be considered there needs to be a sufficient number of patients with a similar condition who can benefit from the educational content of the session. Generally speaking, group learning can be a useful tool for providing basic knowledge to patients with similar conditions or needs. It is the nurse's responsibility to make explicit at the start of the session that he is only able to provide the group with 'general' information regarding the topic, and that these details will be expanded upon according to specific needs on an individual basis. According to Dean-Baar (1996) (cited in Hoeman 1996), 'Even in a situation where it is appropriate to include clients in group activities, it is always important to provide an opportunity for clarification of content and application of the content to the individual.' There are few disadvantages reported regarding group learning. Smallegan (1982) suggested that, 'A serious problem in group discussions occurs when the content to be covered is inappropriate or ill-focused.' It is important that the content is seen to be familiar enough to all involved in order that each individual patient can make a contribution. The implication behind this is that this method of teaching may be of no use to a 'mixed' group of patients all of whom have different conditions. For example, group learning may be of little value if carried out on a busy medical or surgical ward where everyone has a different educational priority, whereas such a strategy may prove extremely useful for a group of cardiac rehabilitation patients or diabetic patients. Patients need to have a sufficient background knowledge with enough potential for development so that they can learn from each other (Smallegan 1982).

Attending a group session allows the patient to meet and interact with other patients who are undergoing similar changes to their lifestyle. Wilson Barnett (1988) states a belief that, 'Those who have the same type of problems may well seek comfort from fellow sufferers.' Knowles (1980) supports this theory, and identified group learning as having richer resources and possibly motivating more effectively than individual learning. Studies carried out with regard to group learning in a rehabilitation setting have produced extremely positive results. A study by Raleigh & Odtohan (1987) reported that in a group of cardiac patients who had received a structured teaching programme the result was greater learning and less anxiety on discharge. Further studies by Nishimoto & Schunk (1987) provided results demonstrating that increased socialisation and camaraderie through groups had been linked to an increase in cognitive functioning of rehabilitation patients.

In order to be successful, the learning environment during group learning sessions should be seen to be non-threatening and should encourage patients to share information with others, therefore helping to promote a supportive atmosphere, and reduce feelings of isolation in patients. Brookfield (1986) identified that learning in a group can provide feedback and support for the patients that encourage reflection, subsequent actions and the sharing of ideas. In group learning, the nurse should be present in order to facilitate learning and provide guidance to the patient group. As part of this role, factual information surrounding the topic being examined should be delivered, and then discussion within the group should be encouraged. The concept of learning through experience is supported by many (Burnard 1989, Knowles 1980). It allows patients the opportunity to learn from and share the things with their peers which health professionals cannot tell them.

Leading a group learning session is not as straightforward and easy as it may at first appear. The art of facilitating a group session is one that is not learned quickly, and therefore a lot of preparation and practice is required if a group session is to be of value. It is important that the nurse pre-plans the session in order to ensure that the focus is correct. Notes should be made regarding points for discussion. A structured teaching session is probably more useful in the clinical setting than is a free-form discussion group. Here, the nurse prepares a list of topics and questions to be discussed based around pre-defined objectives. The content can then be controlled by the nature of the questions asked, while the nurse ensures that the discussion does not become fragmented. The choice of discussion points becomes the nurse's framework for making sure that the session covers what he intended it to cover.

A further advantage of group learning is that it is a cost-effective way of ensuring that a large proportion of patients receive education, while using a minimum of staff and time resources. In the author's experience, the easiest way to organise a session is to ensure that it takes place at a set time on a set day that is agreeable to all concerned. There is little use organising the session to take place when it is known that there is a consultant ward round or there is a therapy session taking place. A good time may be during a shift handover, when there is normally an increased number of staff available. The nurse facilitating the session has the responsibility of organising a patient education timetable and informing the patients and the ward manager of the details. The ward manager can then ensure that the identified nurse is on duty for that particular time and that they are not issued with additional responsibilities for that period. One way of ensuring that the patients are informed of the details is to produce a whiteboard, which can be positioned in full view of the patients and has the main details written in permanent ink and a space for the additional information to be altered accordingly (Fig. 3.3).

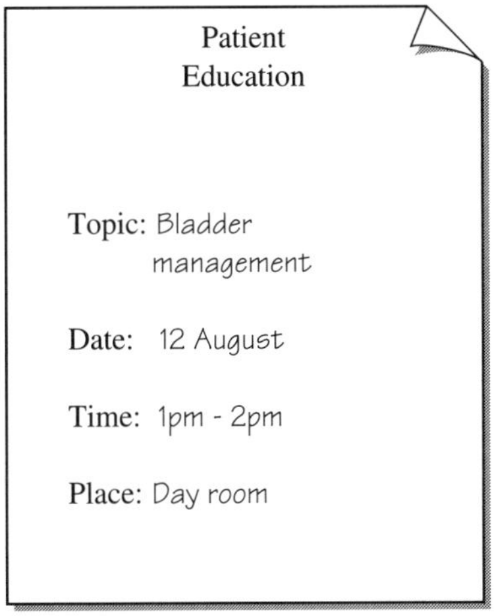

```
Patient
Education


Topic: Bladder
        management

Date:   12 August

Time:   1pm - 2pm

Place:  Day room
```

Figure 3.3 Notification of a patient education session.

As stated previously though, the nurse must be aware that not all patients are candidates for group learning. There is little point in forcing someone who is withdrawn and shy or someone who is disruptive or distracted easily into a group learning environment. This will only lead to problems, and could easily cause the patient in question to become more withdrawn or more disruptive. These are patients who would definitely benefit more from an individual one-to-one teaching session.

Table 3.1 summarises the advantages and disadvantages of the group learning approach.

WRITTEN INFORMATION

Introducing written material into the patient education programme may be more complex than it first appears, and can either help to enhance the

Table 3.1 Advantages and disadvantages of group learning

Advantages	Disadvantages
Cost effective use of staffing resources.	Nurse needs familiarity in managing group sessions.
Most topics lend themselves to group learning.	Only the 'generic' facts can be covered. Individual needs may have to be revisited on a one-to-one basis.
Increases motivation amongst group members – helps goal setting.	Individuals can become discouraged if they see their peers progressing more quickly than themselves.
Provides peer support and increases socialisation and camaraderie.	Needs good group interaction to work successfully.
Helps reduce stigma surrounding certain conditions – allows patients to share experiences.	Session needs pre-planned objectives in order to prevent fragmentation.
Helps to reduce isolation in patients.	

learning process or help to destroy it. Various factors have to be examined when considering producing or distributing such material. First, the information contained in the material has to be correct and consistent in its content; and, secondly, it has to be written in such a way that it is easily readable by all the patients who will receive it.

According to a survey conducted by the Audit Commission (1993), 'Individual patients have different needs, preferences and expectations in relation to clinical information,' and when asked about their experience in hospital it was declared that 'The theme that recurs most frequently is their desire for more information about clinical matters.' Within the context of rehabilitation nursing, the use of written patient information is a vitally important one. It can be used to reinforce and recap on what has been taught in either individual or group sessions. It can also be used by the patient and carers as a source of reference if problems arise following the patient's discharge home. Through considering the following points, written information can be produced that will serve its purpose to individual readers within each particular rehabilitation setting.

FORMAT AND DESIGN

It is important to decide how the finished product will be presented. In some settings it may be that all relevant information is combined together in book form. If this is the case, then it is important to consider how often the information contained in the book will be subject to change. For example, information regarding benefits for disabled persons may alter annually. Therefore, it may be beneficial and more cost-effective to produce the information in a loose-leaf format rather than a bound format, so that sections can be updated as necessary and replaced with ease. In addition, relevance must be considered, (i.e. how much of the information is relevant for the majority of those who will be provided with the book). It is of little use to produce a large, expensive book if only one or two of the sections apply to most of the individuals. It may be advisable to have a more compact handbook containing general information regarding a particular condition, accompanied by several smaller pamphlets relating to specific topics. For example, all patients who have sustained spinal cord damage will need general information regarding bowel, bladder and skin management, but not all patients in this group will require information relating to assisted conception or the use of walking braces. These are topics that apply to some individuals and could be produced as an add-on series of pamphlets that could be referred to as and when necessary. If too much information is given to patients at one time (especially in the early stages of rehabilitation) it could lead to 'overload', and it is possible that patients will miss out on reading the sections that are relevant to their needs.

When producing information books or pamphlets, it is worth checking if the rehabilitation centre uses any logos or follows a particular design used by the rest of the hospital. Using a consistent design to that used for any other literature produced for patients from your centre ensures a corporate image and allows a more professional presentation of the finished product.

Graphics can be used to enhance the text. Patients may remember more easily points that have cartoon-type characters associated with them than those encased in pages of 'boring' looking text.

Whatever the chosen method, all the information must be presented in a clear, easy to read format. The information should be split into small sections rather than given as many pages of solid text. It is sometimes advisable to use subheadings or a question and answer format. This enables the patient to find the answer to their question easily, without having to plough through the whole book.

CONTENT

It is essential that the content of patient education material is up to date and correct. It is advisable to use a multiprofessional approach when producing literature applicable to rehabilitation, in order to ensure that all areas of the speciality are included. This is an important point to consider when deciding who writes the material. It is useful to have a panel of individuals considered to be experts in their subjects who can oversee the content and offer their 'seal of approval', thereby giving credibility to the work produced.

LANGUAGE

A key factor to bear in mind is that the average patient may not understand medical terminology or technological jargon; therefore, these should be avoided at all times. If it is essential to include such terms, then they need to be clarified in lay language.

When embarking upon writing patient information material, it is worth analysing what the 'average' patient is like. For example, take into account the age, gender, social status, etc., of patients. This will help the writer to focus the content and structure of the material on the client group it is aimed at, and help prevent the use of language within the text that is inappropriate to the reader. After all, complicated, jargonistic words will be off-putting to the majority of patients, and may lead to a decrease in compliance by patients who do not understand the information given to them.

It is much better to write using short, sharp sentences that are straight to the point than to use sentences that are long-winded and contain complicated grammar. It is recommended by Boyd (1987) that sentences should contain no more than 60–70 characters. It is better to try to limit the words used to those containing no more than two syllables and to use longer words only if they are absolutely essential to the content.

Written material for patients should be reader-friendly. It should use the active rather than the passive voice, as this is usually shorter and more direct and is in the first rather than the third person. This makes the language more personal to the reader. Sentences should be written using lower case rather than upper case characters. The excessive use of capital letters makes reading difficult on the eyes and will result in the patient missing out on important facts. According to Albert & Chadwick (1992) the misuse of capitals can have 'a harmful effect, by slowing the reader, intruding in the text and giving unnecessary prominence'. The font and typeface are also important considerations. Guidelines set by the Royal National Institute for the Blind recommend 12 point as the minimum size for a readable typeface and do not recommend the use of italics, but rather a simple, clear type.

READABILITY

A simple way to check whether the information that has been produced is reader-friendly is by completing the fog test. This test has been reproduced in a variety of ways over the past five or so decades (Albert & Chadwick 1992). It has been used many times in auditing communication details within the health service. The test assists the writer in determining the complexity of the text that has been produced. In general, the lower the fog score, the easier the piece is to read.

The following is based on the Gunning fog test given in Albert & Chadwick (1992).

1. Choose a piece of writing of approximately 100 words in length. The piece must end in either a full stop, a question mark or an exclamation mark.

2. Determine the average sentence length by dividing the number of words by the number of sentences contained within the piece.

3. Count the number of words in the piece that are made up of three syllables or more. Do not count combinations of easy words, proper nouns, commonly used jargon or verbs that become three syllables when '-ed', '-ing' or '-es' are added.

4. Add together the average sentence length and the number of long words ((2) and (3) above).

5. Multiply the value obtained in step (4) by 0.4 to obtain the 'reading score'.

An example of the Gunning fog test is given in Box 3.1.

To conclude, after writing any patient information literature it is important that the information is evaluated. A simple and effective method is to distribute the completed work to several patients within the same rehabilitation setting who have a similar educational need. Choose the patients from a variety of age groups and a variety of social backgrounds. Decide upon a range of questions to ask the chosen group and study the answers. All answers should be provided anonymously, as this will appear less threatening to the patients and provide a more truthful series of answers.

COMPUTER-ASSISTED EDUCATION

One way to enhance patients' learning is through the use of computer-assisted learning (CAL) packages. These packages have been in use over the past decade, and reports surrounding their use have proven favourable

---

■ **BOX 3.1 Example of the Gunning fog test**

Consider the following passage (from Smith & Brain (1980), p 39):

'Such a change of interstitial volume may occur when a reduction of plasma albumin leads to a fall of oncotic pressure in the plasma with a consequent "shift" of volume into the interstitial compartment. This results in a small but persistent fall in plasma volume which activates a series of regulating systems that result in retention of salt and water by the kidney. So long as the plasma albumin remains low, however, volume will continue to shift out of the plasma compartment and produce ever-increasing interstitial expansion. The persisting small change in plasma volume may produce no apparent effects of itself but the interstitial oedema which results may be overwhelming to the patient.'

Fog test
(a) Total words   115
(b) No. of sentences   4
(c) Average sentence length $115 \div 4 = 28.5$
(d) No. of long words   14
(e) (c) plus (d) $28.5 + 14 = 42.5$
(f) Reading score $42.5 \times 0.4 = 17$

(Luker & Caress 1989, Noble 1991). There is much optimism about their value in patient education in the future. According to Noble (1991), 'CAL has been demonstrated as being superior to both written and verbal formats in promoting recall and in performance in the undertaking of clinical procedures.'

There are many potential advantages to be considered in the use CAL for education purposes, especially in the rehabilitation setting.

1. Patients can work at their own pace. They are not placed in a position where they can be made to feel 'stupid' or 'ignorant' if they are unable to grasp basic principles surrounding a chosen topic. CAL allows patients to revisit points over and over again until they gain an adequate understanding.

2. Computers can be used by patients of all ages. Even the elderly have been found to prefer this method of receiving information to that of the written text (Daerdorff 1986). The use of graphics can also prove to be an incentive for the younger patient to enjoy learning. As it is possible in today's technological world to produce computer packages that can be used even by those who lack computer literacy, these packages lend themselves to a wide audience.

3. CAL packages can also be accessed by those patients who have sight or hearing impairments that restrict them from participating in verbal or demonstrative sessions. Microchips that allow the computer to 'speak' to the patient and allow the patient to 'speak' to the computer are now used widely in rehabilitation settings. Computer switches are available that

enable even the most severely disabled individual to access programmes (Taira 1994).

4. There is potential for the use of CAL packages in the education of those individuals who lack ease of mobility. For example, a patient requiring continuous assisted respiratory ventilation due to head injury or high spinal cord trauma still has education needs. These patients still need access to information regarding the general implications of their condition (e.g. skin, bladder and bowel management). Problems may arise if they are hindered from attending organised group teaching sessions because of lack of personnel to accompany them in case they need assistance. The majority of these patients are familiar with the use of computers to meet their everyday environmental demands, and therefore using computers to aid learning could add to their independence and provide them with an increased feeling of self-worth and empowerment.

5. Mello (1992) makes a point for consideration when she discusses the vast number of adults (more than 200 000) living in the UK who do not have a full command of the English language. She also emphasises the importance of developing health services to meet the needs of all who use them. If a person has difficulty with the English language, how are they supposed to cope within a rehabilitation setting that promotes group learning (spoken in English) because there is a lack of resources to carry out individual teaching sessions. This person will be immediately disadvantaged in the amount of information they receive regarding their condition. CAL packages have the potential to be reproduced in a vast number of languages and could easily be used by individuals who, finding themselves in this position, would otherwise be at a disadvantage.

Despite these advantages, CAL is only as good as the packages that are produced and the way in which they are used. They should not be seen as an alternative to face-to-face teaching, on either an individual or a group basis. These programmes have their use as accompanying material used to enhance the more formal teaching strategies. They can be accessed by a wide variety of patients in many clinical settings. As computers are becoming a part of everyday life for many of us, the author's personal view is that they deserve to be given a chance within the rehabilitation setting.

EVALUATING THE TEACHING AND LEARNING PROCESS

Evaluation is seen by many as the forgotten part of the teaching and learning process, yet it should be seen as the most important. It is the process that enables the nurse to assess the effectiveness, efficiency and usefulness of what has been accomplished by his teaching. It is a way of measuring whether initial learning outcomes have been met, and whether they have been met successfully enough to have led to a significant change in the patient's behaviour in order for the nurse to assume that learning has taken place. No learning experience should be considered entirely significant if it is not characterised by a positive shift in the learner's attitude to either the subject or to learning in general (Davies 1971). The degree of learning attained should be measured using an objective set of data that can be used to determine the degree to which set goals have been achieved or not achieved.

Unless the full concept of evaluation is understood the benefits will never be appreciated. The results of the evaluation process should be used by both the teacher and the learner. Evaluation is the way by which the teacher is encouraged to improve on his professional skills and by which the learner receives feedback that acts to reinforce whether he is doing things correctly or incorrectly.

There are four main reasons for performing an evaluation.

- It measures the inclination of the patient in terms of whether or not they have appreciated the goals or outcomes that they have set.
- It determines which goals or outcomes have not been appreciated, so that suitable action can be taken.
- It informs the nurse of the appropriateness of the chosen teaching strategy, so that its strengths and weaknesses can be identified and acted upon.
- It indicates whether any additional resources are required to improve learning.

CRITERIA FOR SUCCESSFUL EVALUATION OF LEARNING

There are three criteria that must be met for any evaluation process to be successful.

- It must be *appropriate*. The chosen method of evaluation must be appropriate to the chosen subject, the goals and outcomes that have been set, the chosen teaching strategy and the patient.
- It must be *effective*. The evaluation strategy must measure what it intends to measure. In this way reliability and validity of the chosen strategy are ensured.
- It must be *practical*. The chosen evaluation strategy must be acceptable to both the nurse and the patient. It must be cost- and time-effective and be sufficiently flexible that it can be re-used again and again for similar situations.

METHODS OF EVALUATING LEARNING

There are many strategies that can be employed by teachers in order to evaluate whether appropriate learning has taken place. Five of the more common strategies are identified and briefly discussed below.

Self-evaluation

If the patient has been a major participant in setting the outcomes for the learning experience, then he should also be a major participant in the evaluation of those outcomes. Being actively involved in the evaluation process adds to the patient's self-esteem and gives him a sense of pride in accomplishing the task he set out to achieve.

Oral feedback

This method of evaluation offers great flexibility as it can be used quite well by those individuals who can express themselves verbally but have physical difficulties or do not like completing written evaluations. The patient is able to recall information that has been taught and a problem-solving, scenario-type evaluation can be carried out verbally between the nurse and the patient to ensure that information has been absorbed and can be adapted to situations. A disadvantage of this method is that the patient may feel intimidated by the nurse asking questions. He may feel that he is being placed under scrutiny, and his confidence may be affected if he cannot answer a question when he has been 'put on the spot'.

Observation/demonstration

This is an invaluable method of evaluation in assessing whether or not a patient has managed to learn a psychomotor skill correctly, allowing immediate feedback from the nurse to the patient. The nurse may notice that a patient is turning in bed a little more often in order to avoid the formation of pressure sores, or that a diabetic patient is taking a more active interest in his diet. Continuity, through having a named nurse educator or primary nurse, may facilitate the detection of smaller improvements in practice.

Feedback from relatives and carers

This can be achieved through formal or informal discussion with relatives, carers, etc. The nurse must remember that these people often know the patient better than anyone else, and therefore are a valuable source of information to the nurse with regard to the patient's preferred ways of learning, general acceptance of their condition, and how learning is influencing their behaviour.

Patient notes

Evaluation of patient progress may be assessed by the nurse involving the patient in certain record-keeping exercises. For example, a diabetic patient could be taught how to complete her urinalysis chart, or a paraplegic patient could complete his skin assessment chart. How accurately this documentation is completed will give the nurse an indication of how motivated the patient is, as well as an indication of the patient's progress. There may be concerns if it is thought the patient may be supplying inaccurate and misleading data, therefore occasional 'spot checks' by the nurse to check the accuracy of data may be wise. This method of evaluation

Table 3.2 A framework for evaluating patient teaching

Area	Points to note
Format	Was the method chosen appropriate to the content of the session? Was the format one-to-one, group, etc.?
Content	Was the content presented at the correct educational level? Were the facts presented clearly?
Audio-visual aids	Were they used appropriately? Were they clear and simple?
Patient satisfaction	Were they happy with the session? Was the content appropriate to their needs? Was the timing satisfactory (was it too long/too short)? Were they able to understand any diagrams, etc.?
Activities	Were practice examples used at appropriate times to support theory? Was there adequate encouragement for questions? Was appropriate feedback offered to the patient?
Recommendations	Were you satisfied with how the session went? Were any follow-up activities incorporated into the teaching plan? Did you receive any suggestions for improvements? Would you be happy to incorporate any suggestions into your future sessions?

could also be incorporated in the contract learning approach described in Chapter 2.

As a summary, a framework for the evaluation of teaching is given in Table 3.2. This could be completed by the nurse, a nursing colleague or (for the brave) by the patient.

BARRIERS TO EDUCATION

Although nurses often understand their responsibilities and the need for educating clients, much of the literature indicates the fact that patient education is not being carried out (Close 1988, Luker & Caress 1989, Tilley et al 1987). It is suggested that there are three main factors that influence whether or not a proposed learning experience will be successful (Luker & Caress 1989) (Fig. 3.4), namely:

- the organisation
- the nurse
- the patient.

THE ORGANISATION

It is all too common for nurses to give staff shortages and a high workload as the reason why a patient education programme is not being carried out. It is important that nurses seek support from peers and the hierarchy

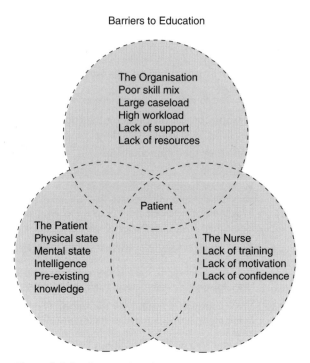

Figure 3.4 Barriers to education.

within the clinical area. Nurses must support each other, and see education as being as a part of their job that is as important as everything else. Systems of work must be altered to ensure that routine times for educating patients can be set and implemented. Indeed, the dependency that the patient has on the nurse for certain procedures can only be reduced if the patient is taught the correct way to carry out that procedure independently. In the author's experience, the easiest way to organise a group session is to ensure that it takes place at a set time on a set day. In this way, everyone knows that, for example, at 1–2 pm each Wednesday there will be a patient education session. This also helps to emphasise the importance of the session to the patients, as it becomes part of their rehabilitation timetable.

Another problem that may be encountered is a lack of available resources. As long as patient education is given a low priority this will remain a problem. Although the organisation of a programme may initially involve some financial outlay, most establishments have access to funds where it may be possible for nurses to put forward a 'case of need', and by emphasising the importance of the education programme may receive funding towards resources.

THE NURSE

It is fundamental to this essential nursing role in rehabilitation that nurses are competent and confident to teach. It is not reasonable to expect a nurse who has had no training to have the ability to address a patient education group and teach successfully. Therefore, nurses must attend one of the many courses now becoming available within institutions, for specific training in facilitating learning within the clinical environment.

It is also essential that the nurse has substantial knowledge of the subject he is about to teach, and feels confident in his own knowledge base. Wilson Barnett (1988) suggests that if the nurse is not confident then he will not teach; what he will actually do is provide the patient with less information than is required, and this information may be inaccurate. As Jenny (1978) points out, 'The critical factor in the patient's acceptance of the help offered will be his perception of the nurse's credibility as an authentic, authoritative source.'

This is not intended to imply that it is only more senior nurses who can become involved in the education process. As previously stated, each nurse has a personal responsibility for educating patients. Therefore, junior staff can become involved by working with their seniors, observing the assessment and the education process. As the more junior nurse gains the knowledge base he needs, he should then be encouraged to become actively involved in the process, which will help to enhance his teaching skills and confidence. The senior nurse acting as mentor can supervise until the nurse is ready to take on this role completely.

THE PATIENT

There are many variables that can influence whether or not a patient is going to gain from the education process, many of which have been covered earlier in this chapter when discussing assessment of learning need and readiness to learn. To reiterate, the key factors from a patient's perspective are:

1. The patient's physical condition may not be conducive to absorbing information at that particular time.

2. The patient may not be psychologically prepared to receive information referring to the longer term effects of their illness or disability.

3. The patient's pre-existing knowledge may cause them to become bored and to 'switch off' if they are included in a session covering information that they are already familiar with. The problem in this situation may be that they may miss a vital piece of information that they were not familiar with.

4. Elderly or very young patients have different ways of learning and differing needs, therefore it is not advisable for them to be involved in the same teaching session. In addition, such patients may find it difficult to sit for a set period of time without becoming irritable or tired.

5. Literacy or language problems may also provide a barrier to the patient being educated. Such patients present with special needs that a nurse may not be familiar with. The use of pictures or models may often be beneficial. It is also the responsibility of the nurse to contact interpreters if necessary, and to ensure that any information produced is in the appropriate language and jargon free.

SUMMARY

Nurses in rehabilitation should class themselves as part of the multi-disciplinary team, and should consider their role as patient educator alongside and equal to that of the therapists and medical staff. This chapter has taken the reader through the assessment of learning needs and suggested strategies and processes through which education programmes can be delivered. As a summary, the following framework is designed to act as a checklist.

A STEP-BY-STEP GUIDE TO PLANNING A TEACHING PROGRAMME

1. *Assess*
   - **The patient:**
     - Is the patient physically and mentally ready to learn?
     - What is his prior experience of the subject?
     - What is the progress in rehabilitation reported by other disciplines?
     - What does the patient want to learn?
     - What does the patient need to learn?
     - What are the outcomes for the session?
   - **The environment:**
     - What type of rehabilitation setting are you teaching in?
     - Does the timing of the sessions fit in with other activities?
     - Do the sessions form part of the patient's rehabilitation programme?
     - Is there a suitable location in which the sessions can be held?
     - Does the chosen location have access for wheelchairs, beds, etc.?
     - Are there sufficient resources available for your teaching session?
   - **Yourself:**
     - Do you have sufficient in-depth knowledge relating to the subjects and skills you have chosen to teach?
     - Do you feel enthusiastic, confident and motivated?
2. *Plan*
   - **Learning outcomes:**
     - Has the patient been involved in setting the learning outcomes?
     - Is the patient aware of your intended specific outcomes within the programme?
   - **Time:**
     - Is the chosen time convenient?
     - Does the time interfere with other rehabilitation sessions?
     - Does the time impinge on the patient's free time/visiting time?
     - How long are sessions going to last?
   - **Area:**
     - Is it quiet with no distractions?
     - Is it easily accessible?

   – Is the room temperature too hot/too cold?
   – Is there adequate lighting?
- **Aids:**
   – Are your teaching notes accurate and up to date?
   – Do you need models, an overhead projector, books, charts, etc.?
- **Patients:**
   – Who is attending?
   – Have you assessed their prior knowledge about their condition?
   – Have you informed them of when and where the session will take place?

3. *Implement*
- **Skills:**
   – Perform the demonstration.
   – Supervise practice.
- **Knowledge:**
   – Test the patient's prior knowledge.
   – Keep 'new' information to an acceptable number of facts, so as to avoid overload.
   – Use aids as required.
   – Speak clearly and slowly.
   – Never assume that patients know what you are talking about.
   – Do not use medical jargon and complicated terminology.
   – Use plenty of repetition.
   – Involve patients in discussion of points. Discuss experiences (good and bad.).
   – Encourage questions.

4. *Evaluate*
- **Skills:**
   – Can the patient perform the skill safely?
- **Knowledge:**
   – Can the patient answer questions correctly?
   – Can the patient discuss potential complications, safety factors, etc., with you?

5. *Feedback*
- Encourage the patient at all times.
- View any mistakes as part of learning, never as failure.
- Is there any noticeable change in the behaviour of the patient?
- Is the patient still motivated?
- Is there positive feedback from other members of the multiprofessional team?

REFERENCES

Albert T, Chadwick S 1992 How readable are practice leaflets? British Medical Journal 305:1266–1268
Antrobus S 1997 Developing the nurse as a knowledge worker in health – learning the artistry of practice. Journal of Advanced Nursing 25:829–835

Audit Commission 1993 What seems to be the matter? Communication between hospitals and patients. HMSO, London

Boyd M D 1987 A guide to writing effective patient education materials. Nursing Management 18(7):56–57

Brookfield S D 1986 Understanding and facilitating adult learning. Open University Press, Milton Keynes

Burnard P 1989 Experiential learning and andragogy – negotiated learning in nurse education: a critical appraisal. Nurse Education Today 9:300–306

Close A 1988 Patient education: a literature review. Journal of Advanced Nursing 13:203–213

Coles C 1995 Educating the health care team. Patient education and counselling 26:239–244

Daerdorff W W 1986 Computerised health education: a comparison with traditional formats. Health Education Quarterly 13(1):61–72

Davies I K 1971 The management of learning. McGraw-Hill, London

Department of Health 1992 The health of the nation: a strategy for health in England. HMSO, London

Department of Health 1995 The patient's charter and you. HMSO, London

Drench M E 1994 Changes in body image secondary to disease and injury. Rehabilitation Nursing 19(1):31–35

Felton G 1976 Pre-operative nursing intervention with the patient for surgery: outcomes of three approaches. International Journal of Nursing Studies 13:83–96

Fleming V E M 1992 Client education: a futuristic outlook. Journal of Advanced Nursing 17:158–163

Gagne R M 1970 The conditions of learning. Holt, Rinehart & Winston, New York

Hoeman S P 1996 Rehabilitation nursing – process and application, 2nd edn. Mosby, St Louis

Jenny J 1978 A strategy for patient teaching. Journal of Advanced Nursing 3(4):341–348

Knowles M S 1980 The modern practice of adult education. Follett, Chicago

Linderman C A 1972 Nursing intervention with the pre-surgical patient. Nursing Research 21:196–209

Luker K, Caress A L 1989 Rethinking patient education. Journal of Advanced Nursing 14:711–718

Mello M 1992 Plugging the gap. Nursing Times 88(43):34–36

Nishimoto T, Schunk C 1987 Group therapy: an alternative treatment approach. Clinical Management in Physical Therapy 4(7):16–18

Noble C 1991 Are nurses good patient educators? Journal of Advanced Nursing 16:1185–1189

Ozbolt Goodwin J 1979 Programmed instruction for self care following pulmonary surgery. International Journal of Nursing Studies 16:29–40

Price B 1986 Mirror, mirror on the wall. Nursing Times 83(39):30–32

Raleigh E, Odtohan B 1987 The effect of a cardiac teaching program on patient rehabilitation. Heart & Lung 16:311–317

Rogers C 1983 Freedom to learn for the 80s. Bell & Howell, Ohio

Roper N, Logan W W, Tierney A J 1980 The elements of nursing. Churchill Livingstone, Edinburgh

Smallegan M J 1982 Teaching through groups. Journal of Nursing Education 21(1):23–31

Smith K, Brain E 1980 Fluids and electrolytes: a conceptual approach. Churchill Livingstone, London

Spicer J 1982a Teaching the patient. Nursing Mirror 155:51–52

Spicer J 1982b Teaching to a plan. Nursing Mirror 155:48–49

Taira F 1994 Computer use by adults with disabilities. Rehabilitation Nursing 19(2):84–86

Tilley J D, Gregor F M, Thiessen V 1987 The nurse's role in patient education: incongruent perceptions among nurses and patients. Journal of Advanced Nursing 12:291–301

United Kingdom Central Council of Nursing, Midwifery and Health Visiting 1992 The scope of professional practice. UKCC, London

Wilson Barnett J 1988 Patient teaching or patient counselling? Journal of Advanced Nursing 13:215–222

The education of the family and carers

Kathleen Dean

INTRODUCTION

This section focuses on the role of the family within rehabilitation. If it is accepted that the family will play a part in coming to terms with the effects of injury and illness to their loved one, it seems somewhat obvious to state that their need for education, as well as that of the individual client, is paramount. The basic premise of this section is that, bearing in mind the potential influence on the client, without the appropriate information the family may not only be unable to fulfil their role in rehabilitation, but indeed they may be detrimental to the rehabilitation process. It is worth emphasising that if this is the case it is not through malice or simply a desire to cause trouble (as may often be anecdotally stated), but more commonly due to a lack of understanding. Such a barrier may be overcome with an appropriate nursing plan. It is the aim of this section to provide the reader with appropriate frameworks to meet the needs of the family and, therefore, ultimately to influence positively the rehabilitation process.

THE FAMILY AND REHABILITATION

The family can make an important, positive contribution to the rehabilitation of patients (Brillhart & Stewart 1989). In support of their role and contribution with regard to cardiac patients, Price et al (1991) note that families can provide:

- important historical data
- psychological support
- encouragement in progress.

In addition, families provide social support and, often, a common link between the professional and the patient. Youngblood & Hines (1992) recognise the involvement of a supportive family as an indicator of successful rehabilitation. It is appropriate, therefore, to consider who the family is. The traditional or conventional nuclear family is no longer considered to be the predominant family type (Haralambos & Holborn 1995). Family units are more diverse, and include groups such as single-parent families, extended families living together, extended families living apart, second-family units and adult-only families. We need to take account of this when we identify the patient's family. Our perceptions of family and those of the patient may not be the same, and therefore those whom the patient considers to be significant in his life may be different to our own expectations.

The family represents a more permanent feature in the patient's life, being there before the onset of illness (Satir 1972, cited in Youngblood & Hines 1992), and given the right circumstances they will continue to be there long after any employed carer. Therefore the family can provide stability and continuity for the patient, whether in a 'hands-on' caring capacity, or in their usual familial relationship.

For the purposes of this chapter and framework, the family is considered as that network of people whom the patient himself considers to be significant in his life and environment. Therefore, identification of who the family is, is an essential fundamental issue when involving them in the patient's rehabilitation. This aspect is discussed further in the section on family assessment.

WHY EDUCATE THE FAMILY?

Care and rehabilitation is much more community focused than ever before. Evidence for this is apparent in early supported discharge (Audit Commission 1995) and hospital at home schemes (Peter & Torr 1996). It seems that this is a trend which will continue to expand. Nowadays patients are in hospital for shorter periods of time, and there is less institutionalised convalescence available. This inevitably means that the family becomes more involved and is more at the forefront of the patient's needs than ever before, whether providing hands-on care or not. If nursing is to be truly holistic, we must consider this issue as part of the overall care strategy. Whatever level of involvement the family members take on, healthcare education for the family is increasingly important if their input is to be effective (Mayo 1993). In consultation with the patient, the family needs to acquire the relevant knowledge and develop the appropriate skills to enable them to understand the nature of the patient's condition, and offer the appropriate support.

This preparation can begin as soon as patients are admitted to hospital, or even before this if their need for rehabilitation is on a planned basis (e.g. for elective surgery). Traditionally, care has focused on the needs of the individual patient, rather than the family unit. Nurses provide patient-centred or patient-focused care, which traditionally may not have viewed the family as an integral part. The exception here is, notably, in the case of children. In recent years many paediatric units have adopted a family-centred philosophy and approach to nursing. Adult nursing could learn a great deal from the philosophies of paediatric care, and there is emerging evidence that the family is gaining significance in relation to adult nursing. With the focus of care in the community, the needs and role of the family are coming under greater discussion. Studies have been undertaken on aspects such as family-focused care (Titler et al 1995), assessment of family needs (Price et al 1991) and family coping needs (Nolan et al 1995). Indeed, if one goes back to Chapter 1 of this book, which promoted the concept of rehabilitation in the context of societal function rather than physical function, the influence of the family is clearly significant. Not only are there the more obvious aspects of social integration and relationships, but also there are key issues surrounding other potential roles such as 'provider' in the employment domain, and the potential role of a family member as carer within the physical independence area.

As the evidence indicates the potential positive influence of the family in successful rehabilitation, then nursing must focus more on the family and the patient as a unit of care. The family should be a part of the rehabilitation team (Wright 1983, cited in Youngblood & Hines 1992), and be seen to be working in partnership with the patient, nurses and other healthcare professionals (Fig. 3.5).

Whatever the reason for rehabilitation, the family will react in some way to it. Families may be anticipating a need for their increased involvement, such as with someone who has multiple sclerosis or motor neuron disease. However, the increased role may not be anticipated, for example the supportive role required in helping a child cope with diabetes and self-administer insulin. Alternatively, there may be a need for more long-term direct care and support, such as with a patient with trauma following a head injury, spinal cord injury or amputation. It may result from a medical emergency following a myocardial infarction, cerebral embolism, or chronic respiratory problem. The client may be a baby, a child, an adolescent, a young adult, a mid-life adult, elderly or old. Equally, the family will vary considerably. All these factors may have an influence.

It is well documented that the family's response to the situation can affect the rehabilitation outcomes (Evans et al 1992). Family-systems theories suggest that, while the family exists over time, it can often be overwhelmed by illness (Satir 1979, cited in Youngblood & Hines 1992). It is important, therefore, that the family is offered support, and in some situations counselling if such a need is perceived. Families often feel isolated and alone when their relatives are ill and in hospital. They may feel quite useless when they see everyone dashing around and they can do nothing for their family member. They cannot comprehend what has happened. Their need

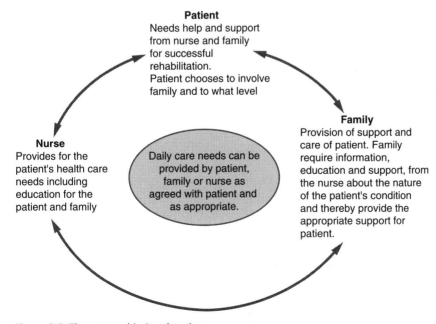

Figure 3.5 The partnership in education.

for care at this time is every bit as important as the patient's needs. All that may be required is gentle reassurance that everything possible is being done to help the patient, along with simple explanations about the care their relative is receiving. Family-needs analyses have shown these two factors to be the most highly rated needs referred to by family members (Leske 1986, 1992, Molter 1979, Price et al 1991, Titler et al 1995). Recognition of these needs and early intervention by the nurse can be fundamental in developing early trust and bonds between himself and the family. Such therapeutic relationships are important. They have been shown to enhance effective coping strategies and positive adaption by the family to stressful situations (Mayo 1993).

If patients come from families who were supportive and close before rehabilitation, there is no evidence to suggest that this will be any different afterwards. Likewise, if family ties were distant and unsupportive before rehabilitation this is not likely to change. The available evidence strongly suggests that it is the patients with supportive families who fare better in their rehabilitation (Evans et al 1992).

Registered nurses are accountable for the care they provide (United Kingdom Central Council of Nursing, Midwifery and Health Visiting (UKCC) 1992). It is in the patient's interests that the family is educated. There is an expectation that family (and friends) will be kept informed of a patient's progress, with the patient's consent. This is part of the patient's charter (Department of Health 1995). Therefore, in view of such evidence, nurses would be failing in their responsibility to the patient if they did not respond to the information and educational needs of the family.

ASSESSMENT OF EDUCATIONAL NEEDS

An assessment of learning needs should occur before an educational programme is implemented. Lorig (1992) observes that one of the most common problems when developing patient education programmes is that there is a failure to consider the needs of all those involved, including, among others, the family. Everybody's agenda in terms of what they want from the education programme may be very different. The nurse may have one set of ideas, the patient another and the family's needs and concerns may be completely different still. If the family see no relevance to the programme for themselves, or if it does not fit in with their beliefs and values, then they are more likely to reject it. If they do accept the programme, it will be executed grudgingly, and consequently little learning will take place (Nolan et al 1995, Youngblood & Hines 1992). In addition, Maklebust & Magnan (1992) maintain that learning will not occur unless the learner is interested. Knowles (1984) recognises that adults learn best when they know why they need to learn and when they are motivated to do so. In view of this it seems essential that the first practical stage in family education is actually to highlight the need for it in the first place.

When the assessment remains patient centred, the philosophy of family involvement can be incorporated. The assessments can be completed over a period of time as more information becomes available. In this way a profile can be built up of the patient and family, and this will form the basis of an educational programme which will suit the family's needs.

It is essential to look at the structure of the family and how family members relate to the patient. Spending time getting to know the family and building a relationship with them is an important first step in any assessment process. Although this may happen with nursing more than any other discipline, often this may be as a side-effect of dealing with the patient, rather than through a direct, more formal approach. Formal time should be set aside to explain to the family what is happening with their relatives in terms of treatment and care. It is probable that this will require re-inforcement rather than just simply being a one-off exercise just after they are made aware of the potential diagnosis or prognosis. When a patient assessment is being carried out, it may be appropriate to include the family. This may be a controversial and complex notion, and should be approached in accordance with the patient's wishes. The patient's own abilities should also be a major consideration here. Answer questions promptly and honestly, and be attentive to the family's needs. Allow the family members to participate in care if they wish, and with the patient's consent. Often this can help to demystify what happens to the patient, and can be an excellent learning opportunity in itself.

It is often through the building of such relationships that the most significant family member is identified. Clearly, in many rehabilitation situations the patient can identify who it is that they wish to be their primary support person or carer. It should not be for the nurse to make such a decision but, armed with appropriate evidence, gleaned through assessment, the nurse can certainly facilitate the process to ensure that family and client are happy. Consider the following example. If a 17-year-old youth is suddenly paralysed following a spinal cord injury, the option to have his mother care for him may not be the most appropriate. This is significant, especially where intimate physical care is required. In reality she had not cared for him in this way for many years. The result may be embarrassment for both. While it must be the patient's choice in this or any situation, the health professional can ensure that all parties are aware of the possible implications of whom they choose as carers.

Dean-Baar (1996) proposes four categories or areas of need that should be considered when undertaking a learning-needs assessment. These are physical, social, psychological and vocational. These needs are expanded upon below, in order to highlight their relevance to the assessment and educational needs of the family. Psychological needs are discussed first, as the factors related to this area need to be addressed before any educational programme can be initiated.

PSYCHOLOGICAL NEEDS

This considers the stresses resulting from the patient's illness or disability, and highlights the potential need for counselling in cases of severe stress before any learning can take place. Under the area of psychological needs, Dean-Baar (1996) considers the attitudes of the patient and the family to their condition. This raises questions about individuals' health beliefs, and prior knowledge and experience of ill-health, disability or any situation where another individual is in need of assistance. Cultural factors must also be taken into account. What is acceptable practice in one culture may be taboo in another. Cultural differences may also strongly influence the way in which the family responds to the individual's illness, condition or disability. Intellectual impairment or ability needs to be considered, in relation to both the patient and the family.

Significance for family assessment and education

Psychological factors will clearly have implications for family carers, and must be addressed within the assessment and educational process. Evans et al (1992) highlight the significance of counselling, rather than education only, in reducing the risk of family breakdown during the rehabilitation process. Therefore, in some situations the recognition that some form of counselling may be required before any educational programme can be implemented must be in the mind of the nurse. It is clear that many of these factors will have an impact on the family member's desire or ability to learn.

Some of the issues discussed above will provide indicators about the level at which to pitch any educational programme. Caring for someone can be lonely and stressful, so it is useful and important to find out how individuals cope under stress, how they relax and what or who are their support mechanisms. There are separate tools that have been developed to assess such coping strategies (Nolan & Grant 1992, cited in Nolan et al 1995). Ensuring these support mechanisms are up and running could be an important part of the educational process.

PHYSICAL FUNCTIONING

This considers the limitations of the patient's current condition, and how these differ from before the onset of their condition. It focuses, therefore, on physical activities of living (eating, washing, writing, dressing, etc.)

Significance for family assessment and education

This aspect features primarily the condition of the patient, and how much physical help will be required. The family may be instrumental in providing information about previous abilities. However, it may also be necessary to assess the ability of family members to assist the patient in carrying out activities of living if this is to be part of their role. For example, what happens if the family member or carer has a known back problem, a rehabilitating cardiac patient has a family member who himself has a heart condition, or the patient requiring insulin injections is unable to administer to himself and the family member has almost phobic tendencies about such a procedure? Again, cultural and religious beliefs may also dictate what and who may or may not carry out certain aspects of care.

SOCIAL NEEDS

Social needs cover areas such as finance within the family, identification of who the family members are, and their roles and relationships. Cultural and religious factors could be considered here too. Social needs also include issues such as ownership of the home and the physical structure of the home.

Significance for family assessment and education

The focus for learning here is related to how the above factors affect both the patient as an individual and the family as a unit, as a result of the patient's condition. This is especially important in relation to relationships and roles within a family (as discussed at the beginning of this section). This category may particularly highlight areas that nurses cannot actively address, but which they can refer on to other professionals. Cultural norms and taboos can raise a whole series of issues that must be addressed if the family are to be able to participate in the programme.

VOCATIONAL PROBLEMS

This area considers the working role of the patient and/or family members. If the patient is an adolescent, it may address how their school or college education is going to continue.

Significance for family assessment and education

The focus here is on learning needs to maintain vocation or retrain and learn new skills. There is a need to consider the employment needs of the family as well, and how this is affected by the situation. This will obviously depend on the care role that the family member takes on.

SUMMARY

Once the assessment is complete the nurse can begin to plan an educational programme which will address the needs of all those concerned. It is not suggested that the nurse is expected to address all of these educational needs himself, but from the assessment he can identify those areas where he has the expertise and is in a position to plan and implement a teaching programme. The nurse is then well placed to refer the patient and family on when other areas of learning are evident, which are considered to be within the sphere of expertise of other professionals.

PLANNING THE PROGRAMME

Once the assessment is complete the nurse can begin to plan the programme of learning. Knowles (1984) asserts that adults learn best when:

- they know why they need to learn
- they can be self-directed

- they can use their own life experiences
- there is a link between what they need to know and their real lives
- learning uses a more problem-solving, life-centred approach
- they are motivated to learn (e.g. effect on own life, quality of life, self-esteem).

These are factors that are well worth keeping in mind when considering the development of any teaching and learning programme that is to include the family.

Whatever method of teaching is employed or resources used, it is highly probable that there is a core level of knowledge and skill that is expected. It is very useful, therefore, to devise local protocols on what educational input is required, and identify what the expected learning outcomes are. This provides an insight as to the level of teaching required, allays fears about what to teach, and offers a guide to ensure that all nurses are teaching in the same way. Lorig (1992) points out that, while nurses are comfortable with their own knowledge base, they are often unsure about the essential content and level when teaching patients. This is unlikely to be any different when teaching families. The result is that the nurse either teaches everything in too much depth, or may omit it altogether. Maklebust & Magnan (1992) suggest that families can be overwhelmed by often unnecessarily in-depth knowledge. What they want to know are the practicalities of how to deal with a hypoglycaemic attack, or how to make their family member more comfortable when breathing is difficult for them.

MAINTAINING INTEREST AND MOTIVATION

Finding a way to maintain the learner's interest is vital, otherwise learning is unlikely to occur. At all stages of the educational programme the learner must be an active participant in any planned programme. Setting individualised learning outcomes, in addition to the core outcomes discussed earlier, can be very useful here. When learning outcomes are set they must be what the learner wants and not what the professional decides they should want. Maklebust & Magnan (1992) recommend the use of teaching strategies that incorporate the use of audio-visual aids which 'involve the learner emotionally' as a way to enhance and promote learning and maintain learner interest.

TEACHING AND LEARNING METHODS

How the educational package is structured and delivered will depend on a variety of factors. Suitable teaching aids can be devised, such as lecture notes, slides and overhead transparencies, that can be held centrally for all nurses to use. Although this may appear to take away the individuality of a programme, it does help to ensure that all those teaching are focusing on the same areas. There is nothing to prevent the content being individualised by, for example, changing the order of teaching or the method used to teach, if the family members learn better in a different way, and by linking the content much more closely to the family's individual learning outcomes.

GENERAL WARD VERSUS SPECIALIST ENVIRONMENT

For the families of patients on a general medical or surgical ward where there is a broad range of conditions, educational packages may have to be predominantly, if not exclusively, of the one-to-one teaching type. This could be the case in newly diagnosed diabetics, or asthmatics for example, or clients requiring surgery for conditions as diverse as inguinal hernia or repair of cholecystectomy. This may provide a very individualised teaching and learning experience, being paced at a level to suit the family. However, the negative side of this method is that the family may miss out on finding out how other families have learnt to deal with issues that arise. The input from 'experienced' family members can clarify many issues for 'new' families, and raise ones that as nurses we may not have had to deal with. Such experiences support the learning that occurs through real-life incidents, and develop the ability to problem-solve, through peer support.

Within the field of spinal cord injury there are educational packages that involve the individual family and patient working with the nurse and the multidisciplinary team on a one-to-one basis, with a supplementary family day every few weeks. Educational goals and strategies are decided during goal-planning sessions (Kennedy et al 1991). The areas identified in goal-planning are those on which the family and patient work together. The family day involves several families coming together in a group. There is a timetable of speakers on generic topics about spinal cord injury, and the opportunity to discuss issues with team members, a person who is already living in the community and with each other. This day is for the families only, so patients are not invited. It is planned away from the ward area, and is well rated by families as being a time to share experiences with peers. It is also a time when they can explore anxieties which they may not wish to voice in earshot of their relative. It also provides the opportunity to consolidate some of what they have already learnt on the individualised programmes.

This is a system that can work well in specialised areas where there are patients with similar conditions. Clearly it is not so easy to set up in ward settings where the patient group may be very diverse. It is in these situations that formal support groups or 'buddy' systems can be very useful and influential.

Other ways in which family education has been addressed have been described by Houtts et al (1996). They have developed a problem solving approach to family education. The model uses the acronym COPE (creativity, optimism, planning and expert information). Care-giver manuals have been developed which the family members work through. Case studies are given from which the family members develop their problem-solving skills. Learning in this way, it was suggested, has been found to empower the family and patient and help in alleviating a moderate degree of care-giver stress.

Easton et al (1994) developed a programme for stroke patients and their families. Their programme was developed after it was decided that there was clearly a deficit in knowledge levels once patients had been discharged. Patient education had been carried out on an informal basis, but, judging by the number of calls from relatives and patients, a knowledge deficit was evident in specific areas. This led the nursing team to develop a more standard education programme, which included the family. Following research into the primary areas of concern, the nursing team developed a 6-week group programme of lectures, based on the average length of patient stay. Attendance by both family members and patients was excellent, and the programme has been implemented on a more permanent basis, with regular review and evaluation.

A common trend in many of the educational programmes explored in the literature is the use of videos (Brillhart & Stewart 1989, Easton et al 1994, Houtts et al 1996, Maklebust & Magnan 1992). These can have significant benefits for the learner. They can be used when the client is on his own, at the learner's leisure, to recap on information, in one-to-one sessions with the nurse, or within small groups and used as the basis for discussion and questions.

SUMMARY

In this section I have endeavoured to provide a practical framework for education that will enable you, the nurse, to meet the needs of the family. Ultimately this will have a positive influence on the rehabilitation outcomes of the individuals in your care. The four elements within the framework have been explored in order to provide a theoretical backdrop, and included issues around:

- who the family is
- why we need to educate the family
- assessment of educational needs
- planning and delivery of a programme that meets these needs.

It is worth emphasising the importance of evaluating the success of educational programmes, both on an individual family basis and as a whole. This can be achieved using a number of methods:

- by observing the way in which the family relates to their loved one, both from a hands-on perspective and emotionally
- by providing problem-solving activities for the family and observing results
- by talking to the family and requesting information about what they have learnt and whether this has prepared them adequately in relation to needs identified.

Finally, the relationship between nurse, client and family should be seen as a partnership if successful rehabilitation outcomes are to be achieved. Any educational strategy used should be evaluated against such criteria and adjusted accordingly to ensure continuing success.

REFERENCES

Audit Commission 1995 United they stand. HMSO, London
Brillhart B, Stewart A 1989 Education as the key to rehabilitation. Nursing Clinics of North
    America 24(3):675–680
Dean-Baar S L 1996 Outcome directed teaching and learning. In: Hoeman S (ed)
    rehabilitation nursing: application and process, 2nd edn. Mosby, Missouri
Department of Health 1995 The patient's charter and you. HMSO, London
Easton K L, Zemen D M, Kwiatkowski S 1994 Developing and implementing a stroke
    education series for patients and families. Rehabilitation Nursing 19(6):348–351
Evans R L, Griffith T, Haselkorn J K, Hendricks R D, Baldwin D, Bishop D S 1992 Post
    stroke family function: an evaluation of the family's roles in rehabilitation. Rehabilitation
    Nursing 17(3):127–132
Haralambos M, Holborn M 1995 Sociology: themes and perspectives, 4th edn. Collins
    Educational, Bath
Houtts P S, Nezu A M, Nezu C M, Bucher J A 1996 The prepared caregiver: a problem
    solving approach to family caregiver education. Patient Education and Counselling
    27:63–73
Kennedy P, Walker L, White D 1991 Ecological evaluation of goal planning and advocacy
    in a rehabilitation environment for spinal cord injured people. Paraplegia 29:197–202
Knowles M S 1984 Andragogy in action: applying modern principles of adult education.
    Jossey Bass, San Francisco
Leske J S 1986 Needs of relatives of critically ill patients: a follow up. Heart and Lung
    15(2):189–193
Leske J S 1992 Needs of adult family members after critical illness: prescriptions for
    interventions. Critical Care Nursing Clinics of North America 4(4):587–596
Lorig K 1992 Patient education: a practical approach. Mosby, St Louis
Maklebust J A, Magnan M M 1992 Approaches to patient and family education for pressure
    ulcer management. Decubitus 5(7):18–20, 24, 26, 28
Mayo A M 1993 Teaching family/significant other nursing. Journal of Continuing
    Education in Nursing 24(1):27–31
Molter N C 1979 Needs of relatives of critically ill patients: a descriptive study. Heart and
    Lung 8:332–339
Nolan M, Keady J, Grant G 1995 CAMI: a basis for assessment and support with family
    carers. British Journal of Nursing 4(14):822–826
Peter S, Torr G 1996 Paediatric hospital at home: the first year. Paediatric Nursing
    8(5):20–23
Price D M, Forrester A, Murphy P A, Monaghan J F 1991 Critical care family needs in an
    urban teaching medical centre. Heart and Lung 20(2):183–188
Titler M G, Bombei C, Schutte D L 1995 Developing family focused care. Critical Care
    Nursing Clinics of North America 7(2):375–385
United Kingdom Central Council of Nursing, Midwifery and Health Visiting 1992
    Guidelines for professional practice. UKCC, London
Youngblood N M, Hines J 1992 The influence of the family's perception of disability on
    rehabilitation outcomes. Rehabilitation Nursing 17(6):323–326

The nurse as psychological support in rehabilitation

Psychological implications and assessment following illness and injury

David Thomas

INTRODUCTION

The potential effects of illness and disability on the psychological status of a client may be profound. Nurses are in a unique position of being present as rehabilitators in the clinical area for 24 hours per day, and therefore are not only in a position to be able to continually observe a client's behaviour, but also are frequently the recipients of that individual's anxieties and concerns relating to all aspects of his psychological well-being. It is due to this indisputable fact that, in practice, the nurse is the client's source of first-line psychological support. Fundamental to effectively addressing these psychological needs, as with any healthcare intervention, is the first stage of assessment. The level or depth of the assessment will depend on the expertise and training of the nurse involved, as well as the scale and type of psychological problem involved. It is this aspect of provision of psychological care that forms the major basis of this section. In addition, some commonly occurring diagnoses that the nurse may wish to use following assessment are suggested, and the potential treatment goals for each are outlined. More general issues that may impact on the assessment process involved in psychological care, notably managing expectations of rehabilitation, compliance, and breaking bad news to a client, are briefly examined.

ASSESSMENT

To give effective psychological support we must first understand the potential psychological implications of illness and disability for both clients/patients and their significant others (i.e. relatives and carers). While formal psychological assessment often remains in the traditional domain of the psychologist, within some rehabilitation settings (e.g. in traumatic brain injury) this often tends in reality to be reserved for the client with major psychological disturbance. Clearly, this position, and the need of nursing to respond positively, has implications for the training and extension of

■ **BOX 4.1 Factors impacting on individual well-being**

- Adaption, adjustment and coping
- Perception of goals, potential barriers to achieving goals, and possible strategies to overcome barriers
- Cognitive and communicative status
- Economic resources
- Environmental factors (in places such as the workplace, home and school)
- Family dynamics
- Functional ability (in areas such as self-care, elimination and mobility)
- Patient's knowledge about the nature of his own disability or chronic illness
- Level of impairment
- Physiological status
- Safety

the role of nurses (Elliott & Jackson 1996). Indeed, in meeting appropriate standards of rehabilitation nursing practice (American Nurses Association 1991), a minimum level of psychological assessment skills is required in all qualified nurses active in this area. The priority of the information to be gathered in the assessment phase is determined by the client's immediate condition and/or needs. Depending on the specific set of circumstances there may be many influencing factors on an individual's psychological well-being. A thorough assessment, incorporating all potential variables, would therefore seem essential. A suggested list of what these factors may be is given in Box 4.1 (Hoeman 1996).

UNDERPINNING PRINCIPLES OF PSYCHOLOGICAL ASSESSMENT

As the reader will no doubt recognise, if all these factors should be considered in psychological assessment, there may be difficulty in separating physical factors from psychological well-being. Secondly, it will often not be possible to obtain this information as part of a 'one-off' assessment, particularly in those with complex disability whose problems may be multifactorial. More commonly, obtaining the full picture will be a slower process over a period of time, involving liaison with the client's significant others and, perhaps, previous healthcare providers. Although the pace of physical rehabilitation is accelerating with modern technology, it is worth emphasising at this early stage that the pace of psychosocial adaption is slow in comparison (Zejdlik 1992).

Deciding what measurement parameters to use is also time consuming. Assessment guides may be available (Hoeman 1996), but these may need to be adapted, depending on the specific client group with which we are dealing. Combined with this, training in the use of such assessment tools may be needed. Such tools may also form the basis of evaluation relating to the success or otherwise of interventions to address psychological needs. The escalation of health costs and the increased awareness of clients and their significant others about quality issues such as length of stay and frequency of individual therapies increase the pressure on rehabilitation nurses to demonstrate effectiveness and provide quality nursing care.

NURSE ASSESSMENT OF PSYCHOSOCIAL NEEDS

Nursing assessment can be divided into two distinct areas. First, a comprehensive history needs to be taken; and, secondly, continual assessment of psychological strengths, weaknesses and progress must take place, as mentioned above.

In taking a comprehensive history a pre-injury profile of the patient and family will provide a base record of some of the key issues. Clearly, many of these may be potentially difficult for the individual to discuss, and so a sympathetic and non-threatening approach must be used by the nurse. The establishment of a non-judgmental relationship between the rehabilitation nurse and the family/significant others of the client is of the highest importance.

Key factors that are important in psychological assessment include those described below.

CULTURAL INFLUENCES

Gestures may be culture specific. For example, the movement of the hand as in 'thumbing a lift' is acceptable in England, but may be considered obscene in Greece. Similarly, many cultures do not indicate 'yes' by a nodding movement.

EDUCATIONAL AND VOCATIONAL BACKGROUND

There may be a potential effect on the ability of the individual to perform in the same way as previously in the working environment. Key questions around this may include:

- Does the client have the ability to absorb written information?
- Is the injury likely to force a vocational change?
- Will the client be able to work at all?
- Will re-training be required?
- How does the individual feel about the above?

FAMILY POSITION OR ROLE

Existing and potential changes in family dynamics may be of great importance. For example, an injury may change a breadwinner into a long-term recipient of care. In addition, pre-existing difficulties between the patient and his family may be exacerbated by the new disability. Acquired brain injury may produce the scenario where 'He's not the man I married.' Aspects of the effect on relationships are considered later, in the section addressing the promotion of sexual health. There may also be concerns regarding other family roles, such as parenting, which will require exploration.

INTERESTS

Existing preferred interests and hobbies may no longer be physically possible. Krause (1992) wrote that there was a limited amount of research looking at life satisfaction after spinal cord injury. Spinal cord injury eliminates or reduces many activities, occupations and vocational pursuits that have been a source of intrinsic pleasure prior to disability. The predominant interests in most persons at injury involved physical strength and manual dexterity, so spinal cord injury was particularly devastating, and its aftermath was denial of many commonly enjoyed pursuits and interests. The prospect of facing the transition from participating in an activity, for which the individual has had a passion, to becoming solely a spectator may be difficult and painful psychologically. It is often a good tactic to inquire about other recreational activities that the individual may not yet have tried but would be interested in pursuing.

INTERPERSONAL RELATIONSHIPS

Not only may there be an effect on the family dynamics, but interpersonal relationships within that individual's established social circle may also be affected. The ease or difficulty (i.e. whether we like or dislike a person) of interpersonal relationships has been examined (Hayes & Orrell 1995) and broken down into several component areas.

- *Familiarity*. We tend to like people that we see often. We also tend to like people who we trust and whose behaviour we can predict.
- *Similarity of attitudes*. If we approve of another person's attitudes we are more likely to like them.
- *Physical attraction*. This may play an even stronger part than similarity of attitudes in initially forming a reason for liking someone.
- *Reciprocal liking*. This can be seen as liking someone because they like us. It is, however, influenced by how good we feel about ourselves.

RECENT LOSSES OR DIFFICULTIES

The effects on an individual of a recent major life change or a loss (e.g. a bereavement) prior to the current injury or illness may be compounded further by the additional stress of major injury.

RELIGION

Religious beliefs may be a source of much comfort, but it is important that individual beliefs are known, and so not compromised by inappropriate statements or failure to appreciate particular aspects. In either case the potential result could be counterproductive to the psychological state of the individual, exacerbating any direct effects of the injury. The offering of inappropriate nutrition might be an example.

SOCIO-ECONOMIC BACKGROUND

The socio-economic background of the client has a direct bearing on his future life in the community. It may also affect client education, understanding of treatment goals and compliance generally.

VALUE AND BELIEF SYSTEMS

It is important that an understanding of the client's values and belief systems is achieved in order to synchronise client, significant others, and healthcare providers in the rehabilitation effort (Hayes & Orrell 1995). One will often find that these systems are created by a combination of the above factors. Clearly, myths and misunderstandings, relating either directly to a disability or the potential impact of this on the client's life, will not contribute well to the programme as a whole. Even at the early stage of assessment the nurse can begin to remove some of these.

NURSING DIAGNOSIS IN PSYCHOLOGICAL SUPPORT

Following on from assessment, the use of a nursing diagnosis centred approach may be useful, both as a framework to ensure systematic management and also to ensure that standards of care are met (Hoeman 1996, p. 704–707). In addition, it may facilitate the documentation of psychological care, something we as nurses often have difficulty doing. In these days of having to justify and outline what we do, it is worth strong consideration. We cannot simply ignore documenting the psychological care we provide; it is no longer sufficient to say that we do it anyway. To take this approach can only be detrimental to rehabilitation nursing.

A 'typical' list of nursing diagnoses related to psychological support might include:

- altered role performance
- altered sexuality pattern
- hopelessness
- impaired adjustment
- impaired social interaction
- ineffective individual coping
- powerlessness
- body-image disturbance
- self-esteem disturbance.

These are not listed in any particular order. Clearly their individual importance will vary uniquely from client to client.

For each of the above diagnoses, a summary statement of the potential effect on the client and a list of suggested brief treatment goals is outlined below. In addition, two of the more common diagnoses that the rehabilitation nurse may encounter (i.e. body-image disturbance and self-esteem disturbance) are explored in a little more detail. Clearly, there is not space in this chapter to explore all these issues in great depth, and the reader is encouraged to supplement the information given here with further reading.

ALTERED ROLE PERFORMANCE

There may be a disruption in the way the client's role is perceived (e.g. as a parent or provider).

Suggested treatment goals. The client:

- identifies a realistic perception of his role
- states his personal strengths
- acknowledges his problems related to carrying out the current role and suggests solutions
- states new/altered responsibilities, and verbalises acceptance.

ALTERED SEXUALITY PATTERN

This is discussed in detail in Chapter 4 Part C and, therefore, is not addressed here.

HOPELESSNESS

The client perceives that he has no available alternatives or choices in his life.

Suggested treatment goals. The client:

- is able to verbalise feelings
- makes positive statements (e.g. 'I can' and 'I'll try')
- makes eye contact and focuses on the speaker
- has an appropriate appetite and sleep time.

IMPAIRED ADJUSTMENT

The client shows an inability to modify his previous lifestyle consistent with his change in health status.

Suggested treatment goals. The client:

- states acceptance of his health change
- states personal goals when dealing with his health change
- lists behaviours required to adjust, and moves towards independence.

IMPAIRED SOCIAL INTERACTION

The client may experience insufficient or ineffective quality of social exchange. Often, such individuals will become almost entirely socially isolated. Although there may be physical and environmental barriers to mobility, the focus here is on a self-imposed isolation.

Suggested treatment goals. The client:

- identifies barriers
- discusses feelings
- states comfort in social situations
- is able to communicate/participate in social situations.

INEFFECTIVE INDIVIDUAL COPING

The client shows impaired adaptive behaviours and problem-solving abilities.

Suggested treatment goals. The client:

- verbalises his ability to cope and asks for help when needed
- demonstrates an ability to solve problems
- is free of destructive behaviour towards himself and others
- is able to discuss potential strategies to be used.

POWERLESSNESS

The client may actually lack control over a situation, or perceive that his actions will not affect the outcome. One could strongly suggest that it may well be the hospital regime that is the causative factor in actual lack of control.

Suggested treatment goals. The client:

- states a feeling of powerlessness
- identifies things over which he has control
- participates in his care and makes decisions
- questions whether prescribed care meets his personal goals
- verbalises a hopeful future.

BODY-IMAGE DISTURBANCE

The patient with an altered body image may have to navigate tense social interactions stemming from the stigmatising effects of visible disability. Adaption to a new body image is influenced by societal attitudes, which may be affected by many factors, including media representation. The 'ideal look' as portrayed in modern society is a body free of physical disability, perfect in complexion, hairstyle and fashionable attire (French & Phillips 1991). Marini (1994) cited three common factors in most of 302 films depicting disability:

- the disabled person was victimised
- the disabled person was unemployed/unemployable
- the disabled person had an abnormal personality.

Little effort was made by the producers of these films to educate about the disability or to correct misconceptions.

In addition, there are identifiable social barriers to those persons with disabilities, and these may contribute negatively towards the feelings of being 'disabled'. Clearly, prior to acquired disability an individual may well have had such attitudes and behaviours towards people with a disability. These will almost certainly be carried over into the initial post-injury period, and be the source of often severe distress. Research has indicated that an individual's life satisfaction is linked to social judgments of comparisons with others (Krause & Crewe 1991), and has suggested that the following three issues were key indicators.

- Interactions between those persons with disabilities and able-bodied people tend to be strained and uncomfortable.
- Able-bodied people tend to reject relationships with persons with disabilities.
- Even those attitudes that are perceived as superficially positive in the disabled were correlated with the more underlying negative attitudes.

Body image is an amalgam of continuous sensory feedback between an individual and his environment and a psychological process including the individual's feelings and attitudes about his body. When the flow of information between the individual's body and the environment is disrupted (Beeken 1978, cited in French & Phillips 1991), a disturbance in body image is created. Rapid, unexpected, uncontrollable and unwanted changes in body image are particularly difficult to accept (Piotrowsky 1982, cited in French & Phillips 1991). Moreover, clients with injuries, such as spinal cord injury, that result in both external and internal physiological changes are especially susceptible to negative effects on body image (Perry & Sutcliffe 1982). It is worth noting that those individuals most susceptible to injuries which may have an effect on body image are often those individuals most concerned with appearance (i.e. those in their late teenage years or early adulthood). Having said this, cross-sectional studies have suggested that persons who are younger at the time of a chronically disabling injury are more likely to have better long-term adjustment when measured in terms of adjustment ratings, distress ratings and employment status. Hohmann (cited in Krause & Crewe 1991) believes that a certain amount of time is necessary to adjust to the initial problems caused by disability, and that, with increasing age a new set of problems may appear which produces a decline in adjustment.

The stress caused by any injury or illness may precipitate any number of compensatory and self-protective behaviours in response to a threatened body image (Box 4.2). However, a definition of 'normal' responses to losses following injury or illness is not possible, as the individual response is almost infinitely variable in nature.

Phases of body image recovery may be divided into four categories.

1. *Impact:* recognising change. The initial experience of discovering that the old body has vanished and has undergone a devastating change can be intolerable. The emotional shock of the injury may cloud the patient's ability to evaluate his condition realistically and he may even question whether life is worth living. The carer's role during this phase may simply be to

---

■ BOX 4.2 Behaviours associated with stress following illness or injury

- Anger and hostility
- Rebelliousness, such as refusing care or refusing to get up
- Refusal to socialise (fearing rejection, the person shuns others, including family and friends)
- Depersonalisation; avoiding or disowning altered body parts
- Refusal to participate in activities

---

provide physical care. Teaching is not recommended during the impact phase because the client has not yet come to grips with the implications of the changes. The nurse should listen to the client and encourage him to share his feelings. False reassurance is most detrimental to the patient's recovery of a healthy body image, and must be avoided at all times.

2. *Retreat:* withdrawing from the loss. Emotional withdrawal occurs when the patient begins to recognise the significance of the injury and the implications of the change. Mourning, withdrawal and depression are common behaviours in this phase and the carer should recognise that these behaviours are normal during this phase of adjustment. Self-care should be encouraged, but the patient may not be emotionally ready for extensive involvement in personal care.

3. *Acknowledgment:* realism begins, rehabilitative efforts are effective, and the patient should be included in self-care activities. The patient's accomplishments should be praised and reinforced. This not only instills hope but also supports an optimistic outlook for the future.

4. *Reconstruction:* living with reality. At this stage, patients are enthusiastic about their rehabilitation, and may work hard to achieve the best function possible. They use prosthetic and adaptive devices to improve their appearance and functioning. The individual consciously attempts to integrate the former body image with the new body image created by the injury. The optimistic patient sets his own realistic, future-orientated goals.

SELF-ESTEEM DISTURBANCE

Self-esteem is one's personal feeling of value or worth, and is largely based on feedback from others in our lives. The way in which we deal with feelings (anger and aggression in particular) stems from limitations imposed by others in our upbringing. Overall, the individual with self-esteem disturbance may either negatively evaluate his self-worth as a person or underestimate his capabilities.

Some of the more common specific manifestations of low self-esteem include:

- expressions of self-deprecation or self-dislike
- sensitivity to criticism or self-consciousness

- anorexia or overeating
- a tendency to be a listener rather than a participant
- withdrawal from activities
- decreased motivation, interest and concentration
- seeing oneself as a burden to others.

Treatment goals are, as in the other cases, a staged set of behavioural responses to overcome self-esteem disturbance, rather than a focus on the manifestations of the problem. The client:

- identifies personal strengths
- states personal strengths
- is able to accept compliments
- accepts responsibility for his own actions
- accepts constructive criticism and attempts to correct problems.

MANAGING EXPECTATIONS OF REHABILITATION AND RESULTING BEHAVIOURS

Synchronising expectations of the rehabilitation outcome between the patient/family and the rehabilitation staff is a difficult process, as briefly mentioned earlier when discussing value and belief systems. Staff expectations are largely based on objective data such as the level of injury in the spinal cord injured, co-existing conditions and the previous experience of staff in similar injuries. Initially, the patient and family may lack sufficient knowledge to grasp the probability of permanent paralysis in complete spinal cord lesions or the uncertainty of prognosis in stroke or heart disease (Caplan & Reidy 1996).

There are a number of recurring themes in managing the expectations of the patient and family. One example is in the early phase of rehabilitation, where the patient and family (although obviously not in all cases) see recovery as being directly linked to walking. This has the practical effect of promoting participation in physiotherapy and reducing interest in other therapy areas, such as occupational therapy. The acceptance of the permanent changes caused by the injury is a difficult process and may involve 'giving up' on walking. In my experience many patients after spinal cord injury signal their non-acceptance of the injury's consequences by resolutely stating, 'I am going to walk out of here whatever you say.' In this scenario the onset of muscle spasm or the presence of 'sacral sparing' giving non-functional sensation or movement may be seen as a very positive sign, albeit an inaccurate one. The nurse who constantly tries to introduce realism has a difficult task in balancing appropriate hope against an ill-founded euphoric optimism.

Whatever system or model of care is used, it is easily seen that specific treatment aims agreed by both the patient/family and the rehabilitation team are essential to ensure that all are striving for the same targets. Such agreed aims should be subject to negotiation and be written down, as the patient/family may wish to strive for targets not considered practical by the rehabilitation team. Potential conflicts are of very real concern in the

■ BOX 4.3 Potential sources of conflict

Staff versus patient	Family versus patient	Family and patient versus staff
• Attendance at therapy	• Responsibility for the accident	• Prognosis
• Timing of analgesia	• Eventual destination	• Staff inattentiveness
• The need to lose weight		• Slow response to patient requests

rehabilitation process and may involve any or all of the participants (Caplan & Reidy 1996). Potential sources of conflict are outlined in Box 4.3.

In the real world it is often productive to be strong willed, even stubborn, and to question authority. Some independence behaviour (e.g. verbal assertiveness) may challenge hospital policies and the hospital culture. It is worth recording that such behaviours (albeit within reasonable boundaries) may be most valuable and adaptive after discharge. It is important to the mental health of the individual to have a solid sense of self-efficacy and to believe that their efforts can produce the desired result. Indeed, many personal experiences of disability link self-reliance and emotional resilience to overcoming obstacles and physical limitations.

Possibly the most valuable and often the most underused resource available in the development of a positive attitude towards disability is the experiences and peer support of those who have experience of living with a similar illness or injury. Spooner (1995) found that it was talking to other patients and their families in the ward that proved to be the best way for patients to cope with a totally changed life. In a survey of 'consumer satisfaction', 30% felt that being able to speak to someone who had suffered the same injury (a year ago or longer) would have been useful. This resource, generally considered useful, could be extended to family members (Holicky 1997). Within the rehabilitation area, group learning may have a substantial place in contributing to the necessary education of patients. Group learning can provide feedback and support, as well as a non-threatening environment (Payne 1993). The merits of and methods involved in the group learning approach are discussed in Chapter 3.

PERCEIVED NON-COMPLIANCE

It is reasonable to believe that shrinking healthcare resources will lead to increased calls for efficiency from purchasers and the government, thus provoking institutional efforts to promote greater compliance (Caplan & Reidy 1996). Non-compliance in the form of treatment refusal lengthens stay in many situations. In the form of verbal or physical abuse non-compliance may adversely affect recruitment or retention of nursing staff. Treatment refusals during rehabilitation are often characterised as non-compliance. Such refusals may take the form of refusing medications, non-cooperation with physiotherapy, refusal to discuss placement and failure to cooperate with bowel or bladder management programmes.

The ethics of patient non-compliance were considered by Coy (1992, cited in Crozier et al 1992). She identified four basic assumptions that may be prevalent in healthcare workers.

- All non-compliance is a problem in need of a solution.
- The solution to non-compliance is compliance.
- All compliance is non-problematic.
- Non-compliance is the patient's problem.

ALL NON-COMPLIANCE IS A PROBLEM IN NEED OF A SOLUTION

The key issue is whether the patient's decisions are competent. Autonomy is a patient right and a decision by the patient is not incompetent simply because it does not agree with the nurse's or therapist's view. The often complex nature of disability and the subsequent psychological sequelae (e.g. emotional shock, denial or depression) may prevent true autonomy, at least in the early stages. If the patient's decision (however ill-informed or apparently nonsensical) is overridden by the rehabilitation team, the treatment given and the patient's ability to resume autonomous decision-making must be formally measured and recorded to prevent treatment disputes or recrimination (Crozier et al 1992). During this time a degree of 'paternalistic' care may be necessary, but the individual *must* retake control at the earliest opportunity, becoming increasingly autonomous, for rehabilitation to have succeeded. Strategies to enable this may include the patient beginning to manage his own care and organise his own daily routine (Graham & Royster 1990), rather than being entirely at the mercy of the hospital routine.

This is clearly fundamental to empowerment and independence, as discussed in detail in Chapter 1. It is this which is the essential difference between traditional medical models of rehabilitation and truly client/patient-centred models (Table 4.1). The influence of the traditional medical model has caused individuals in wheelchairs with a long-term disability to be regarded as 'patients' and, therefore, as passive. Attempts to change this perception on a societal level may require a militancy that potentially may erode public sympathy.

Table 4.1 Comparison of the medical and client-centred models

	Medical model	**True client-centred model**
Role of patient	Passive	Participatory
Knowledge	Shared or withheld at doctor's discretion	Fully shared
Autonomy	No	Yes
Right to refuse treatment	No	Yes

THE SOLUTION TO NON-COMPLIANCE IS COMPLIANCE

This assumption is influenced by the nurse's or therapist's ideas of what the outcome should be and, revealingly, what the route to get there should be. Patient choice is paramount because the therapist or nurse will not have to live with the outcome.

ALL COMPLIANCE IS NON-PROBLEMATIC

Overcompliance represents dependence and is ultimately a poor treatment result on discharge, as it poses potential problems for the client on re-integration into the community.

NON-COMPLIANCE IS THE PATIENT'S PROBLEM

If we overlook explanations of basic care because we expect cooperation, if we set goals that the patient does not agree with or want, if we get the patient's opinion but do not actually incorporate it into their care, then refusal may be the only form of control the patient has. Why rehabilitate to give maximum autonomy and then fail to respect such decisions? Making mistakes (i.e. experiential learning) is how everyone learns in life, not just the disabled, and certainly not just the able-bodied.

TREATMENT REFUSALS: PRACTICAL STEPS

DEFINE THE REFUSAL

- *Type:* selective or complete refusal.
- *Length:* occasional or persistent (acute or chronic).
- *Causes:* failure to understand the importance of the intervention/activity due to:
    - cognitive deficit
    - inadequate education by staff
    - patient–staff personality conflict.
- *Reasons stated:* e.g. pain, fatigue, hopelessness.
- *Staff responses:* coaxing, demanding, withdrawal, etc.
- *Family:* do family members see the behaviour as consistent with pre-morbid behaviour?

INITIAL STEPS IN MANAGEMENT

- patient education
- pain management
- sleep-disturbance management
- supportive counselling.

FURTHER STEPS: PSYCHOLOGICAL AND EMOTIONAL ASSESSMENT

These are measured to assess the impact of potential psychological and emotional deficits on the level of compliance. The question of whether a patient is 'competent' to make his own decisions is integral to acceptance by the rehabilitation team of treatment refusals. Psychological assessment should not be used as a tool to prove 'incompetence' in a patient who refuses treatment or who does not agree with some treatment goals but should be used as a precursor to treatment that improves the patient's decision-making abilities. However, in an American study, 76% of referrals to a psychiatrist were for the purpose of investigating staff–patient conflicts around treatment refusals (Farnsworth, cited in Crozier et al, 1992).

COMPETENCE

Competence is essentially the patient's ability to make an informed decision about the benefits and risks of certain aspects of his rehabilitative care. Caplan & Reidy (1996) urge great caution in challenging a patient's competence. While it may be possible to prove incompetence legally or clinically, such challenges are likely to produce antagonism and alienation, and this will ultimately adversely affect the end goals of the patient's rehabilitation.

DOCUMENTATION

Open lines of communication between all those involved in the rehabilitation process are always necessary, but particularly so when the patient is refusing care. Careful documentation will provide a record of treatments given in the event of overriding the patient's wishes about care, and will also play a part in a swift return to patient autonomy. The careful initial documentation of treatment targets agreed between the patient and the team will allow for discussion, education programmes and a shared perspective.

The development of flexible guidelines for necessary medical care will allow an increased sense of control in the patient. Some procedures may be considered necessary (e.g. endotracheal suctioning), but the scheduling could be decided or influenced by the patient.

MEETINGS

Regular meetings in a variety of settings and with varying combinations of participants are necessary to provide the following:

- the patient and family with opportunities to express their needs, wishes, opinions and fears regarding treatment
- the patient with the opportunity and time to voice concerns in private
- the staff with the opportunity and time to express and discuss treatment-refusal concerns as well as concerns about their professional roles.

Effective communication between the patient, the family and the rehabilitation team is essential at all times, but especially when care is refused. Although the move towards a model of rehabilitation care that involves total patient participation in the setting of agreed treatment goals may be difficult to set up, the potential rewards are undoubtedly worth the effort required.

GIVING PATIENTS THE DIAGNOSIS/PROGNOSIS (BREAKING BAD NEWS)

Breaking bad news is never easy. Although this may often be done by the medical staff, it appears that nursing staff are often the bearers of bad tidings also. Even in the former case, it is usually within the remit of the nurse to reinforce what the client has been told. Conflict between the patient/family and staff regarding prognosis is common (Caplan & Reidy 1996), and may lead to resentment towards nursing staff. Although somewhat difficult for the nurse to deal with on occasion, it may in some cases be a necessary part of the client's adaption to a new set of life circumstances. Family support is necessary in providing effective advocates to challenge and, perhaps, eventually confirm the diagnosis in the patient's mind prior to acceptance. The key to minimising the degree of conflict is for a consistent approach to be taken, not only by the rehabilitation nursing team, but by other team members also. It is therefore essential that the information given to the patient and family is recorded. Not only is this of benefit for future reference in enabling reinforcement of the same information, but it can also be used as a cue to encourage the person to talk. For example, a question relating to how the information made the individual feel, or perhaps the less direct, 'What are your thoughts on what you were told about your illness?' The provision of effective emotional support is essential as a fundamental component of all care in rehabilitation (Caplan & Reidy 1996). Such support, however, begins in earnest at the time when the client is told the prognosis. Through creating a clear, unambiguous picture of what the future may hold in the mind of the individual client, his emotional readiness to take on the various aspects of his rehabilitation will be, at best delayed, and even potentially absent. The long-term life effects of this may, obviously, be significantly detrimental.

REFERENCES

American Nurses Association 1991 Standards of clinical nursing practice. ANA, Washington, DC
Caplan B, Reidy K 1996 Staff–patient–family conflicts in rehabilitation: sources and solutions. Topics in Spinal Cord Injury Rehabilitation 2(2):21–33
Crozier K, Reidy K et al 1992 Treatment refusals during rehabilitation: ethical considerations of the interdisciplinary spinal cord injury rehabilitation team. Spinal Cord Injury Psychosocial Process 5(2):44–51
Elliott T, Jackson W 1996 Psychologic assessment in spinal cord injury rehabilitation: benefitting patient, treatment team, and health care delivery system. Topics in Spinal Cord Injury Rehabilitation 2(2):34–45
French J, Phillips J 1991 Shattered images: recovery for the spinal cord injury client.

Rehabilitation Nursing 16(3):134–136

Graham C, Royster V 1990 Rehabilitation of a paraplegic prisoner: conflicts for patient and nurses. Rehabilitation Nursing 15(4):197–201

Hayes N, Orrell S 1995 Psychology: an introduction. Longman, London

Hoeman S (ed) 1996 Rehabilitation nursing – process and application. Mosby, New York

Holicky R 1997 What consumers tell us. Topics in Spinal Cord Injury Rehabilitation 2(3):118–123

Krause J 1992 Life satisfaction after spinal cord injury: a descriptive study. Rehabilitation Psychology 37(1):61–70

Krause J, Crewe N 1991 Chronologic age, time since injury, and time of measurement: effect on adjustment after spinal cord injury. Archives of Physical and Medical Rehabilitation 72:91–100

Marini I 1994 Attitudes towards disability and the psychosocial implications for persons with Spinal cord injury. Spinal Cord Injury Psychosocial Process 7(4):147–152

Payne J 1993 The contribution of group learning to the rehabilitation of spinal cord injured adults. Rehabilitation Nursing 18(6):375–379

Perry P, Sutcliffe SA 1982 Conceptual framework for clinical practice. Journal of Neurological Nursing 14:318–321

Spooner A 1995 A personal perspective: the psychological needs of spine-injured patients. Professional Nurse 10(6):359–362

Zejdlik C 1992 Management of spinal cord injury, 2nd edn. Jones & Bartlett, Boston

Providing psychological support

Susan Tripp

INTRODUCTION

In discussing the nurse as first-line psychological support in rehabilitation, the following statements are proposed as key underpinning principles, and will be the focus for exploration in this section.

- Nurses are ideally placed to provide first-line psychological support.
- Effective communication skills provide the foundation for this.
- Knowledge of the psychological response to illness, trauma and loss enables the nurse to support the patient effectively.
- Increased self-awareness enhances the ability to provide psychological support.

This section follows on from the previous section, where the concepts underpinning assessment of psychological need were briefly discussed, and has the aim of providing practical advice to the nurse in a rehabilitation situation in dealing with some of those psychological needs. In addition, further information is given specifically on what could be considered to be two major issues often present in the rehabilitating setting: management of aggression, and the client with chronic pain.

Most nurses are very skilled in identifying and assisting the patient in meeting their physical needs, by providing expert technical care, advice and information. However, it is recognised that each individual experiences illness and disability within many different spheres:

- the biological and physical sphere (the actual physical processes that occur as a result of trauma or disease)
- the individual emotional and psychological process that occurs in response to the physical situation
- the responses that occur within the social context of that individual (i.e the implications within their immediate social system – family, friends and colleagues)
- the implications of life changes within the broader social context of the individual and his family (e.g. roles and responsibilities as a parent, husband, wife or child).

If we are to practise 'holistically', as many areas within rehabilitation claim, (Barnitt & Pomeroy 1995) it is necessary to take all these areas into account. Most models of care routinely acknowledge the psychological needs of the patient as being an important part of the rehabilitation process, but nurses often appear reluctant to address these, perceiving emotional response to trauma, disability and loss as being outside the norm, something that should be addressed only by therapists with specialised training. Motyka et al (1997) studied the response of a group of nurses to the expression of anxiety by a patient. They found that the most common responses were cheering the patient up, collecting information about the symptom and offering explanations. One of the least common responses was that of showing empathy towards the patient and actually facilitating emotional expression. Nichols (1984), after reviewing many studies that have shown that physical illness and associated change and loss are frequently accompanied by psychological disturbance or disruption, concluded that 'serious illness, disability or disfigurement *inevitably* cause psychological reactions or psychological disturbance, for which psychological care is necessary.' If we accept Nichols' statement that emotional disruption is inevitable, it follows that these needs should be recognised and addressed as a matter of routine, as part of the care package offered by nurses. When emotions are viewed as a problem, as an abnormality to be treated rather than a normal response to illness or disability, the patient is encouraged to view his appropriate feelings as unacceptable, shameful and something to be hidden.

Working within a multidisciplinary setting, there are likely to be many others attempting to meet the psychological needs of the patient, all claiming to some degree to have more expertise in this area. This, in effect, causes the nurse to question and doubt his own skill. Why, therefore, should nurses be the first-line support?

1. There are currently about 650 000 nurses registered in various fields with the United Kingdom Central Council of Nursing, Midwifery and Health Visiting (UKCC 1997), many of whom are present on a 24-hour shift basis within hospitals, and who are therefore far more readily accessible than many other professionals.

2. By the nature of their role, nurses spend a far greater proportion of their time with the individual, frequently developing a very close and intimate relationship when giving personal care, often over an extended period of time.

3. Nurses have the opportunity to meet with the significant others in the patient's life, and observe the interaction between them, as well as providing education and guidance when appropriate.

Why then do nurses sometimes appear reluctant to take on this role? I would suggest that it is perhaps the nurses' own fear that prevents them from doing so. The nurse may fear that through allowing the patient to focus on his emotions, particularly when difficult emotions such as anger and grief are being expressed, these emotions will overwhelm both patient and nurse, and the nurse will be unable to contain them for the patient. There is also the fear that the nurse will 'get in too deep' and will not know what to say, or will not have the answer. With physical problems, we are taught to identify the problem and take action, which is designed to answer the problem. It can sometimes be very difficult for nurses to realise that in order to provide psychological support, their role is not to provide the solution but to facilitate the expression of a 'normal' emotional response and allow the patient to be heard. I am not suggesting that the nurse is in a position to provide the *only* psychological care required, but rather that nurses should, as a regular part of their role, be aware of the psychological response of individuals to trauma and disability, as well as understanding what constitutes an expected or normal response and that which requires the intervention of a team member with different, perhaps more developed, skills.

Working as both a nurse and a counsellor, I often feel that colleagues think that I have one special technique, a key that enables these areas to be dealt with. Of course, when working with patients in a very defined counselling relationship, it *is* necessary to have a deeper understanding of psychological processes. One must also know where and when it is appropriate to apply particular skills, as well as when it is appropriate to refer on to others. However, not all of this is necessary in order to provide immediate first-line support. In areas where there is awareness of the potential for nurses to utilise their unique role, there have been attempts to distinguish the different professional roles in which listening and counselling skills might be used, as distinct from the more defined psychological care that might be given by a professional who has undergone more extensive training. There is general agreement that when these skills are used by the nurse to enhance communication, establish a therapeutic relationship and maintain and promote the physical and psychosocial safety of the patient, the relationship can facilitate the achievement of goals and the resolution of problems (British Association for Counselling, 1997). Therefore, it is worth exploring what these basic interpersonal and communication skills actually consist of.

COMMUNICATION SKILLS

One of the fundamental requirements for acknowledging, identifying and addressing psychological needs is the ability to communicate those needs and have that communication heard and understood. We communicate in many different ways, both verbal and non-verbal. Non-verbal behaviour refers to anything that is not speech, and should not be regarded as a separate form of communication, but rather as an enhancement of what is being said. We all use non-verbal communication to give emphasis to what we say, to signal to the other party that we are listening, to show our approval, or to contradict what is being said. Non-verbal behaviours include such things as eye contact, posture, hand gestures, facial expression, distance between communicants and head movements, and we often use them to make very quick judgments on people when we first meet them. It is important for the nurse to be aware of not only the patient's non-verbal behaviours or body language, but also of his own habitual body language, and the additional messages he is giving by it, which may be understood differently by different people. By attending to his own non-verbal messages, the nurse can use his body to communicate more effectively. Egan (1994) uses the mnemonic SOLER to remember the basic skills of effective non-verbal communication:

S   face the person squarely, to indicate involvement
O   open posture (crossed arms and legs can indicate unavailability to the patient)
L   lean appropriately towards the patient

E   eye contact, as a way of saying 'I am with you' (but be aware not to stare, which can be read as threatening)
R   relaxed (be natural and comfortable with yourself and the patient).

Verbal communication embraces speech. This incorporates an awareness of the tone of voice, rapidity of speech and loudness, as well as the style of speech adopted, through which we make assumptions about the other, and their level of knowledge and understanding. Through this method we can each establish our position and status – for example, by giving elaborate, technical explanations, when we have assumed that the recipient has little or no knowledge of the subject.

NON-JUDGMENTAL ACCEPTANCE

Non-judgmental acceptance is one of the conditions essential to creating an effective support system. It means more than just an acknowledgement of the patient's response in the here and now; it means accepting that response as valid for the patient, and valuing that individual's unique humanness. Rogers (1990) also calls this 'prizing and unconditional positive regard'. This allows the other person to have his own feelings and experiences, with no 'ifs or buts', and means accepting the patient's negative, bad, painful feelings as well as positive, mature and confident feelings. Acceptance also involves the nurse questioning his own value judgments and assumptions that he makes about what is right or wrong. It does not mean that the nurse has to accept the other's moral and ethical codes as his own, but rather that he acknowledges the other's right to hold them, and does not seek to impose his own views and codes upon the patient.

ACTIVE LISTENING

Within all two-way communication, the aim is to be heard and understood. We are all able to listen and to repeat back exactly what has been said. This does not necessarily mean that we have heard and understood the message being communicated. In order to listen actively, we need to be present physically and emotionally. This involves an awareness of the patient's non-verbal behaviours and their context within verbal behaviour, as well as hearing the words said within the current situation. Active listening also means sometimes tolerating silence, without having the need to fill it with helpful suggestions or wondering what should be said to break it. It means letting go of the usual rules of conversation, whereby we take turns at speaking, and allowing the patient to lead in this. It is often helpful to use such skills as open-ended questions and reflecting back to facilitate emotional expression, showing the patient that he has been fully heard. Reflecting does not mean merely repeating back parrot fashion what has been said, but is a paraphrasing and summarising of what has been said. It is a skill that takes effort to learn, but is extremely valuable. Essentially, I view active listening as being *present* with the patient, primarily as one human being to another, before being there as a professional. Being present with the patient requires a further condition, that of empathy.

EMPATHY

Empathy is described by Rogers (1990) as the ability to enter the private perceptual world of the other and being thoroughly at home in it, experiencing the flow of emotions that he is experiencing. Egan (1994) proposes that empathy is the skill that enables helpers to communicate their understanding of the patient's world, and that it is impossible genuinely to respond with understanding unless you are empathic. A good empathic response involves an awareness of behaviour (non-verbal and verbal), experiences and mood, reflecting the patient's world as he sees it. It also involves an understanding of the other's frame of reference, the way he understands and finds meaning in the world. In order to provide effective care, it is important for the nurse to maintain a separate sense of himself as an individual, and not to feel swallowed up by the other's inner world, and unable to leave it behind. A helpful way of providing this boundary between self and other is through allocating time.

TIME

By giving allocated time to the patient to address his needs for psychological support, both parties are able to have a clear beginning and a clear ending. It is unsafe and difficult for both if there are no firm time boundaries between the different roles. It gives conflicting messages to the patient if, when a nurse is attempting to hear him emotionally, he is whisked away, perhaps to perform a physical task. On the one hand, the nurse is recognising the importance of this to the patient, but on the other he is stating that it is not important enough to stay with.

Neither is it appropriate that emotional support be planned at a time when other physical tasks are being carried out. Many nurses claim that they are able to develop a very emotionally supportive relationship while carrying out such care as blanket baths. This is not appropriate, when you consider the position of the patient. They may often be feeling very vulnerable and exposed at that time, with the nurse in a very powerful, mother-like position. It is appropriate to acknowledge any fears or needs expressed at these times, assuring the patient that he has been heard, but making more formal arrangements to discuss the issues at a more appropriate time. When time is allocated, neither the nurse nor his colleagues should regard it as a moveable feast, as this will diminish the importance of psychological care. Neither should the nurse get so caught up in the patient's inner world that he allows the time to be extended.

Clear time boundaries act as a container for patient's feelings, and I have found that most patients are well aware of this and will reduce the intensity of expression for themselves, when they know that the time is coming to an end. It is perfectly acceptable to remind the patient that there are 5 or 10 minutes left and to arrange the next meeting. I imagine many nurses throwing up their hands in horror, saying that they are far too busy to allocate specific time for psychological care. If we are to take a holistic view of rehabilitation, surely we must allocate time for this aspect of care.

SELF-AWARENESS

Before attempting to provide any of the above conditions, it is necessary that the nurse reflect upon himself. Reflection seems to be a buzzword at the moment, but it is an important element in providing a safe environment for addressing the psychological needs of the patient. If a nurse is not able to question his own value judgments, acknowledging his own emotions, such as anger, fear, happiness, as well as his likes and dislikes of certain patients, he is unlikely to be able to tolerate the expression of these from another. The probable result will be that of the nurse taking avoiding action when the situation occurs. Nurses are easily able to take avoiding action, by looking rushed and busy, answering patients 'on the hoof' and never appearing to have the time. Referring on to others might also be seen as taking avoiding action, by refusing to acknowledge the skills that he does have. It may often be the individual nurse's own fear of emotional expression that is preventing him from allowing the patient to express emotion, not his lack of skills.

There are many research articles within the counselling field that identify the most important part of the relationship as feeling heard, not the use of special techniques and tricks. By using active listening skills, we are all able to hear. It is important that each individual nurse identifies his own support systems, both professional and personal. In any area of health care we are likely to have experiences that generate emotions within ourselves. Sometimes these are areas that we have not dealt with successfully on a personal level, and this can lead to difficulty when encouraging patients to express their own emotions. We may have feelings of failure and incompetence, frustration, anger, grief and sadness, as well as feelings of joy and achievement when things are going well. It is important to realise that, if we have not acknowledged these feelings in ourselves, this can lead to increasing levels of stress and anxiety. You cannot expect to be present with a patient in an area that you are unable to be present in yourself. Where nurses are attempting to provide psychological support, at whatever level, it is essential that they are able to explore their actions and the feelings that are generated by them in a safe and non-judgmental environment. This may be in the form of clinical supervision, either as an individual or within a peer group, where both positive and negative experiences are discussed. Skilled supervision enables nurses to reflect honestly on their actions, and helps to identify any areas that are likely to present both professional and personal difficulties, as well as identifying knowledge deficits.

MANAGING AGGRESSION

- Aggression usually occurs as a result of a combination of factors, which may be patient, environmental or professional related. Removal of any such factors may contribute positively to outcome.
- Self-presentation, both verbally and non-verbally, may escalate or defuse a situation.

- Reporting and reflecting on incidents is vital to enable staff to manage aggression safely.
- Staff should honestly acknowledge their limitations and identify their training needs, as well as their personal and professional support systems.
- Personal safety is paramount.

Working within the healthcare setting, we are fortunate indeed if we never have to care for an aggressive patient or relative, or deal with an aggressive colleague or situation of conflict. There can sometimes be a fine balance between submission, assertion and aggression:

Passive.................................Assertive..................................Aggressive
(You count, I don't)   (I have rights, you have rights)   (I count, you don't)

Patients are often encouraged by the system to become passive receivers of care. After suffering trauma, illness and disability, they are under tremendous physical and emotional threat.

- Patients may be admitted to a very busy and confusing area, of which they have no previous knowledge or understanding.
- Patients are often subject to very intimate and invasive questions and examination by strangers.
- Patients may be stripped of the external trappings that identify who they are (clothes, make-up, jewellery, family and work roles) and asked to wear a label in order that they might be identified.
- Patients are often told things that they do not want to hear.
- Patients' view of themselves as powerful and independent beings that are able to make their own choices is challenged by the professionals who are deciding care.

In effect, the recipient may become depersonalised and disempowered, and it can be difficult for the patient to take an active part in rehabilitation, remaining instead in a submissive, passive role.

Many individuals regard themselves as assertive, when in fact others regard their actions as aggressive. Assertion can be defined as getting your own needs met without violating the rights or needs of others. It is not always about getting your own way, but having your standpoint acknowledged without feeling humiliated or disempowered. There are certain skills and strategies that can be used by both participants within the helping relationship:

- owning (making 'I' statements such as 'I feel … when you say … because')
- stating clearly and calmly what you want from the other person
- avoiding blaming, apologising or exaggerating
- acknowledging the other's feelings
- using SOLER to transmit non-verbal signals
- not taking responsibility for the outcome if the other person reacts badly.

Within a potentially aggressive situation, the rights of others *are* being violated, and either party can view the situation as a struggle to achieve power.

Aggression takes many forms, from non-verbal and verbal behaviours, such as ignoring attempts at communication, challenging eye contact, verbal mocking or arguing, through to attempted or actual physical aggression. Why are some people aggressive towards those who are in the helping role? Using aggression to get needs met is often a learned response. As children, we learn to get our needs met by behaving in a certain way. We learn what is acceptable or unacceptable within our own social situation, and generally take the simplest, quickest and most effective route to achieving our goals. If our goals are met by this route, there is no reason not to use the same methods on other occasions when we have similar needs. As adults, we start to learn that old methods are not always acceptable, and we often modify or change our behaviour accordingly. However, when we are under threat, we can forget the new behaviours and revert back to previous, more child-like ways of coping. All of us also have an instinctive aggressive or conflict response, which if used appropriately can be instrumental in us fulfilling our goals.

Aggression is usually accompanied by the same physiological arousal as anxiety, that of the 'flight or fight' response, where adrenalin levels rise, heart beat increases, breathing becomes rapid and muscles become tense. This response may be recognised as anger by the individual, and not as the response to anxiety. Mastery, defined as an individual's ability to be in control of his own life and life events, over the perceived threat, causes a reduction in those responses. Thus it is frequently the sense of loss of control and power that accompanies the illness process that leads to frustration and conflict. Feelings of powerlessness are increased when the individual feels that his concerns are not being acknowledged or are invalid. Frustration can lead to disagreement and conflict, which, if unresolved, leads to anger and the potential for more serious aggressive behaviour. If the individual is not assisted in recognising those feelings of anger as a response to anxiety, frustration, fear and loss of control, and their concerns validated, the situation can continue to escalate.

As a first step in preventing and managing conflict and aggressive feelings, it is important to identify the usual coping strategies of the individual, preferably prior to any dispute. This can be done simply by asking the patient how they normally manage anxiety-provoking situations. Within this it is then possible to assess the level of assertiveness, and the patient's methods of recognising stressors. Clear, concise and consistent information, identifying the patient's expectations and explaining any differences in yours, as well as inclusion in any decision-making process, helps to reduce the level of anxiety, powerlessness and fear. Patients can be encouraged to take an assertive role in their care in order to get needs met, which may involve both themselves and the staff in negotiation and compromise, with each party encouraged to listen to the other's view. Compromise can be reached without making things worse for one or other of the parties, and can at the very least prevent deterioration of the status quo. Characteristics of destructive coping and means through which effective coping can be facilitated are outlined in Box 4.4.

■ **BOX 4.4**

Destructive coping	Effective coping
• Loss of control and power	• Nurse acknowledges these as normal response
• Increase in anxiety	• Nurse assists patient in identifying those feelings; helps patient develop effective coping strategies
• Physiological arousal (flight or fight response)	
• Recognised as anger	• Physiological arousal reduced
• Angry, rejecting behaviour	• Nurse supports patient in taking active role in decision-making
• Increased isolation and fear	
• Higher physiological arousal	• Patient regains sense of control
• Loss of control; aggressive, abusive behaviour	• Effective communication established; patient feels heard and supported
• **Violates rights of others**	• Compromise and negotiation possible
	• Nurse and patient meet on a level position
	• **No rights violated**

Within the handling of potential conflict or aggressive situations, it is important that the nurse understands and recognises her own bodily responses. Nurses can react to the threat of aggression by increasing levels of anxiety and arousal, leading to anger. A calm and assertive approach to the situation, with constant repetition if necessary, and an awareness of non-verbal behaviours, posture, breathing and eye contact, can all assist in defusing a difficult situation.

Unfortunately, there will undoubtedly be occasions when situations escalate into potential or actual violence, despite the best endeavours of those involved. It is then necessary to look at other factors that might be influencing the situation (Box 4.5). When situations do escalate, safety of self is paramount.

SELF-PRESERVATION

Your response may depend on the severity of the incident and the particular individual involved. If it is safe to do so:

- Be supportive, using effective communication skills.
- Avoid situations that might result in loss of face for the aggressor (this may promote escalation).
- Ask if there is anything in the environment that might be contributing (e.g. an audience).
- Be respectful and courteous.
- If there is no resolution, get out of the situation, and either return later with support or refer the patient on.

Because there is potential for violence within any healthcare setting, it

■ BOX 4.5 Factors that contribute to the occurrence of conflict

Patient factors

- Loss of control, powerlessness
- Perceived threat to self
- Knowledge and understanding
- Mental and physical state

Environmental factors (may influence both patient and nurse)

- Ward facilities (lack of privacy and dignity)
- Influence of others (is there an audience?)
- Structure of the day (is the patient given choices?)
- Staffing issues (do the patient and nurse feel that the needs for support of each can be met?)

Nurse factors

- Self-awareness
- Interpersonal skills
- Attitudes
- Stress (makes overreaction more likely)
- Lack of knowledge
- Personalises abusive behaviour without recognising other influences

■ BOX 4.6 Long-term measures to control, contain and review conflict incidents

Staff

- Reporting details of incident
- What happened (antecedents)
- Details of response (behaviour)
- Outcome (consequences)
- Reflection and supervision on incident

Patient

- Arousal reduction: assist patient in recognising triggers (external events and internal beliefs that occur when angry)
- Internal reminders: use of key phrases such as 'keep calm'
- Use response reducers (deep breathing, counting backwards, visualising peaceful scene)
- Self-evaluation (assist patient to reflect on incident)

is important that each area develops its own policy on the handling of threatening or violent incidents, which should include long-term measures to control, contain and review incidents (Box 4.6).

By assisting patients to develop their assertion skills and reduce the aggressive response, it may then be possible to negotiate a contract with those who are likely to respond with abuse or violence, so that they agree

■ BOX 4.7 Factors to consider when reviewing abusive or violent incidents

Antecedents

- What led up to the incident?
- What was going on at the time?
- What did particular individuals say or do?
- What environmental factors may have contributed?
- With hindsight, was this incident predictable?
- How did I feel?

Consequences

- How did I/we react?
- Whose safety was compromised?
- How did the episode come to an end?
- Was the outcome satisfactory?
- How do I feel now?

Behaviours

- What exactly did the aggressor do?
- What body language was exhibited?
- What did I and other staff do?
- Was anything said that may have indicated the reason for the behaviour?
- Were any other people implicated?
- Was or could any aspect of the incident have been minimised by preventive measures?

Decisions

- Do we have all the relevant information?
- What decisions need to be made now?
- Do we need to change current policy, and if so how?
- Do we need to change aspects of the environment?
- What support do the individuals involved require?
- Are there unmet educational needs?

to take certain actions when they recognise their arousal response. These may include using relaxation techniques, taking time out, or using music, smell, colour or distraction to reduce the physiological arousal state.

Environmental factors can be altered, audiences reduced and privacy and dignity maintained. Positive reinforcement of non-aggressive behaviour and playing down aggressive incidents can help to establish an improved therapeutic environment. Finally, it is important for patients and staff, both current and future, that all abusive or violent incidents be reviewed (Box 4.7).

CHRONIC PAIN

Management of chronic pain is based on the following principles.

- Chronic pain is a life situation not an event.
- Chronic pain has wide-reaching psychological, social and

occupational consequences, affecting many areas of the sufferer's life.

- Chronic pain does not respond successfully to the methods used to treat acute pain.
- Recognition of the above factors can assist the patient in managing chronic pain.

Whatever area we work in within health care, but especially within the rehabilitation field, we are likely to meet patients who are suffering from chronic pain. Despite the fact that chronic pain affects 10% of the population of Great Britain, and 2.5 million of these sufferers are severely disabled by their pain (The Pain Society 1996), many nurses have little understanding of the emotional and psychological implications for the sufferer, and often become very frustrated at their failure to relieve the pain. The physiological mechanisms thought to be responsible for acute and chronic pain have been well described elsewhere (Melzack & Wall 1988), but it is worthwhile spending a little time looking at the differences between the two pain categories.

ACUTE VERSUS CHRONIC PAIN

Clinically, pain is divided into two separate groups, which can be seen as distinct from each other.

Acute pain is generally defined as 'pain with a purpose', that is present in response to trauma, injury or disease. It alerts the sufferer to the biological process or it occurs as part of a treatment, as in surgery. Hoskins Michel (1985) describes it as a warning that the function or structure of the integrity of the body is threatened. Patients can relate the acute pain to the context in which it occurs, and can expect it to have a beginning and an end. Melzack & Wall (1988) suggest that acute pain encompasses the hope of future recovery, and that part of its purpose is to encourage the sufferer to take the most effective steps in ensuring appropriate treatment.

A body of literature relating specifically to chronic pain has developed over the past few years, with some dispute over the time-scale involved for the pain continuum to move from acute to chronic. It is often described as pain lasting for more than 6 months, as it is supposed that any injury to the body will have healed by this time, although some authors argue that any damage will have healed by 3 months. Melzack & Wall (1988) describe the chronic pain syndrome as being pain that persists after all possible healing has occurred, or long after pain can serve any useful function and is no longer a symptom of injury or disease. It is ineffective to attempt to treat chronic pain as an event, as acute pain is treated; it is more productive to view chronic pain as a situation (Twycross 1984). Within this situation, the sufferer and his family may frequently undergo major changes to their lifestyles.

EMOTIONAL ASPECTS

As with all pain, chronic pain is recognised as a subjective experience. The resulting disability can have wide-reaching psychological, social and occupational consequences, affecting many areas of the sufferer's and his family's life. Many chronic pain patients have undergone years of investigation and treatment, often to little avail. Failure to resolve the problem may frequently lead to the sufferer feeling disbelieved, the inference being that their pain is imagined, exaggerated and 'all in the mind', or being maintained for 'secondary gain' (i.e. the sufferer receives the rewards of attention, sympathy and tender loving care). Patients suffering chronic pain can frequently be observed to be grimacing, limping and generally dramatising their pain. However, this does not imply that the problem is imagined. It is rather more helpful to consider whether the dramatisation and 'abnormal illness behaviours' are exhibited in an effort to have the problem dealt with effectively, and the fear and anxiety relieved (McCaffrey & Beebe 1989).

Sufferers who recognise the disbelief sometimes shown by professionals often start to doubt themselves, and find it impossible to explain and understand the sometimes massive losses that accompany the chronic pain syndrome. Loss of appetite and libido, insomnia, irritability, reduced range of interests, reduction or cessation of activity and feelings of hopelessness and helplessness (in effect the symptoms of depression) are frequently identified as common elements of the chronic pain syndrome. Some may suggest that there are certain 'neurotic' personality types that predispose to the failure to cope with the pain. However, there is little evidence to support this; rather more evidence suggests that, once the problem has been effectively dealt with, the 'neurotic' aspects will disappear. The life changes that accompany chronic pain frequently occur very gradually and insidiously, and it is often not until the patient has been given the opportunity to reflect on his life as a whole that he is able to recognise these and can be helped to take effective action.

THE CHRONIC PAIN CYCLE

A natural response to any pain is to attempt to protect the painful area by limiting the activity that increases pain. Any reduction or major limitation in activity very quickly results in loss of muscle strength and endurance, as well as reduced cardiovascular fitness. When muscle strength is reduced, any attempt to resume usual activities frequently results in increased pain and rapid fatigue, thereby reinforcing the original anticipation of pain. Within an acute pain episode, the problem is normally of a short enough duration that any losses can be recovered quickly. With chronic pain the situation is very different (Fig. 4.1). If there is no ending in sight to the problem, and activity continues to result in more pain, there is little encouragement for the sufferer to attempt to resume or maintain a healthy activity level. Over the longer term, other underused joints will become painful on exertion and, as a result of the reduced cardiovascular fitness and muscle inactivity, tissue repair will slow down, particularly in the peripheral areas. Ultimately this inactivity may result in reduced bone density.

The fear of activity causing more pain may encourage an overreliance

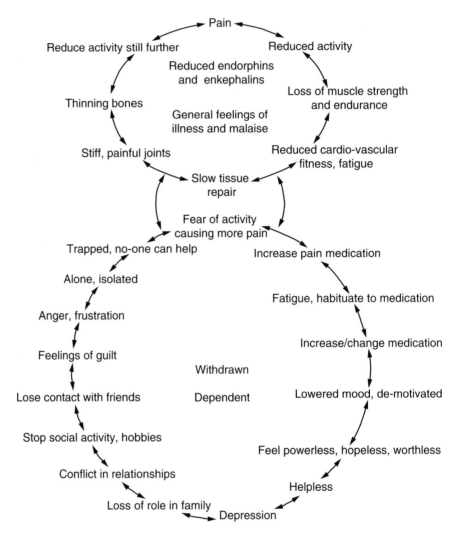

Figure 4.1 The chronic pain cycle.

on analgesic medication. Long-term use of analgesics leads to habituation, and causes changes in brain chemistry and mood, with loss of concentration and demotivation. Lowered mood, inactivity and overuse of medication all reduce the natural production and secretion of the body's own painkillers and 'feel good hormones', the endorphins and enkephalins.

The sufferer may experience major role changes within his family situation, with an increased dependence on partners for assistance, and perhaps a loss or change of occupation and subsequent financial changes. He may lose his role as a parent who was able to plan for and spend time with his children. Frequently, there is also a reduction in social activities, hobbies and contact with friends, which we all need in order to maintain balance in our lives. The person trapped in a chronic pain syndrome is often unable to plan ahead, with activity being dependent on the level of pain at the time. With all this going on, it is hardly surprising that the sufferer is depressed, isolated and feels angry, helpless and powerless to change anything. The healthcare professionals such patients have turned to for help are frequently unable to give them hope, leaving them feeling trapped in the situation.

THE NURSING ROLE IN CHRONIC PAIN MANAGEMENT

As acute pain may be regarded as an event, it is more likely to be managed successfully within the traditional medical model. Analgesic medications, in conjunction with appropriate support and information from the nurse, as well as the use of pain measurement scales and adjustment of medication if required, can enable the patient to regain some sense of control. This will lessen any associated anxieties and enhance recovery. In contrast, the management of chronic pain does not respond well to this type of approach. Patients have frequently experienced failure to contain or manage the pain when offered traditional treatments, which has led to increased anxiety, muscle tension, fear and despair.

In historical terms, the management of chronic pain is still in its infancy, although there are now well-recognised components that should be available within a structured pain-management programme. These programmes are multidisciplinary, utilising the skills of medicine, nursing, counselling, psychology, physiotherapy and occupational therapy, and generally use a cognitive–behavioural approach. This approach assists the patient in challenging and changing thoughts about their pain, identifying negative thought patterns and encouraging the sufferer to find alternative, more helpful ways of managing their life around the pain. It does not seek to offer complete pain relief. The belief within the cognitive approach is that thoughts affect feelings, and therefore that feelings can be altered by thinking different thoughts. This method is usually, to a greater or lesser extent, combined with a behavioural component, whereby the sufferer is given positive feedback or reward for activity that reduces the focus on pain, and is given negative reinforcement for increased pain focus (Flor et al 1992).

This type of programme is not readily available to all chronic pain sufferers and, even if it were, it would still not help the nurse in a general setting who is finding it difficult to support the patient suffering from chronic pain. However, some component parts of such a programme can be utilised. As discussed earlier, many patients feel that they are disbelieved by healthcare staff, who are unable to realise the broader impact of chronic pain. I believe that the most essential role that the nurse can play is to listen to and believe the patient.

Listen to and believe the patient

In order to do this effectively, it is necessary to use the communication skills discussed previously (active listening, non-judgmental acceptance and empathy). When the chronic pain sufferer is telling you about his physical pain, he is also telling you about his fears, anxieties, losses and changed relationships, and until these are acknowledged with him, he may be unable to move on. The containment offered by time can be useful in preventing both the patient and yourself being overwhelmed by his experience. It is also important to reflect upon your own attitudes to pain.

- Do I make assumptions about another person's level of pain?
- Do I believe that people in pain behave in a certain way?
- What basis do I have for that belief?
- Do I stereotype patients in pain according to gender expectations?
- What beliefs do I have about the effects of medication, particularly narcotic medication, and the patients that request this?
- What basis do I have for that belief?
- What knowledge and understanding do I have about pain, particularly chronic pain?

Obviously, any identified false beliefs or assumptions need addressing, on both a personal and a professional level.

Breathing and relaxation

Chronic pain can fit the definition of chronic stress, which includes such symptoms as reduced immunity to disease, sleep disturbance, fatigue, headaches, lack of concentration, shortness of breath, increased muscle tension and anxiety and depression (Caudill 1995). Therefore some techniques commonly used in stress management can be helpful in pain management, and are frequently used in structured pain management programmes. The patient can be supported in using these by the nurse, albeit in a limited way. The release of adrenalin from the sympathetic nervous system (the 'flight or fight response'), which occurs as a result of perpetual stress, results in increased physical tensions, which in turn lead to an increase in pain. It has been shown that practising a relaxation technique can reduce the arousal response and sympathetic activity. While many relaxation techniques require that the trainer undergoes a comprehensive training in order to teach them to others, as well as requiring the long-term commitment of the patient to practising them, there is a simple technique that may be suggested by the nurse.

When the stress response becomes a permanent state, people frequently become 'chest breathers'. This occurs due to anxiety, when tension is increased in the abdominal area, preventing the diaphragm from contracting or the abdominal wall from moving out on the in-breath. This results in short, shallow breaths. Recognising this, and encouraging the patient consciously to breathe using the diaphragm can bring about a feeling of calmness and relaxation.

1. Assist the patient in finding a comfortable, well-supported position.

2. Ask the patient to place one hand on his sternum and one hand over his umbilicus.

3. Ask the patient to close his eyes and become aware of what is moving when breathing in and out.

4. If his chest moves up and down with each breath, he is not breathing diaphragmatically.

5. Ask the patient to place his hand just below his umbilicus and imagine a balloon inside his abdomen.

6. Ask the patient to imagine the balloon filling with air when he breathes in, and collapsing when he breathes out. If the patient feels light-headed or dizzy, he may be breathing too fast or too deeply. Suggest he stop practising for a minute and breathe normally until the feeling passes.

Once the patient is able to recognise the calming response to this technique, he can be encouraged to scan his body and notice any particular tensions being held in different muscle groups, and to make a conscious effort to let these tensions go.

Distraction

Many people find that distracting themselves with an activity that they enjoy can be helpful in reducing anxiety and pain. There are many different ideas that might be suggested to a patient to encourage him to use distraction, for example listening to favourite music, joining in with the conversations of others, taking a walk around, getting involved in hobbies, such as painting, drawing or knitting, or setting up a game with other patients involved. It might seem a rather simplistic suggestion to make, but it can be very effective in allowing the patient a 'window' in his pain, as well as encouraging socialisation with others.

Paced activity and realistic goal-setting

There is not the space available here to discuss fully the principles behind paced activity, but in a non-specialised setting it is likely to mean that the nurse offers support and encouragement to the sufferer to maintain some activity level, which must be set at an achievable level and gradually increased. This should normally be done in conjunction with any physical therapy. Any goals or aims that are identified must be realistic and achievable, as setting unrealistic goals is doomed to end in failure, causing further reinforcement of the sense of hopelessness. Pacing will also ensure that the sufferer gets adequate rest and sleep, as well as appropriate nutritional input, which may have been lacking due to depression.

Summary

The nurse can help the patient by recognising the complexities of the chronic pain situation and ensuring appropriate referral on to others with more specialised skills.

SUMMARY

In concluding this section, the reader is encouraged to revisit the key principles outlined at the begining. As a nurse, you are essential to the psychological well-being of the clients in your care, and in rehabilitation you indisputably provide that individual's first-line psychological support. There are clear deficits not only in the way we work but also in the preparation of nurses to undertake this vital role effectively. These problems must be resolved. Psychological support is not an optional extra, to be offered when and if we have the time, but is as fundamental to the client as is nursing of physical needs. As a profession it is time to stop paying lip-service to how vital it is, and develop the appropriate systems and support to ensure its delivery.

ACKNOWLEDGEMENTS

The author is grateful to Mike Smith for giving his permission to adapt his model for managing aggression.

REFERENCES

Barnitt R, Pomeroy V 1995 An holistic approach to rehabilitation. British Journal of Therapy and Rehabilitation 2(2):87–91
British Association for Counselling 1997 Code of ethics and practice for counselling skills. BAC, Rugby
Caudill M A 1995 Managing pain before it manages you. Guildford Press, New York
Egan G 1994 The skilled helper. A problem managed approach to helping, 5th edn. Wadsworth, Belmont, California, ch 5, p 91
Flor H, Fydrich T, Turk D C 1992 Efficacy of multidisciplinary pain treatment centres: a meta-analytic review. Pain 49:221–230
Hoskins Michel T 1985 Introduction and state of the art. In: Hoskins Michel T (ed) Pain. Churchill Livingstone, Edinburgh
McCaffrey M, Beebe A 1989 Pain: a clinical manual for nursing practice. Times Mirror Publishers, London
Melzack R, Wall P 1988 The challenge of pain, 2nd edn. Pelican, London
Motyka M, Motyka H, Wsolek R 1997 Elements of psychological support in nursing care. Journal of Advanced Nursing 26:909–912
Nichols K A 1984 Psychological care in physical illness, 2nd edn. Chapman & Hall, London
Rogers C 1990 Speaking personally. In: Kirschbaum H, Henderson V L (eds) The Carl Rogers reader. Constable, London
The Pain Society 1996 Pain management programmes. Communication to The Royal College of Nursing, London
Twycross R G 1984 Control of pain. Journal of the Royal College of Physicians 18(1):32–39
United Kingdom Central Council of Nursing, Midwifery and Health Visiting 1997 This is the UKCC. Protecting the public through professional standards. UKCC, London

FURTHER READING

Casement P 1985 On learning from the patient. Tavistock Routledge, London
Hawkins P, Shohet R 1989 Supervision in the helping professions. Open University Press, Buckingham
Keable D 1997 The management of anxiety. Churchill Livingstone, Edinburgh
Robertson S E, Brown R I 1992 Rehabilitation counselling: approaches in the field of disability. Chapman & Hall, London

The nurse as promoter of sexual health

Mike Smith

INTRODUCTION

Until relatively recently, the topic of sexuality and sexual health has received minimal attention in the nursing and rehabilitation literature, with the exception of the predominantly medical focus on issues surrounding erectile and ejaculatory function. In addition, and somewhat disappointingly, since the publication of *The Health of the Nation* (Department of Health 1992), I would suggest that, as a term, in the UK 'sexual health' has almost become synonymous with HIV and AIDS. This belief stems from a recent literature search, performed on CINAHL, of UK nursing articles written in the last 8 years. This revealed that out of the articles listed that related to sexual health, over 75% concentrated on HIV or AIDS, and a further 12% on more general sexually transmitted diseases.

In addition, anecdotal evidence from the areas in which I have worked and the literature suggest that sexual health issues tend to be neglected somewhat in assessment of patients and in care planning. So often, only brief reference, if any at all, is made to sexuality issues, perhaps incorporating only whether someone has a partner, children or is HIV-positive. If the reader were to look at the nursing documentation within his own area, it would not be suprising if he found this to be the case. Surely one would have to acknowledge that there is significantly more to sexual health than these factors. After all, sexuality is recognised within currently used nursing models (e.g. as part of an individual's activities of living) (Roper et al 1985).

In a survey involving rehabilitation nurses and occupational therapists, Novak & Mitchell (1988) found that there were large inconsistencies between sexuality counselling actually performed in practice and recommendations cited in the literature. It was suggested that there is a lack of knowledge and skills in dealing with clients with sexual health problems. The poor emphasis on and delivery of education and counselling regarding sexual health issues has also been outlined in other studies (Kreuter et al 1994, Tepper 1992). Such evidence would suggest that nurses are either:

- ill-equipped to deal with such issues, due to lack of knowledge, training or supervision, or perhaps a combination of all three, or
- nurses do not consider sexuality as important.

One would hope, and indeed strongly suggest, that it is likely to be the former reason.

The aim of this section is to explore the nature of sexuality and sexual health, identify potential sexual health problems with which patients may present following illness or injury, and suggest practical advice in dealing with these.

SEXUALITY

There appears to be some degree of consistency in the literature related to the definition of what constitutes human sexuality (Bancroft 1994, Cole & Cole 1990, Masters & Johnson 1986a, Savage 1987), indicating clearly identifiable similar threads. These key common threads relating to sexuality include the following.

- Although they are a component, sexuality is significantly more than just the biological aspects of the sex act.
- Sexuality also encompasses the very characteristics (physical, psychological and social) relating to gender, which identify an individual as a man or a woman.
- Sexuality is specific in nature to that individual within his or her unique setting within society and culture.
- Sexuality is a dynamic feature of being a person throughout one's life, in that it will be subject to change due to personal circumstances and experiences, including those resulting from health changes.

GENDER ROLE

Although all of the above issues will be referred to throughout this chapter, it is worth exploring the concept of gender role in a little more detail at this stage, as an understanding of this is key to appreciating some of the issues discussed later.

Gender identity and role within an individual's life, originating in and developing throughout childhood and adolescence, usually become more stable in adulthood. Although the individual nature of sexuality was stressed above, Fairburn et al (1993) suggest there may be a degree of predictability in some of these changes to the constitution of a person's sexuality which occur throughout life from childhood to old age. As the remit of this book is to give a discussion of rehabilitation in adult nursing practice, this chapter obviously focuses on changes that may occur in the client from adulthood to old age.

The role within and related to the home, be it husband, wife, partner, or parent, will contribute significantly to one's sexuality. In addition, other roles, such as provider to dependents through earning at work, form an integral part of gender role. The social roles one plays in the company of others, either at work or with friends or aquaintances, often have a gender-orientated component. One need look no further for an example than the many discussions relating to male nurses over the years, or the differences in the content of all-male and all-female discussions. Therefore, expectations and personal behaviour when with friends and others in the individual's social circle can demonstrate, and develop further, the individuality of a person's sexuality (Savage 1987). The influences on this are too complex to discuss in great detail within this chapter, but are many, and include those of peers, culture and the media.

SEXUAL HEALTH

As well as the physical aspects of injury or illness, changes in any of the sexuality issues discussed above can be thought of as potential influences on the perceived sexual health of the individual (Spica 1989, Woods 1987). Masters & Johnson (1986a) suggest that sexual health is closely interwoven with the total health of the individual, and may be influenced by and is dependent upon a freedom from both physical and psychosocial limitations and barriers. Therefore, the influence on and potential disruption of all aspects of sexual health subsequent to an acquired illness or disability may be profound (Rieve 1989, Weinburg 1982).

Reflecting this opinion, three distinct factors that comprise sexual health have been defined by the World Health Organization (WHO 1975). An individual should possess:

- a capacity to enjoy and control sexual and reproductive behaviour in accordance with a social and personal ethic
- a freedom from fear, shame, guilt, false beliefs and other psychological factors inhibiting sexual response and impairing sexual relationships
- a freedom from organic disorders, diseases and deficiencies that interfere with sexual and reproductive functions.

Arguably, however, this definition seems to suggest that the individual with a physical disability following illness or injury will be unable to attain sexual health. Certainly I would personally strongly refute this suggestion. Rather, I would propose that, through rehabilitation and education, the physiological limitations that may exist as a result of a disability may be overcome, and the objective of sexual health may still be attained.

In view of this, the following alternative criteria are proposed for ascertaining sexual health status. These could be broadly used to measure the success or otherwise of sexual health rehabilitation approaches:

- the presence of sexually appropriate behaviour in accordance with a social and personal ethic
- a freedom from psychosocial issues that result in an unwelcome reduction in or absence of engaging in sexual relationships
- an ability to engage in sexual activity through adapting to changes in physical status that may interfere with sexual function.

These three criteria are explored below, and potential areas for nursing assessment are suggested for each. Key aspects of the criteria are developed further later in the chapter when examining nursing interventions related to sexual health.

SEXUALLY APPROPRIATE BEHAVIOUR

Aspects of this that may be relevant to a nursing situation may include dealing with cultural issues and issues of personal choice of the individual as regards his sexual behaviour. Neither of these may conform to the beliefs and choices of the nurse, and so may be the cause of potential conflict or discomfort for either party if not respected by the other.

Assessment within this aspect could include ascertaining who the partner of the individual is, indicating sexual orientation, and the status of the relationship as regards marital or living arrangements. If the individual is from a culture or religious background unfamiliar to the nurse, it is worth investigating these issues and recording them.

PSYCHOSOCIAL ISSUES

There are five major issues that may lead to a reduction in or an absence of engagement in sexual relationships (Fig. 4.2).

Relationship problems

Although it is true that problems with a relationship may have an adverse effect on sexual function, this is usually far from being the inevitable cause of sexual health problems. Relationship problems are often secondary to other issues, or are a general difficulty in the person or partner in adjusting to the implications of the injury or illness. In addition, if some care must be provided in the community and responsibility for this falls on the partner, this may impose further strain on a relationship (Hall et al 1994). However, as a primary cause of sexual health problems is often poor communication between couples, one would suggest that effective communication is essential for a mutually satisfying sexual relationship. Conversely, poor communication may have the opposite effect. Some couples may find communication difficult, viewing sex talk as 'dirty', and may not possess the vocabulary to express their needs, desires and hopes to their partner

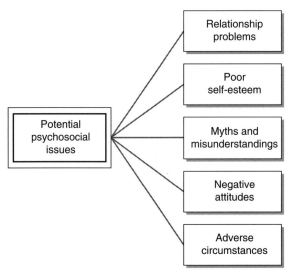

Figure 4.2 Potential psychosocial issues affecting sexual health.

(Chicano 1989). Such problems may often have already existed prior to the illness or injury, but are exacerbated by the new set of circumstances. However, even in the confines of a secure, trusting, apparently 'healthy' relationship, difficulties may arise following the change in general health status.

Formal assessment of this may be possible to some degree through asking the client how his partner feels about what has happened, and whether they have discussed the potential implications of the illness or injury. However, as much information will be gained through informal means, as nurses will be the professionals who will see the interaction between couples in the rehabilitation environment, and will deal with the distressed relative. It is often on such occasions that the nurse has the opportunity to initiate discussion of such matters in greater detail, either with the client on an individual basis or with the couple.

Poor self-esteem

People who are depressed and feel inadequate may often have difficulty in giving and receiving pleasure (Teal & Athelston 1975). There are multiple causes of low self-esteem. It may be historical, relating to events in childhood and adolescence, or related to recent life events, either physical (illness) or psychological (bereavement, loneliness or conflict). Actual or perceived changes in body image, commonly associated with disability, may result in the individual feeling unattractive, and be further compounded by the views of others and society in general (Goddard 1988). Disability of any degree, lacks congruence with the standard media portrayal of what constitutes 'normal', desirable or ideal, through images that are reinforced continuously in television and newspaper advertising (Savage 1987). Indeed, an American study showed that a person with spinal cord injury often feels less of a man or woman (Althof & Levine 1993) because of the effects of their injury. A man may perceive that he does not 'measure-up' sexually, and this can result in feelings of embarrassment, confusion or depression over his situation (Masters & Johnson 1986b). Consequently, he may avoid sexual activities, invent excuses, or attempt to place the blame on something or someone else. Other aspects of sexuality relating to gender role may also be affected, for example the perceived impact on the ability of the individual to act as a good father or mother. Gray & Schimmel (1990) suggest that no body of scientific evidence has been accumulated that addresses the fundamental questions which people with disabilities have regarding parenting. Recognising the limitations of previous work, Buck (1990) has discussed the impact of disability on families and parenting, and has suggested that the problems may be significant and require counselling and educational programmes. He has proposed that such programmes should assist parents with disabilities to overcome their concerns and anxieties and to use their strengths, thus enabling them to parent more effectively.

Again with reference to assessment, a significant part of the nurse's role will be that of observing the behaviour of the person. Behaviours that may indicate low self-esteem include apparent withdrawal from, or even total absence of, social contact with others in the rehabilitation environment. The individual is often unlikely to be very positive in what he says about any aspect of his situation, and again may avoid voluntarily discussing the future. Specific verbal cues relating to relationship prospects may be given, suggesting that a perception that they have become unattractive (e.g. 'no-one will be interested in someone in a wheelchair'). The nurse could also explore how the person feels others are reacting, or may react, to any change in their body image. In addition, if appropriate, the nurse could explore the feelings the client may have regarding being a parent.

Myths and misunderstandings

Many myths and taboos exist regarding sex, which will differ according to a person's cultural background and the extent and quality of sex education received. The myths and taboos may stem from childhood and adolescence, and therefore many people enter adult life and sexual relationships having little or incorrect information about sex. A poor understanding of anatomy may be present regarding the sex act (e.g. role of foreplay) or faulty expectations may exist (e.g. always experiencing simultaneous orgasm).

When faced with illness or disability the individual is also subjected to, or may carry with him, a barrage of further myths specific to sex and disability (Chicano 1989). Masters & Johnson (1986b) have described the myths held by the public in their American study (Box 4.8).

In attempting to address these problems, the nurse must assess existing knowledge and preconceptions that the individual may have, not only regarding general aspects of his change in health status, but also specifically relating to relationships and sexual health. In addition, it is worth pointing out that nurses must examine themselves to explore any preconceptions they may have, and use the support of others to deal with these as appropriate.

■ **BOX 4.8 Myths regarding sex and disability**

- Disabled people are asexual.
- Disabled people are dependent and child-like, so they need to be protected.
- Disability breeds disability.
- Disabled people should stay with and marry their own kind.
- Parents of handicapped children do not want sex education for their children.
- Sexual intercourse culminating in orgasm is essential for sexual satisfaction.
- If a disabled person has a sexual problem, it is almost always as a result of their disability.
- If a non-disabled person has a sexual relationship with a disabled individual it is because he is unable to attract anyone else.

Negative attitudes

Negative attitudes to sexuality are commonly cultural or religious in origin. Attitudes are fashioned according to the expectations of the society in which one lives (Drench 1992). Sexual attitudes relating to self and others have a basis in the environment in which one lives and develops. Negative attitudes towards sexuality that exist before illness or injury are likely to be carried over after the event, and may include generalised beliefs that sex is dirty or bad in some way and should not be discussed.

Other negative attitudes may relate to some traumatic sexual experience. These may originate from any stage of life, the obvious extreme examples being those of child abuse and rape. Needless to say the intervention required in such cases is complex, often takes many years and is beyond the scope of all but the specialist. In such a case immediate referral must be made.

Adverse circumstances

There are many circumstances, often beyond the control of the individual or couple, that may be either primary causes of or contributors to sexual health problems. The physical environment in which couples interact and share their relationship may be responsible. This may include an inability to obtain privacy or the presence of uncomfortable surroundings, neither of which are conducive to the development and maintenance of sexual health (Chicano 1989, Goddard 1988). Creation of sufficient time to share feelings about and problems with both the sexual and general aspects of the relationship may be difficult due to family and work pressures. A preoccupation with other aspects of the life of the individual, frequently associated with work and financial concerns, may also be a causative factor. The documented low level of employment in people with a physical disability may exacerbate this situation further (Weinburg 1982).

As the aspect of sexual health usually becomes apparent only on return to the community, it is an issue that may be picked up either by community professionals or at outpatient appointments. However, it is essential that, during the assessment of the client, the nurse ensures that he is able and given permission to create some 'space' to obtain the privacy needed to discuss sexual issues with his partner. The psychosocial aspects related to sexual health that should be considered when assessing clients are summarised in Box 4.9.

ABILITY TO ENGAGE IN SEXUAL ACTIVITY

Sexual health problems that are primarily physically based following illness or injury can be divided into three categories (Bancroft 1994): interference with either sexual appetite, sexual behaviour or sexual response.

Interference with sexual appetite

By their very nature, illness and disease can result in malaise and lethargy, and thus can affect sexual appetite. Often this will return once physical

■ **BOX 4.9 Assessment sexual health: psychosocial factors**

- Culture
- Religion
- Whether discussion has taken place with partner about the change in circumstances
- Observation of interaction with partner
- Observation of social interaction with others within the rehabilitation environment
- Voluntarily verbalised comments relating to prospects following injury/illness
- Knowledge and attitudes towards the impact of illness/injury on sexual activity
- How the person feels others may react to him
- Ability to obtain privacy

health has been restored. However in chronic illness, the time-scale may be lengthy. Alcohol and certain types of medication, notably antidepressants, antispasmodics, diuretics and steroids, may have an adverse effect on sexual appetite.

Assessment of general physical health will be undertaken as a matter of course and the medication which the person is taking noted. If deemed significant, the side-effects of medication should be discussed with the client and documented as regards the potential effects on sexual health.

Interference with sexual behaviour

Frequently, interference with sexual behaviour results directly from physical conditions or is due to symptoms of the disease or disability (e.g. immobility, pain or spasticity) (Drench 1992). In addition, changes in behaviour may be enforced due to medical advice, albeit often on a temporary basis. For example, some patients who have undergone back surgery may be instructed to wear a brace, which will limit movement. Other forms of enforced immobilisation particularly prevalent in orthopaedic conditions include wearing of splints and plaster of Paris, either in the form of jackets with halo traction or used to immobilise limbs. Those with acquired disability often need to adopt alternative approaches to sharing a sexual experience with another compared with their sexual behaviour prior to disability (Weinburg 1982). Couples may need to experiment with new ways of pleasuring one another. For some this may be exciting and an adventure, whereas for others it may be perceived as a disappointing and frustrating chore (Althof & Levine 1993). Indeed, any motor deficit resulting from illness or injury may affect the ability to hug, caress or hold a partner, these being considered to be the most basic of physical interactions during the sex act. Other 'technical' problems that may result from reduced motor function include undressing, transferring to a bed or other suitable place, and assuming desired positions.

The presence of a neurogenic bowel and bladder may result in 'accidents' during the sex act unless there is associated planning and preparation. The lack of spontaneity that this preparation engenders may be an initial cause of upset for the couple concerned.

Therefore, assessment can be based again on the potential implications for sexual behaviour of the individual's specific circumstances, and this can form the basis of intervention through discussion and education at an appropriate time.

Interference with sexual response

Interference with the sexual response itself may occur due to disturbance in bodily organs and systems. This has generated a significant proportion of the work done in the area of sexuality and disability. Three factors influence what is considered to be a 'normal' physiological sexual response: the nerve and blood supply must be intact; the cardiovascular and respiratory systems must be able to react to the physical demands of the sex act; and the genital organs must be healthy.

Disruption in the neural supply to the sexual organs and the resulting consequences for the client will depend on both the level and severity of neurological damage. In women, vaginal lubrication is thought to be also controlled via these same spinal nerves (Szasz 1992). In men, erection may be affected, and may be either totally absent or insufficient for penetration.

Ejaculation in the course of the sex act rarely occurs in men with complete neurological damage to the spinal cord. It has been suggested that such individuals may also have reduced numbers of or no mature spermatozoa, thus further complicating potential fertility (Seager & Halstead 1993).

With regard to the physiological demands of the sex act, neurological damage to the cervical portion of the spinal cord, or any respiratory or cardiovascular pathology may necessitate changes in behaviour, with the individual taking a more passive role.

An obvious threat to healthy genital organs, as with any individual, is that of sexually transmitted diseases (STDs). Effective genital hygiene and 'safe sex' should minimise the risk of STDs. Problems with insufficient production of vaginal secretions during sex may require the use of a lubrication jelly to avoid problems.

The nurse should be aware of the implications for sexual response relating to the particular health condition with which the client presents. If such implications are recorded they can form the basis for appropriate education.

It must be acknowledged that it is oversimplistic to look at each of these issues as separate problems, as it is clearly the interplay between all of them which comprises an individual's sexual health (Bancroft 1994, Woods 1987). For example, a client who has erectile dysfunction due to neurological damage may use alternative methods to attain erection, thus overcoming any physiological dysfunction. However, he may believe that others will perceive his disability as unattractive or repulsive, and may find maintaining relationships problematic. If an individual is susceptible to secondary health problems, such as incontinence, or is not in a position to manage pain effectively, it is not inconceivable that he will refrain from engaging in sexual activity with a partner. A man who has suffered a myocardial infarction and undertaken a cardiac rehabilitation programme, which has resulted in him having the required cardiovascular and respiratory capabilities to participate in the sex act, may not do so due to fear of a recurrence of his condition.

The interrelated nature of the physiological and psychosocial aspects of sexuality suggests that sexual health rehabilitation should encompass all these issues. It must begin with a thorough assessment, as discussed above, without which sexual health needs may be left unmet. It is clear that, as with other psychological issues, nurses are at the 'front-line' of sexual health promotion due to the 24 hour nature of their work, and therefore they may often be the most appropriate team members to carry out such primary assessment.

NURSING AND REHABILITATION RELATING TO SEXUAL HEALTH PROBLEMS

Probably the most vital point to stress regarding intervention relating to sexual health is that the individual nurse must be able to recognise his limitations. It is essential that the nurse is aware of what may be appropriate to deal with himself and what must be referred to specialists. Such specialists may also be nurses, and indeed perhaps should be nurses, but they will have an expanded role due to having undertaken the relevant training and supervision.

There appear to be four possible approaches to sexual health rehabilitation (Fig. 4.3). Emphasising again the interplay of factors involved in sexual health, a combination of any of the four approaches may be required to address sexual health, depending on the specific needs and situation of the individual concerned.

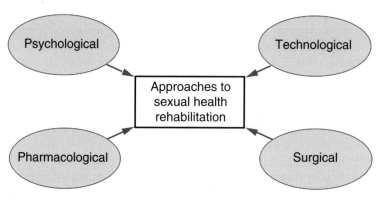

Figure 4.3 Approaches to sexual health rehabilitation.

PSYCHOLOGICAL APPROACH

It has been suggested that this is often the most appropriate primary approach (Szasz 1992). It seems logical that the maximum benefit of the other approaches will only be achieved if there is first an exploration of any sexual health problems of psychological origin. Indeed, Cole (1975) states: 'The knowledge that more sexuality lies within the head than between the thighs helps to set the stage for restoration of a satisfactory sex life.'

If the need to address the issues raised in the previous section is to be met, it is essential that the client is actually able to recognise that a problem may exist. Without this recognition attempts at dealing with a problem may, at best, be fruitless, as the client will not cooperate with prescribed interventions. At worst the client could be offended, and the interaction and trust between the professional and the client could be severely damaged.

Approaches therefore need to be cautious in the initial stage, using evidence provided both by the client's own experiences and the nursing assessment. The ideal situation would be an environment that encourages the client voluntarily to raise questions relating to sexual health. Basic written information regarding the aims and objectives relating to dealing with sexual health, and introducing the roles of the specific personnel involved, may act as means of introducing the topic of sexual health, thereby prompting questions from the client. Such opportunities must be seized early, as this may be less threatening and disturbing than a professional approach. However, if the client does not make an approach, there may often be no choice but to raise the issue. One could broach the topic in the form of the questions raised in the previous section, e.g. 'How does your partner feel about your injury?' or 'Has anyone talked to you yet about sex?' An appropriate dedicated environment, offering privacy to explore such matters, may additionally facilitate undisturbed, comfortable discussion. The nurse should guide the client to such an area as soon as the topic is raised.

There are four main broad objectives of the psychological approach relating to the potential sexual health problems described earlier:

1. Dispelling myths associated with sexual health and disability through reassurance and a programme of education relating to all aspects. With regard to the method of providing education, although didactic sessions in a group situation may be useful, these should be supplemented with time for individual discussion and further exploration of individual issues (Chicano 1989) due to the very personal nature of sexuality.

2. Provision of information enabling increased choice in potential methods to minimise interference with sexual response, appetite and behaviour. Again this may be achieved through a programme of education.

3. Supporting the right to express feelings, and encouraging communication with the partner, both generally and specifically relating to sexual issues.

4. Working through any unresolved feelings and emotions with the individual until there is a recognised acceptance of the new situation through a programme of counselling.

Provision of counselling, both with and without the partner present, is essential (Cushman 1988), and it has also been suggested that general 'communication therapy' or training would be beneficial (Cole & Cole 1990). The use of counselling by peers (i.e. other individuals in similar circumstances) has been proposed as potentially valuable (Althof & Levine 1993), not only in the sharing of a common problem, but also so that advice can be given and suggestions made from personal experience. Aspects of this are dealt with earlier in Chapter 4; however, as previously mentioned, the input of a specialist in sexual health counselling may be required.

PHARMACOLOGICAL APPROACH

The main pharmacological approaches focus on the associated impairments which may impinge on the sexual behaviour aspects of sexual health. These may include, for example, medication to control spasticity thus facilitating mobility, and medication associated with maintenance of the specific bladder and bowel programmes.

Medication prescribed to affect mood and general psychological state may be provided on a short-term basis, but this should be discouraged for long-term use, other methods to manage the psychological status of the client being preferable.

A major part of this approach should be a review of all medication, with particular reference to those drugs that may have a direct or indirect influence on sexual function.

A pharmacological approach may also be used in the management of erectile dysfunction. Intercavernous injections of a vasodilating substance, commonly Papaverine, is now a well-established procedure and should be easily administered by any individual with adequate hand function. There is a risk of prolonged erection, which may lead to ischaemic changes in the corpus cavernosum should it last for 6 hours (Dietzen & Lloyd 1992). In such circumstances a sympathomimetic agent will be required to alleviate the situation.

TECHNOLOGICAL APPROACH

The technological approaches concentrate on erectile and ejaculatory dysfunction, which are often the result of neurological loss. Most of these approaches are beyond the scope of all but the specialist nurse in sexual health, and so only a brief description is given here.

Erectile dysfunction

Vacuum devices to obtain erection are now available in several forms (e.g. Erectaid) and are increasingly used due to the non-invasive nature of the procedure (Aloni et al 1992). A firm cylinder is placed over the penis and the air removed using a hand pump. The vacuum created encourages the penis to become engorged with blood, resulting in erection. The erection is maintained by placing a rubber ring around the base of the penis.

Ejaculatory dysfunction

In those with ejaculatory disturbance, two common techniques are used to obtain semen: vibratory stimuli and electro-ejaculation.

SURGICAL APPROACH

The insertion of either inflatable or rigid penile implants for erectile dysfunction has been described (Linsenmeyer 1991). Potential complications which have been highlighted include infection and dislocation of the prosthesis with subsequent erosion (Dietzen & Lloyd 1992). The nurse's role is restricted to pre- and postoperative care in those specialist centres that undertake this procedure.

STAFF EDUCATION AND SUPPORT

All members of the rehabilitation team should receive basic knowledge regarding sexual health and must be aware of available services, including who to refer to if specialist intervention is required. This should be given as part of an induction programme and through an ongoing in-service development programme (Halstead et al 1977). This will encourage increased individual expertise and develop a team approach to sexual health rehabilitation (Tepper 1992). Principles of education are covered in detail in Chapter 9. However, it is worth stressing that such sexual health education should be focused on the potential client needs within that particular speciality, as well as on the more generic principles of sexuality and sexual health covered earlier in this chapter.

Adequate supervision for all personnel involved is essential to facilitate staff well-being and development. Those who are involved as specialist nurses in the sexual health field, and therefore are involved in some of the more complex and difficult issues, should have an identified supervisor who has experience as a sexual health counsellor.

SUMMARY

It is indisputable that sexuality is a major part of being human, and therefore promoting sexual health in health care should be as vital as any other aspect of daily life. Nursing and rehabilitation generally appear to be falling short of meeting client needs in this area, in comparison to other areas which are addressed more fully. There are several reasons why this may be the case, not least the social taboos that have traditionally surrounded sexuality. We must find ways to overcome these.

Nurses are in an ideal situation, because of their working practices and relationship with clients, to begin to address sexual health more fully. In addition, individuals must be aware of their limitations and make appropriate and prompt referral as necessary.

Clearly, sexual health is a complex interplay of many factors, and thus thorough assessment is essential. This chapter has outlined the potential impact of illness and injury on aspects of sexual health, suggesting means by which client need may be identified beyond the brief or absent references usually made to sexual health.

Individual nurses must not only seek out and demand information and education related to sexual health, but also be facilitated in examining and addressing their own attitudes and perceptions, which may be detrimental to discussing what may be a sensitive topic with clients.

REFERENCES

Aloni R, Heller L, Keren O, Medelsohn E, Davidoff G 1992 Non-invasive treatment of erectile dysfunction in the neurogenically disabled population. Journal of Sex and Marital Therapy 18(3):243–249

Althof S, Levine S 1993 Clinical approach to the sexuality of patients with spinal cord injury. Urological Clinics of North America 20(3):543–548

Bancroft J 1994 The biological basis of human sexuality. In: Human sexuality and its problems. Churchill Livingstone, London, ch 2, pp 12–145

Buck F M 1990 Parenting by fathers with physical disabilities. In: Haseltine F R, Cole S, Gray D (eds) Reproductive issues for persons with physical disabilities. Brookes, Baltimore, ch 15, pp 163–185

Chicano L A 1989 Humanistic aspects of sexuality as related to spinal cord injury. Journal of Neuroscience Nursing 21(6):366–369

Cole S, Cole T 1990 Sexuality, disability and reproductive issues through the lifespan. In: Haseltine F R, Cole S, Gray D (eds) Reproductive issues for persons with physical disabilities. Brookes, Baltimore, ch 1, pp 3–22

Cole T 1975 Sexuality and physical disabilities. Archives of Sexual Behaviour 4(4): 389–402

Cushman L A 1988 Sexual counseling in a rehabilitation program: a patient's perspective. Journal of Rehabilitation 54(2):65–69

Department of Health 1992 The health of the nation: a strategy for health in England. HMSO, London

Dietzen C J, Lloyd L K 1992 Complications of intracavernous injections and penile prosthesis in spinal cord injured men. Archives of Medical and Physical Rehabilitation 73(7):652–655

Drench M 1992 Impact of altered sexuality and sexual function in spinal cord injury: a review. Sexuality and Disability 10(1):15–31

Fairburn C, Dickeson M, Greenwood J 1983 Sexuality from childhood to old age. In: Sexual problems and their management. Churchill Livingstone, Edinburgh, ch 3, pp 23–33

Goddard L R 1988 Sexuality and spinal cord injury. Journal of Neuroscience Nursing 20(4):240–244

Gray D, Schimmel A B 1990 Future directions for research on reproductive issues for people with physical disabilities. In: Haseltine F R, Cole S, Gray D (eds) Reproductive issues for persons with physical disabilities. Brookes, Baltimore, ch 29, pp 339–354

Hall K M, Karzmark P, Stevens M, Englander J, O'Hare P, Wright J 1994 Family stressors in traumatic brain injury: a two year follow up. Archives of Physical and Medical Rehabilitation 75:876–884

Halstead L S, Halstead M M, Joyce J T, Stock D D, Sparks R W 1977 A hospital based program in human sexuality. Archives of Physical and Medical Rehabilitation 57:409–412

Kreuter M, Sullivan M, Siosteen A 1994 Sexual adjustment after spinal cord injury focusing on partner experiences. Paraplegia 32:225–235

Linsenmeyer T A 1991 Evaluation and treatment of erectile dysfunction following spinal cord injury: a review. Journal of the American Paraplegia Society 14(2):43–51

Masters W H, Johnson V E 1986a Perspectives on sexuality. In: On sex and human loving. Macmillan, London, ch 1, pp 3–31

Masters W H, Johnson V E 1986b Sexual disorders and sexual health. In: On sex and human loving. Macmillan, London, ch 19, pp 503–530

Novak P P, Mitchell M M 1988 Professional involvement in sexual counseling for patients with spinal cord injuries. American Journal of Occupational Therapy 42(2):105–112

Rieve J E 1989 Sexuality and the adult with acquired physical disability. Nursing Clinics of North America 24(1):265–276

Roper N, Logan W, Tierney A 1985 The elements of nursing, 2nd edn. Churchill Livingstone, Edinburgh

Savage J 1987 The nature of sexuality. In: Nurses, gender and sexuality. Heinemann, London, ch 5, pp 28–42

Seager S W, Halstead L S 1993 Fertility options and success after spinal cord injury. Urological Clinics of North America 20(3):543–548

Spica M M 1989 Sexual counseling standards for the spinal cord injured. Journal of Neuroscience Nursing 21(1):56–60

Szasz G 1992 Sexual health care. In: Zedjlik C P (ed) Management of spinal cord injury. Jones & Bartlett, Boston, ch 10, pp 175–201

Teal J C, Athelston G T 1975 Sexuality and spinal cord injury: some psychosocial considerations. Archives of Medical and Physical Rehabilitation 56:264–268

Tepper M 1992 Sexual education in spinal cord injury rehabilitation: current trends and recommendations. Sexuality and Disability 10(1):15–31

Weinburg J S 1982 Human sexuality and spinal cord injury. Nursing Clinics of North America 17:407–419

Woods N F 1987 Toward a holistic perspective of human sexuality: alterations in sexual health and nursing diagnosis. Holistic Nursing Practice 1(4):1–11

World Health Organization 1975 Education and treatment in human sexuality. The training of health professionals. WHO, Geneva, technical report series No. 572

The rehabilitation nurse as technical expert and provider of care

5

The technical skills and caring role of rehabilitation nurses

Part A

Jo Seymour   Mike Smith

INTRODUCTION

As outlined in Chapter 2, one of the key roles of the nurse in the rehabilitation of an adult is that of technical expert and provider of care. This
role incorporates the skills required by the nurse to perform or assist
in the physical care of another person. The techniques may range from
what is considered basic care, such as mouth care, to the perceived more
'technological' skills using the latest in electronic monitoring equipment.
Although it is somewhat false to separate the physical aspects and skills
of rehabilitation from the psychosocial issues which are undoubtedly
interlinked in all of what nursing provides, these have been covered in
depth in Chapter 4. Therefore this chapter focuses on the technical skills
that nurses require in order to provide care initially and then transfer care
and responsibility to the patient and his carers in relation to particular
functional areas of living.

The skills required by rehabilitation nurses can be classified into two
distinct categories:

- those activities and interventions that are prescribed and performed
  by nurses
- those activities and interventions that are prescribed by other
  rehabilitation professionals. In order to provide continuity and to
  monitor the results of these activities and interventions over the
  24-hour period, these activities are also undertaken by nurses.

Rehabilitation nursing creates many challenges, not only for the individual nurse, but also the nursing team as a whole. The nurse who is working
in rehabilitation needs to have many abilities. This requires learning new
skills in order to be able to undertake not only the prescribed interventions
of nursing but also those interventions prescribed by other team members.
This is particularly the case when the client group consists of those with
multiple or complex disabilities, which often require extending of traditional nursing roles. Fundamental to the success of this type of nursing is
the ability to work effectively with the many agencies and other disciplines

which may be involved in rehabilitation provision. Therefore, the ability to deal confidently and competently with internal and external staff, at all levels, from all disciplines, both on a one-to-one and a one-to-many basis is of paramount importance to the rehabilitation nurse.

Interventions prescribed and performed by nurses fit into the nursing process format. However, interventions prescribed by others, and performed by nurses, lend themselves to a slight variation from the standard stages (Box 5.1).

The interventions which may be nurse led include:

- meeting nutritional requirements
- meeting hygiene requirements
- promotion of continence
- control of pain
- promotion of adequate sleep and rest
- promoting health
- promotion of skin integrity
- monitoring physiological function to determine potential health problems.

Nursing interventions led by other disciplines include:

- promoting mobility

■ BOX 5.1 Types of nursing intervention where the nurse is a technical expert

Nurse-led interventions
- Assess individual-need deficits
- Prescribe nursing interventions in the form of a plan of care within a rehabilitation interdisciplinary context
- Be able to provide the relevant technical expertise required to carry out nurse-led interventions
- Evaluate the success or otherwise of such interventions and devise new or adapted plans of care, reporting such evaluation to other team members

Nursing interventions led by other professionals
- Have an understanding of the assessment process and results of other disciplines
- Identify need for the nursing aspect of meeting need deficits prescribed by other disciplines; included in this is the identification and undertaking of required training
- Be able to provide the relevant technical expertise required to carry out nursing interventions led by other team members
- Provide information to others, enabling the effective evaluation of interventions prescribed by other disciplines, allowing them to ascertain if adjustments to such interventions are required

- promoting communication
- promoting physiological function through the administration of medication
- use of aids to assist in the achievement of daily living skills.

It is these interventions which will form the basis of discussion in this chapter. Some topics are covered to some degree in other chapters in this book, and therefore are referred to only briefly here, whereas other areas are discussed in more detail, focusing on the practical implementation of nursing assessment and intervention.

Assessment in each area will be covered, as it is essential:

- as a tool to aid accurate diagnosis
- in order to plan treatment and care through the use of client-centred goals
- as a baseline from which to monitor progress
- as a point of reference for other team members.

Evaluation of rehabilitation nursing is discussed in detail Chapter 7 and is an obvious common thread throughout all areas.

In addition, it is worth reinforcing that common to all the issues covered in this chapter are the general rehabilitation concepts described in Chapter 1. The recognition of a person's right to make his own decisions about treatment and care is central to any rehabilitation programme, the aim being to enable maximum function (physically, psychologically and socially) of the individual in order that they may return to their community and lead an active and productive life.

MEETING NUTRITIONAL REQUIREMENTS

Food is not only a basic necessity, but is often a source of enjoyment for us. Many of us spend time thinking about what we are going to eat, buying the food, preparing the food and cooking the food before finally enjoying our meal. We all have our likes and dislikes, and many of us will crave a particular food from time to time.

Following injury or illness, nutrition becomes of even greater importance. Complications associated with inadequate nutritional intake include weight loss, skin breakdown, increased risk of infection, poor wound healing, dehydration and, ultimately, malnutrition, which may lead to death (Tierney 1996).

The intervention of a nurse who is both able to assess for, and is knowledgeable regarding methods through which to meet, nutritional requirements could prevent the potential complications associated with poor nutritional intake (Robshaw & Marbrow 1995). Despite this fact, nutritional aspects of care often seem to be underprovided for, as many individuals in our care are still reported to be undernourished.

Assessment of the patient is essential in order to establish current and previous eating patterns and to identify specific deficits in that individual. A comprehensive nutritional assessment should include:

- Dietary history.

- Physical assessment, including factors such as the presence of:
  - obesity
  - emaciation
  - body weight
  - poor condition of skin, gums, teeth and lips.
- Current ability of the patient to:
  - obtain food, including the mobility required to buy food
  - prepare food or be able to open containers, and to cook or cut food into manageable size
  - bring food to the mouth, including the dexterity needed when reaching for food and the use of any utensils in order to eat.
- Potential difficulties in eating the food, including the ability to chew and swallow (e.g. injuries, disease or neurological impairment affecting the mouth, throat and gastrointestinal tract).
- Particular dietary likes and dislikes.
- Specific religious or cultural dietary issues.

During the acute phase of any injury or illness, or in some cases on a long-term basis, it may not be possible for the person to eat or drink (Woodward 1996). This may be due to the patient's consciousness status, general ill-health (e.g. severe fatigue, or limitations of hand/arm function) or the patient may be physically unable to swallow. If any of these situations are present, nutritional support will have to be provided by some other means. Options that are available to provide nutritional support in such situations include total parenteral nutrition and enteral feeding, which can be via a nasogastric tube or a percutaneous endoscopic gastrostomy (PEG) tube. Clearly there is no one solution to every problem. Any method of alternative feeding has benefits as well as potential problems (Fawcett 1995).

TOTAL PARENTERAL NUTRITION

Total parenteral nutrition (TPN) involves giving a solution of sterile nutrients, often via a central vein. TPN may be used during the early stages of treatment (Cohen 1996), and in some instances patients may require long-term parenteral nutrition (Holden et al 1996). These people and their families are taught how to manage their treatment at home. Not surprisingly, a key role of the nurse in this situation is that of educator, and appropriate programmes and times must be in place to allow this to happen.

ENTERAL NUTRITION

Nasogastric tubes are commonly used in the first instance, provided that the patient has a functioning gastrointestinal tract. They provide a direct route to the stomach and are relatively easy to pass. However, they are not without their problems (Anderson 1995, Kennedy 1997). The most serious potential problem is that of aspiration. It is necessary to check that the tube is in the stomach before each feed; this is often done by testing the aspirate using litmus paper for acidity, which indicates that the tube is in the stomach. The tube can become dislodged and cause severe irritation and erosions in the nasopharyngeal area. If the patient is agitated or confused, he may pull the tube out. This may result in the frequent repositioning of the tube in order to maintain nutritional status and this may further distress the patient. If the tube is being used to give a continuous feed and it dislodges, it is possible that the feed may go into the lungs, and could cause death by drowning. Nasogastric tubes are unsightly and, if longer term feeding is required, alternatives may need to be considered.

A gastrostomy is another direct method of providing enteral nutrition (Liddle 1995). The tube is situated on the abdomen and is inserted directly into the stomach. The tube is unobtrusive and, therefore, more socially acceptable. Feeds can be given in bolus form or administered slowly over a longer period of time. Once the tube is inserted, gastrostomy feeding may continue for several months or even years if the person requires it (Arrowsmith 1996). The gastrostomy tube has fewer associated problems, and may be becoming the preferred method for providing nutritional support on a long-term basis (Holmes 1996). Many patients are able to manage their own feeding with a gastrostomy tube and this should be encouraged where possible. Feeding overnight frees up long periods of time during the day for therapies to take place, or for social activities. If a patient is tube fed, the social and pleasurable aspects of eating are lost. These drawbacks should not be underestimated. The thought of food, the smell of food cooking and the presentation of food are all part of the culture of eating. The nurse may want to improvise in order to maintain certain social aspects of eating. A few drops of a patient's favourite food may be placed on the patient's tongue or lips as a pleasurable experience and to add to the normality of mealtimes.

ASSISTING THE PERSON ABLE TO TAKE FOOD ORALLY

When considering nutrition with the patient, the nurse may have to be quite creative. During the transition from tube to oral feeding both methods may be employed. Oral feeding may also need to be staged. Food may need to be pureed at first, then minced, and then cut into small pieces. The patient may not progress past one of the stages. Food is difficult to make presentable and loses taste when it is pureed, and therefore additional seasoning may be required for some people. It may be necessary to completely change the feeding regime during the transitionary phase. It should also be remembered that a person may be able to manage food but may still have difficulties with fluids. It may be necessary to thicken fluids using one of the many commercially available products. Fluids can be thickened to various consistencies, using honey, yoghurt and thickening agents.

We all know of situations where patients have received their food and then, when they have not been able to eat it, the food has been removed with no thought of the consequences for the patient. In order to promote adequate oral intake meals should be:

- served at the correct temperature

- what the person has chosen
- within the reach of the person.

If the patient is unable to do any of these, the nurse has a professional responsibility to ensure that he is fed appropriately. This may involve simply cutting up the food or actually feeding the patient.

Positioning of the food or of the person himself to facilitate eating and drinking may be important for some individuals. Issues such as ensuring that the food can be reached, that the patient has appropriate seating and posture (e.g. in an upright position), and that there is sufficient space for the patient to move his arms in order to hold the appropriate cutlery may make the difference between some degree of independence and total dependence on the nurse or carer. The nurse must consider the patient's vision in those with visual impairment, either placing the food where the person can see it or giving a clear explanation of where it is located. Feeding aids are often required to overcome any deficits in physical abilities, optimising independence, often in consultation and liaison with an occupational therapist. It is worth bearing in mind that some equipment, such as feeder beakers, may not be acceptable to an adult.

Finally, in those with identified problems with eating, monitoring is essential, not only to determine the extent of the problem but also to determine progress (Davison & Stable 1996).

MEETING HYGIENE REQUIREMENTS

Most of us take for granted our choices and abilities when it comes to meeting hygiene requirements and desires. If a person is less able than in his normal state, on either a temporary or a permanent basis, the current hospital routines may result in him losing the element of control over his personal hygiene. The often regimented manner in which we assist in the meeting of such needs may not cause the patient undue distress, but can increase dependency on nurses, which can be avoided (Spiller 1992). Clearly, the traditional approach, that the patient must be clean and ready at a time that suits a doctor's ward round or therapist's diary, is not conducive to the rehabilitation of the patient. In addition, the time pressures that such an approach may create may devalue and minimise the opportunities for rehabilitative interventions by nurses. However, it is unfair to place the blame, and the onus to recognise and change such practice, solely on our healthcare colleagues, for we are in many respects our own worst enemies as we often continue to let this happen. Nurses spend a large amount of time performing intimate personal tasks for patients. These tasks include washing, hair care, menstrual care and oral hygiene, to name but a few. The value of the time that a nurse spends on these tasks should not be underestimated.

The nurse in a rehabilitation setting should allow and assist the patient to maintain his previous level of hygiene. When we have just washed and dressed, we feel good and our self-esteem is high. We should be facilitating that good feeling in our patients (Jones 1994).

As part of rehabilitation the nurse should recognise the benefit of encouraging the client's partner to help with bathing, and use any or a combination of the following:

- music
- massage
- hair washing
- head massage
- candles
- wine.

This opportunity may also have the value of being:

- allocated private time
- romantic
- fun
- normal.

Although bathing might be seen as a monotonous task, it seems clear that such time can be therapeutic.

Oral hygiene plays an important part in our own daily routines. It is important for the patient's comfort, well-being and self-esteem, as well as in preventing infection (Holmes 1996). The consequences of poor oral hygiene include tooth decay, infection, halitosis and loss of ability to eat, due to mouth pain and discomfort, which may in turn lead to dehydration and malnutrition. Certain drugs and treatments may affect the condition of the mouth. These include some antibiotics, phenytoin and oxygen therapy. The use of a small, soft-headed, adapted toothbrush and toothpaste of the patient's choice can make what may be a difficult task easier. As with other aspects of hygiene, this may be something that a relative may wish to carry out, and this should be encouraged if desired by the client.

Menstrual care has to be one of the most intimate tasks we ever perform for a patient. The woman should be facilitated to perform as much of the task as she can. The nurse must remain sensitive to the patient's needs at all times. It is not acceptable to use inappropriate aids for menstruation management (i.e. an incontinence pad is not designed for this purpose). The use of mirrors, adapted underwear and adapted positions may all be required, and it may be necessary for the nurse to use all her skills to facilitate independence for the woman.

Shaving is an important aspect of many men's hygiene. Electric shavers may help facilitate independence and prevent accidents in the early stages of rehabilitation. Women may shave their legs and underarms, and this practice should not be overlooked.

The use of deodorants and make-up should be continued if they were part of the patient's previous daily routine.

PROMOTION OF CONTINENCE

Disturbances in patient continence are commonplace in rehabilitation units for many reasons. Depending on the circumstances, individuals may suffer from incontinence of urine, faeces or both. Continence is a skill that we have all learned as small children, and after illness or injury it may have to be re-learned or regained, often through the use of assistive devices. For an adult, to be incontinent may be acutely embarrassing, and therefore a psychologically difficult aspect of an individual's change in health status to deal with. Incontinence is thus far from limited to physical discomfort, and may have major psychological and social effects. As nurses we are expected from our first encounter with patients to deal with incontinence, and many authors have stressed this as clearly within the remit of nursing (Johnson 1995). Nurses have always cleaned people up, and changed clothing and/or bedding from wet or dirty to dry and clean. In the past, the solutions to incontinence were through exclusive use of pads and urethral in-dwelling catheters, but the management of continence has changed beyond recognition over the last few years (Pottle 1992). Incontinence is often neither inevitable nor irreversible. Although the use of a catheter of some sort may be the eventual solution, surely one has a responsibility to look at all possible options. There are now many options available for promoting continence which should make the use of an in-dwelling catheter one of the last options to be considered. However, experience tells us that currently this is often not the case, due to nurses' lack of the knowledge, skills or attitudes required to overcome the situation creatively and effectively.

Examples of some common medical diagnoses and interventions that may threaten continence are given in Box 5.2. It is worth stressing that it is not the medical diagnosis that should be the focus of any nursing assessment, but rather the combination of consequences. Physical, psychological, environmental and social factors may influence continence or the lack of it for many individuals (McGrother et al 1990). Consequently, in order for the nurse to assist the incontinent person, she must recognise the knowledge, skills and physical requirements necessary to achieve continence, and through a comprehensive assessment of all of these issues

---

■ **BOX 5.2 Examples of common conditions that result in incontinence**

- Cardiovascular accident
- Spinal injury
- Conditions resulting in reduced mobility (e.g. back pain, osteoarthritis)
- Trauma to urinary system
- Dementia
- Epilepsy
- Enlarged prostate
- Medical interventions such as drug therapy (e.g. diuretics, anticholinergics, antidepressants, hypnotics)
- Medical procedures (e.g. bladder-neck surgery, hysterectomy)
- Obstetric history (e.g. number of pregnancies)

formulate plans that may make the goal of continence a reality (Abbott 1992, Woodward 1993).

To be continent the individual must be able to do the following:

- recognise the need to pass urine or faeces
- identify and get to an appropriate place to pass urine or faeces
- possess the control to 'hold on' until they reach the appropriate place
- remove clothing in order to pass urine or faeces, and pull up clothing afterwards
- pass urine or faeces when they get to the appropriate place
- clean or dry themselves.

If a person is unable to do all or some of these, incontinence may be the result. It is these aspects which should therefore form the basis of a nursing assessment relating to continence, enabling an effective plan to be developed to promote continence. It is worth stressing the need for sensitivity at all times, both when undertaking the assessment, and when discussing with the person methods through which continence may be achieved.

RECOGNISING THE NEED TO PASS URINE OR FAECES

Broadly speaking, problems with recognising the need to pass urine are either of physiological origin or of psychological origin (Addison 1996, Norton 1996). In those individuals without the necessary 'awareness' due to a problem of physiological origin, the disturbance is invariably related to loss of neurological function (e.g. in spinal cord lesions). Anecdotally, there are some patients who have incomplete damage to neural pathways who may have, or may develop, a 'vague' awareness, which can be used as the basis for a regime to empty the bladder or to know when assistance with bowels is required. More commonly, however, in those who are cognitively intact, awareness of the need for elimination is facilitated through teaching the individual to monitor both intake and output and devise strategies accordingly. For example, recognising that a residual bladder volume of under 500 ml is desirable, the individual is encouraged to monitor his daily intake and use some method to maintain volumes below that level (e.g. a 2 litre intake requires bladder emptying four times daily). In addition, there will be differences in bladder function depending on the level of cord damage, particularly relating to the presence (in upper motor neuron injuries, i.e. to the brain and spinal cord) or absence (in lower motor neuron injuries, i.e. to the spinal nerves that form the cauda equina) of a bladder reflex. It is not within the remit of this text to go into great detail about such factors, as others have covered this extensively. However, it is worth pointing out that involuntary voiding in such an individual is likely to suggest that a reflex is intact, whereas a bladder that keeps filling is not only dangerous, but indicates the absence of a reflex.

Problems of a psychological origin are commonplace in those with major cognitive difficulties (e.g. following traumatic brain injury or dementia). Although some degree of success may be gained with some patients by using a set routine, more often there is a need to rely on others. It may be that an individual is unable to recognise directly that a need is there but it may be apparent from other behaviours that something is wrong (e.g. increased agitation). Little formal work seems to have been undertaken in this area, but it may be possible to interpret such signs, if they are formally recorded. Clearly this reliance on others necessitates training in whatever method is chosen for whoever is going to be the carer when the patient returns to the community.

IDENTIFYING AND GETTING TO AN APPROPRIATE PLACE TO PASS URINE OR FAECES

Identifying an appropriate place to pass urine or faeces depends on the patient's cognitive ability being intact. In addition, those with visual impairments, obviously commonplace in the elderly due to the ageing process, may have difficulty in identifying directions and signs that indicate the location of a toilet. In the home this may not be so much of a problem, as it may be easier to educate the individual regarding the layout of rooms than in a hospital ward situation. However, there are obvious means through which locating a toilet can be facilitated. The use of larger signs to indicate the location of toilets, providing a physical orientation to a ward area, situating that person near a toilet, or quite simply physically escorting the person will all assist such individuals.

The major problem, however, is for those who have reduced mobility. The degree of mobility will merit different approaches, and consequently should form a significant part of any assessment regarding elimination. Again, bed planning relating to the location of toilet facilities may encourage independence, at least while the patient is regaining a degree of mobility. The second element within this relates to the ability to use toileting facilities unaided. Some of the common factors to take into consideration are listed in Box 5.3.

POSSESSING THE CONTROL TO 'HOLD ON' UNTIL THE APPROPRIATE PLACE IS REACHED

Problems related to control are clearly linked to the issues raised above. The urgency with which someone needs to eliminate is specific to that individual and their particular change in health status. Issues in this area

---

■ **BOX 5.3 Factors to be considered regarding toilet facilities**

- Accessibility to patient (e.g. doorway width, wheelchair access, space)
- Physical support required (e.g. assistance from nurse, hand rails)
- Height of toilet seat (e.g. a raised seat may be required)
- Commode (available on demand, privacy)
- Urinal (e.g. available at bedside, needs to be emptied)

■ **BOX 5.4 Assessment of control of voiding**

- Micturition pattern (frequency and volume)
- Maximum and minimum voiding volumes
- Leaking when coughing
- Leaking when going upstairs or downhill
- Leaking when getting up from a chair or bed
- Fluid intake volume
- Length of time for which the person is able to hold-on after urge
- Symptoms of dribble/overflow (e.g. knowledge of leaking, wet all the time)
- Hesitancy or straining when passing urine
- Leaking immediately after thinking voiding is finished

---

may include capacity, presence of reflex, whether the voluntary control to inhibit micturition is intact, volume of fluid intake, gender and pelvic floor muscle strength. An assessment of all these factors will indicate possible remedies (Chance 1994, Addison 1996). Urodynamic studies, which indicate bladder function and capacity, may provide some information, but there are other aspects of monitoring that may aid identification of the related issues. Suggestions for assessment are given in Box 5.4.

Following assessment of the above, liaison with medical staff may be required regarding intervention. Possible solutions using drug therapy or surgery can be explored as part of the plan to promote continence. Other aspects are obtaining information regarding any pattern and developing strategies around the identified bladder function, involving consideration of the location of toilet facilities, the use of other methods of bladder emptying, or the use of external catheters (e.g. conveen) or leg bags between visits to the toilet. It is also essential to bear in mind the possibility of infection, the presence of which may increase the likelihood of bladder urgency. Routine urinary specimens could be taken to identify this. However, the use of antibiotics should be minimised in those who use catheters on a long-term basis, generally treating symptomatic infections only rather than bacteriuria. The rationale behind this is that such individuals may suffer urinary tract infection on a regular basis, and to treat every bacteriuria may increase the likelihood of resistant strains developing. The responsibility of the nurse as advocate may minimise the effect of overprescription of antibiotics by medical colleagues.

REMOVING CLOTHING IN ORDER TO PASS URINE OR FAECES AND PULLING UP CLOTHING AFTERWARDS

Fundamental to the ability to adjust clothing before and after elimination is the degree of manual dexterity which the patient possesses. Deficits in manual dexterity may be neurological (e.g. cardiovascular accident) or musculoskeletal (e.g. osteoarthritis) in origin. The degree of lower limb mobility and balance are also integral elements in the ability to perform this task. Solutions to problems in this area are often developed in liaison with the occupational therapist who can facilitate upper and lower limb dressing. In addition, advice regarding the type of clothing, particularly the use of fastenings (e.g. buttons, zips or Velcro) may be sufficient to regain independence. It is worth bearing in mind the aesthetics of any clothing alterations, as some individuals may feel, as most of us may do, that the acceptability of what we are wearing is important. Again the occupational therapist may prove to be a valuable resource in actioning the above.

ABILITY TO PASS URINE OR FAECES

Commonly attributable to physiological changes, an inability to pass urine or faeces on reaching a toilet may be due to interruption of neural pathways or may indicate the presence of a physical obstruction (e.g. detrusor–sphincter dysinergia (often occurring in the neurogenic bladder), bladder neck obstruction (occurring as a result of an enlarged prostate gland or carcinoma), or loss of muscle innervation to rectal muscles or a bowel reflex). In such cases, if surgical intervention is neither possible nor desirable, other forms or methods of management may be required. In problems relating to micturition, intermittent catheterisation or continual emptying through the use of a suprapubic or urethral in-dwelling catheter are obvious options (Haynes 1994, Pomfret 1996, Webb 1994). A brief outline of the advantages and disadvantages of both options is given in Box 5.5.

The aim of a bowel management programme is to restore a normal bowel pattern for the patient. If the patient is regaining independence a normal pattern may begin to return as the patient's eating patterns are restored and his mobility improves. This, however, is not always the case and interventions may be necessary. Faecal incontinence should be regarded as a curable and therefore preventable problem (Norton 1987). In those who have problems with bowel function the key factor is to re-establish a pattern through maintaining regularity, which suits the individual's lifestyle. Experience has shown that this regularity of routine is fundamental. Essential elements in gaining regularity are monitoring (daily or alternate daily) of bowel results to identify a pattern, and assisting or performing interventions at approximately the same time of day. Once a pattern has been established through the use of remaining muscle function, possible use of suppositories or abdominal massage to facilitate an intact reflex, and use of aperients, it is essential that this is adhered to. Straying from an established routine often results in bowel 'accidents'. The effects of diet and fluid intake should also be noted and form part of both the assessment and any plans formulated as a result.

CLEANING AND DRYING

Causes of and solutions to problems in this area are as for removing and pulling up clothing. Clearly cleaning and drying are essential to facilitate

■ BOX 5.5 Advantages and disadvantages of intermittent and in-dwelling catheters

Intermittent catheter

Advantages
- Low infection rate
- Mimics 'normal' bladder function, allowing filling and limiting chances of bladder atrophy
- No need for external collecting devices, impacts positively on body image
- Does not impinge on sexual activity

Disadvantages
- Fluid restriction
- In those with intact reflex requires suppression with anticholinergics (possible side-effects)
- May be difficult for women due to anatomical differences
- 'Hassle' factor high
- Necessitates intact hand function

In-dwelling catheter

Advantages
- No fluid restriction required
- No additional medication required
- Lower 'hassle' factor, just requires remembering to empty it (or instruct others to do so)

Disadvantages
- Requires external collection devices
- Bladder atrophy likely unless catheter is regularly 'clamped'
- Impinges on sexual activity (urethral catheters)
- Higher infection rate

comfort and to minimise the risk of complications (e.g. excoriation, infection and a feeling of being 'dirty').

PATIENT RESPONSES TO A CONTINENCE PROBLEM

As mentioned earlier in this chapter, any incontinence is likely to have a profound effect on the psychological well-being of the individual (Llewlyn 1992, Thomas 1987). There are many responses that an individual may exhibit (Box 5.6). Information about dealing with the general psychological

■ BOX 5.6 Potential patient responses to continence problems

- Apathy
- Denial
- Anger
- Frustration
- Positive outlook/coping well
- Distress
- Embarrassment

responses to illness and disability is given in Chapter 4, but it is worth reiterating the need to deal with each person individually and sensitively due to the intimate nature of such problems.

Incontinence not only affects the way people feel about themselves, but also from a social perspective, the way in which they lead their lives. Being incontinent may be a barrier to taking part in many activities. People worry about having an 'accident', where the next toilet is, how they will use the toilet on the bus, where they can change their pad, whether they smell and whether people will know.

To conclude, following the initial assessment it may be necessary to observe and record for several days the number of voids or bowel movements and the volume passed. From this period of observation it may be possible to identify a reason for the incontinence at the time when it occurs (e.g. the patient is unable to get to the toilet through lack of mobility or lack of assistance). It may then be possible to restore continence with minimal intervention and a programme of education. Following assessment it may be necessary to carry out further investigations. The nurse should not only ensure that interventions which will promote continence according to the desired lifestyle of that individual are delivered, but should also act as an advocate, ensuring that incontinence is not seen as inevitable by any member of the rehabilitation team. Incontinence is an issue that affects a large number of people using rehabilitation services, and nurses are in a powerful and optimum position to make a real impact.

CONTROL OF PAIN

The presence of pain in an individual is an entirely subjective and individual experience for the person concerned (Clancey & McVicar 1992). Although some pain may be easy to anticipate (e.g. after surgical intervention), the experience and degree of pain is impossible to predict. By the very nature of his 24 hour service, the nurse is not only in the prime position to assess the patient's pain, but also to evaluate the success or otherwise of any interventions designed to control it. There are various methods of pain assessment that can be used (Box 5.7).

It is worth bearing in mind that rehabilitation patients may not be able to articulate that they have pain (e.g. they may have cognitive or language difficulties). Again due to the unique intimate relationship that he has with patients, the nurse may be able to detect behavioural changes (East 1992) that may be a response to pain (Box 5.8).

It is often non-verbal cues that indicate that the patient is in pain. The subjective nature of pain necessitates a supportive rather than a 'critical'

■ **BOX 5.7 Some pain assessment tools**

- Visual analogue scales
- Pain diaries or graphs (Baille 1993)
- McGill pain questionnaire (Melzack 1975)

■ **BOX 5.8 Some behavioural responses to pain**

- Agitation
- Anger
- Poor performance of daily living activities
- Distress
- Withdrawal

---

response by the nurse. Pain should not be ignored or underestimated, and patients should not be labelled or stereotyped according to the pain that a nurse may associate with a particular procedure. The issues surrounding nursing the patient with chronic pain are described in depth in Chapter 4, Part B, and readers are encouraged to turn there for more detailed information. It is worth emphasising that reliance on analgesia as the sole tool of pain management may prove disappointing, and often a combination of methods may produce a more desirable result for the patient (Closs 1994, Walker et al 1990). Possible methods include relaxation, positional change, transcutaneous electrical stimulation (TENS), and heat and cold treatment. On occasion total pain relief is not a realistic goal. In such situations the emphasis should be on minimising the effect of pain on the life of that individual, rather than on the pain itself (Snelling 1994). The nurse is the key player, not only due to his expertise in assessment and interventions relating to controlling pain, but also in effectively communicating with other disciplines as appropriate (e.g. medical staff for medication, and physiotherapy for setting up a TENS machine). It is therefore the responsibility of any nursing team to create effective protocols, strategies and channels to facilitate prompt referral and action with reference to pain control (Cornwell 1994). Readers are encouraged to look at their own clinical areas and critically examine whether these are in place.

PROMOTION OF ADEQUATE SLEEP AND REST

Adults spend approximately one-third of their lives sleeping. The importance of sleep may often not be recognised by some healthcare professionals. Sleep is a natural state, during which the body and brain rest after the activities of the day, and energy levels are restored for the following day (Duxbury 1994). The quality and quantity of sleep can be influenced by various factors (Southwell & Wistow 1995, Willis 1989). The factors resulting in poor sleep can be internal or external to the individual (Box 5.9).

Most of us expect to sleep through the night and feel the effects in the morning if we do not; we are aware of and could describe how we feel if we do not get enough sleep. The effects of sleep deprivation are many, and include daytime sleepiness, frequent yawning, listlessness, lethargy and irritability, confusion and, occasionally, poor short-term memory. Obviously the degree of these symptoms depends not only on the individual, but also on the extent to which sleep has been affected (Hodgson 1991).

■ BOX 5.9 Some factors associated with poor sleep

Internal factors	External factors
• Pain	• Unfamiliar environment
• Anxiety	• Noise from nurses working
• Boredom	• Noise from other patients
• Illness	• Ward/rehabilitation routines
• Confusion	• Overestimation of physical capabilities of patient

As rehabilitation nurses we need to remember that a lack of sleep will affect the person we are working with and how they function through the day.

Once again the fundamental first stage is assessment. It is the 24-hour nature of nurses' unique working pattern that places them in the ideal position to undertake this initial assessment, to determine if a problem exists and to intervene accordingly. Clearly it may be overzealous to undertake a formal sleep assessment on every individual undergoing rehabilitation. However, basic information should be gained, during the admission assessment, of a person's night-time habits and sleep patterns, such as:

- pre-sleep routines
- how often they wake and why
- what time they go to bed
- what time they wake up
- what time they get up.

If a problem is detected through discussion with the patient or as a result of observing some of the behaviours related to lack of sleep described above, a more formal assessment of sleep may be beneficial. Overall, the remit of formal sleep assessment involves comparing the patient's usual pattern of sleep with the current sleeping pattern.

Probably the most effective and practical way in which to monitor the sleep of a patient is through the use of a diary. This should include a note of:

- time of going to bed
- time of going to sleep
- any intervention (e.g. medication taken to enhance sleep)
- times of waking during night
- causes of waking
- qualitative statement of how the individual feels in the morning
- particular problems (e.g. irritability, poor performance) and the on-going effect of these
- the amount and times of sleep during the day.

Clearly this must be a joint venture between the patient and nurse. Such a record can be used to evaluate the effect of any future interventions to improve the quality or quantity of sleep.

It is often through focusing on the reasons for waking or difficulty in getting to sleep that successful interventions are planned. Many solutions to the causes of poor sleep have already been covered in this chapter and elsewhere in this book; Table 5.1 gives a summary of these. It is worth noting that there may be a combination of factors contributing to poor sleep, and so a combination of approaches may be required.

It is also worth bearing in mind that a patient's functional ability may change at night. Dim lights, resting splints and general sleepiness may all affect how the patient functions, and consequently compromise patient safety. Finally, it is worth emphasising that the contribution of the nurse at night is invaluable to rehabilitation. To perform aspects of the nursing role

Table 5.1

Cause	Solution
Pain	Appropriate pain relief methods. Repositioning. Relaxation
Anxiety	Determine cause, dispelling any myths or misunderstandings. Relaxation
Boredom	Reduce daytime napping. Increase physical activity. Increase stimulation
Illness	Treat symptoms (e.g. reduce temperature, maintain comfort)
Confusion	Determine type and cause of confusional state (i.e. acute or chronic) and treat if possible (e.g. ensure adequate hydration)
Unfamiliar environment	Regular explanation of surroundings, familiar items on bedside table from home
Noise from nurses working	Consider changes in working methods (e.g. ensure bed-pan washer does not run at night, soundproofing)
Noise from other patients	Explain effects of noise to particular offending patient. Potential isolation of noisy patient at night. Optimum solution to manage poor sleep in noisy patients. Patients who require toileting through the night should be situated near the toilet facilities and should be assisted with minimum fuss and maximum discretion
Ward/rehabilitation routines	Consider possible changes in routine which may create environment more conducive to sleep
Overestimation of physical capabilities of patient, resulting in excessive tiredness	Consider re-scheduling physical rehabilitation activities in liaison with therapy colleagues. Consider repeat health check liaison with medical staff

at night requires the same skills used during the day, ensuring continuity and consistency of care for the client, ultimately influencing outcomes. In addition, to facilitate sleep through all possible means can only further enhance the success of the rehabilitation experience.

PROMOTING HEALTH

The essential component in the promotion of health is client education. This is covered extensively in Chapter 3 and the reader is therefore encouraged to refer to the information covered there. However, it is worth emphasising that it is essential to have the relevant technical expertise in the particular area of health in order to fulfil the role of educator effectively.

PROMOTION OF SKIN INTEGRITY

The skin is the largest organ in the body, the average adult's skin covering an area of almost 2 m². Skin accounts for 15% of body weight and receives one-third of the body's circulating blood volume. The functions of the skin are many, including:

- protection against cold and heat, bacteria and other organisms and dehydration
- it contains receptors that allow the sensations of pain, temperature, touch and pressure
- synthesis of vitamin D and melanin.

Many factors can lead to changes in the condition of the skin. Consequently, maintaining skin integrity and the prevention of pressure sores is a major challenge and consideration in rehabilitation nursing. Factors that alter the skin's function include age, exposure to the sun, nutritional status, hydration, medication and irritants such as soap. Skin may be damaged by mechanical forces such as prolonged pressure, shearing, tearing and friction. Chemical damage may occur as a result of exposure to urine or faeces, soaps and other cleansing agents. Moisture can cause maceration to the skin. Heat damage, from touching things which are too hot or too cold, and lack of blood supply to the area can also cause severe damage to the skin. Failure to maintain skin integrity:

- Can extend the length of hospital stay and, therefore, have major financial implications. Waterlow (1985) estimated that 95% of all pressure sores could be prevented and that the cost of prevention and treatment is £60 million per year.
- Interferes with the rehabilitation process and can potentially influence long-term rehabilitation outcomes.
- Can, in some instances, be life-threatening, particularly in those pressure sores which are large.

Assessment of a patient's skin is therefore of paramount importance and should incorporate the possible presence of any of the risk factors listed in Box 5.10.

■ **BOX 5.10 Risk factors for pressure damage**

- Incontinence of both urine and faeces (moisture increases skin maceration and increases the effects of shear)
- Immobility
- Mechanical factors (friction and shear)
- Malnutrition
- Presence of fracture
- Increasing age
- General health (all acutely ill patients are vulnerable due to the combination of other risk factors)

There are many pressure sore risk-assessment scales available (e.g. the Norton scale (1987), the Waterlow pressure score (1985) and the Braden scale (1989)). A good risk-assessment tool should be simple to use and demonstrate good predictive value (US Department of Health and Human Services 1992). Various studies examining the reliability and validity of the different pressure sore risk-assessment scales have been inconclusive as to their value in different settings, making the choice of scale difficult. However, there are five things to consider when choosing a pressure sore risk-assessment scale.

- Does it take into consideration the specific needs of your patients?
- Has the validity and reliability been established in your care setting?
- Is it understandable?
- Is it easy to use?
- Will it be used to allocate pressure-relieving resources?

The patient's risk status should be re-evaluated on a regular basis, depending on the patient's individual changing circumstances.

In order to reduce the incidence of pressure sores it is necessary not only to use an appropriate risk-assessment scale but also to implement relevant preventive and treatment strategies as a result of that assessment. The use of protocols relating particular risk-assessment scores to the use of different pressure-relieving devices may well be beneficial. Fundamental to determining the success or otherwise of interventions, including the use of pressure-relieving devices, is the regular inspection of skin condition, with particular attention being paid to bony prominences. The frequency of inspection will depend on the individual circumstances of the patient. However, intervention should not be restricted to the use of pressure-relieving aids. The risk factors identified above should form the basis of a planned series of interventions. For example, it should be ensured that patients who are identified as being at risk of developing pressure sores receive adequate nutrition, with referral to a dietitian if necessary. The importance of repositioning patients as a preventive measure can not be overemphasised.

In those patients who have existing sores the next issue facing the rehabilitation nurse is to choose one of the many wound classification tools that are available (e.g. Lowthian 1987). When using any wound classification tool it is important to ensure that:

- all team members are using the same tool
- everyone, including the patient, understands exactly how to use it
- everyone is aware how to interpret the results
- results are accurately documented
- progress of wound healing is appropriately documented and acted upon.

The other major aspect of rehabilitation related to maintaining skin integrity is that of client education. Programmes that cover the basics of skin physiology, skin checking, the use of pressure-relieving aids and strategies to minimise pressure sore development should be incorporated. In those without the capacity to take on such knowledge and practical skills, the education of carers is clearly vital.

This section is designed to be an introduction to the subject of skin integrity, and the reader is encouraged to undertake further reading. However, there are four clear, practically orientated questions that readers should consider in relation to their clinical area.

- Is there a formal pressure sore risk-assessment tool that is usable by all and is used on all at-risk patients?
- Are there protocols for managing identified risk, including when to use various pressure-relieving devices?
- Is there a formal education programme for patients and carers relating to the maintenance of skin integrity?
- Is there a wound classification tool that can be used not only to guide treatment but also as the basis for audit relating to the incidence and severity of pressure sores, thereby demonstrating the success of rehabilitation nursing in maintaining skin integrity?

MONITORING PHYSIOLOGICAL FUNCTION TO DETERMINE POTENTIAL HEALTH PROBLEMS

There are many situations within rehabilitation that require monitoring of the patient for any potential health problems. Although medical staff perform assessments, nurses have a clear responsibility to inform medical staff of any health situation that may be detrimental to the patient. Some of the more obvious examples include:

- monitoring of cardiovascular, respiratory and neurological function
- monitoring of blood sugar levels
- collection of samples of body fluids for investigations
- response to medication
- monitoring neurovascular status (e.g. colour, warmth and sensation) in the patient with a plaster cast.

Readers will be able to think of many other examples from their own clinical area, which will clearly vary depending on the speciality and particular client group at any one time. Although it may seem rather obvious, there is no doubt of the vital nature of such monitoring, not only in the prevention of potential complications, which may delay or even prevent optimum rehabilitation outcome, but also in promoting patient health, through educating patients in the need to monitor some aspects of their physical status.

PROMOTING MOBILITY

Although some authors have made mobility a central concept in nursing within orthopaedics (Davis 1994), there is no doubt that nurses often play a supportive role to a therapist rather than prescribing interventions in all areas of rehabilitation. Clearly there is a vital role to play in minimising the risks associated with reduced mobility, as in pressure sore prevention, and monitoring deep vein thrombosis and the psychological aspects of reduced mobility.

However many nurses will spend a significant proportion of their time assisting or supervising the mobilisation of people undergoing a rehabilitation programme. Although programmes related to regaining or improving mobility and aids to mobility are usually prescribed by the physiotherapist, there are essential abilities that the nurse must have to undertake this supportive role. He must:

- possess a knowledge of the individual patient's capability and the prescribed programme
- possess a precise knowledge of any assistive devices used
- be able to communicate the evaluation of progress in the clinical area of prescribed programmes.

Without all of the above, we cannot expect to fully facilitate the mobility aspects of an individual's rehabilitation, and indeed we may not only compromise the progress and safety of the patient, but also, and equally importantly, our own safety may be compromised. Surely this implies that formal training should be available to all nurses in every clinical area involved in the mobilisation of patients, though I would severely doubt that this is actually the case.

PROMOTING COMMUNICATION

Communication is obviously a large topic and there is a clear role for the nurse in facilitating positive interaction (see Ch. 4). However, in patients with communication problems that are physiological in origin (e.g. head injury, cardiovascular accident and traumatic neck injury) the role of the speech and language therapist is vital as part of the rehabilitation programme. Again the nurse's role is predominantly supportive in such situations, reinforcing prescribed interventions and reporting back to the relevant therapist. This supportive role is undoubtedly essential as, without the continuity of approach over a 24-hour period that nursing provides, the potential for improvement will not be optimal. Again the need for the development of programmes that meet the educational requirements for nurses to undertake this role effectively is worthy of emphasis.

PROMOTING PHYSIOLOGICAL FUNCTION THROUGH THE ADMINISTRATION OF MEDICATION

The safe administration of drugs is integral to the nurse's role in most healthcare settings. The nurse should have an understanding of the concepts that apply when dispensing medication in order to meet legal requirements and to facilitate patient teaching. Medications are numerous and the nurse should be familiar with the specific drugs commonly used in their clinical area and have knowledge of their actions and side-effects. Component parts of this knowledge include absorption rates, therapeutic range of medication, how the drug is eliminated, whether the drug creates dependency and, if so, what the withdrawal symptoms are.

In many areas it is common practice to dispense medication during a drug round, where one or two nurses give out medication at fixed times to all the patients on the ward. Rehabilitation nurses should be challenging this practice. This traditional method of administering medication does not encourage independence; rather, it creates dependence on the nurse and removes control from the patient. If patients' drugs are dispensed individually there is greater opportunity to teach the patient and his family about the drugs being taken. If the patient or a family member understands what the medication is for, why a particular drug has been prescribed and what the possible side-effects are, then it should follow that the patient is more likely to take the medication when he is discharged. The concept of self-medication is a logical and essential step in a rehabilitation setting, and all patients who are assessed as able should be permitted to take their own medication.

Such a system should be staged and requires the creation of quality time with the patient, to educate them about their current medication and explain any changes that are made. This should eventually lead to patients taking their own medication independently.

Although very worthwhile, creating a self-medication programme is time-consuming. Points that need to be considered include:

- patient, carer and staff education (a self-medication information sheet or booklet may be useful)
- patients may need to give consent to taking part in such a programme (Fig. 5.1)
- local policies must conform to the standards of the United Kingdom Central Council of Nursing, Midwifery and Health Visiting (UKCC) and to drug acts
- procedures should be clear (Boxes 5.11–5.13)
- patient assessment must be carried out (Fig. 5.2).

My team nurse has completed an assessment form for self-medication	
I am willing to take part in the self-medication programme	
My team nurse has told me about self-medication and I understand what I have been told	
I understand that the programme is in three phases	
I will go at my own pace	
My team nurse will direct me	
In Phase 3, it is my responsibility to keep my drug cabinet locked	
I must keep the key with me at all times	
The key belongs to ward	
I must ask my team nurse about any problems with self-medication	

Patient's signature	
Patient's name (PRINTED IN CAPITALS)	
Witness' signature	
Witness' name (PRINTED IN CAPITALS)	
Date	

Figure 5.1 Patient consent form for a self-medication programme.

USE OF AIDS TO ASSIST IN THE ACHIEVEMENT OF DAILY LIVING SKILLS

In this chapter many references have been made to the use of resources and the professional expertise of other rehabilitation team members, in order to have prescribed and to obtain aids that may maximise the patient's functional ability in daily living skills. Obvious examples of aids include feeding straps, specially designed cutlery, mobility aids and communication devices. Whatever the area of function under consideration, it is important to recognise when referral is potentially beneficial, to know how to use the prescribed device, and to report back to the team regarding its use over the 24-hour period.

Patient's name ....   Date ....

Do you take medication	Yes [ ] No [ ]

If yes, what medication do you take? (including dosage, frequency and times)

....

....

Do not know [ ]

Do you know what you take this medication for?   Yes [ ]   No [ ]
What are the side-effects, if any, of this medication?

....

....

Would you like to self-medicate?   Yes [ ]   No [ ]
If no, why?

....

....

If you were self-medicating, how would you identify your medication?

Packaging	Yes [ ]	No [ ]
Label	Yes [ ]	No [ ]
Tablet shape	Yes [ ]	No [ ]
Tablet colour	Yes [ ]	No [ ]

Other (please specify) ....

....

Are you colour blind?   Yes [ ]   No [ ]

Would you have difficulties with the following?

Opening boxes	Yes [ ]	No [ ]
Opening child-proof tops	Yes [ ]	No [ ]
Opening screw tops	Yes [ ]	No [ ]
Opening blister packs	Yes [ ]	No [ ]
Using a dosette box	Yes [ ]	No [ ]
Reading labels	Yes [ ]	No [ ]
Opening the drug cabinet	Yes [ ]	No [ ]
Measuring doses of liquids		
using a spoon	Yes [ ]	No [ ]
using a medicine pot	Yes [ ]	No [ ]

To check the patient's abilities use the assessment box which is available on Langley Ward

Assessment completed by

....

Commence programme at (pease tick):

Phase One	[ ]
Phase Two	[ ]
Phase Three	[ ]

Figure 5.2 Patient self-medication assessment form.

> ■ **BOX 5.11 Procedure for a self-medication programme**
>
> 1. The patient's ability to self-medicate is discussed by the team at the key worker meetings.
> 2. The patient is given the information booklet.
> 3. The team nurse completes an assessment with the patient.
> 4. Before beginning the self-medication programme, the nurse discusses with the patient:
>   (a) their medication
>   (b) the reason for taking the medication
>   (c) dosage and times to take the medication
>   (d) any side-effects to watch out for and what to do about them
>   (e) the nurse records on the assessment form that (a) to (d) have been undertaken and that they are satisfied that the patient understands.
> 5. The patient signs the consent form.
> 6. The patient's own named supply of medication is ordered, stating the required dispenser, bottle top and label types. Legally, the patient can only self-administer named drugs.
> 7. Medication is kept locked in bedside drug cabinets.
> 8. The patient commences the programme and works through the three phases until safe (successfully meets the criteria to move from one phase to the next) and competent.
> 9. Progress is documented in the nursing care plan.
> 10. When the patient has his drug cabinet key he has already signed a consent form accepting responsibility to keep it safe.
> 11. On discharge, the key is handed back to the nursing staff and placed in the key cupboard.

SUMMARY

The principles of rehabilitation are transferable and the nurse as technical expert and provider of care is fundamental to the success of any rehabilitation programme. An overview of aspects of this role has been presented, although it is clear that different specialities will require additional information related to the specific client group. There are texts available on many of these; such supplementary reading is essential, and reading as extensively as possible about your speciality is to be encouraged.

Here an attempt to offer practical advice at a basic level on all the topics covered has been made. The chapter title itself emphasises just how much nurses do each day. Nurses have the skills required to positively influence all aspects of the rehabilitation process, either through nurse-led interventions or through implementing interventions prescribed by other members of the team. Nurses must value the skills they have and seek the education necessary to practise such skills effectively.

■ **BOX 5.12 The three phases of a self-medication programme**

Phase 1
- A self-medication assessment is completed by the team nurse with the patient, using the assessment form and assessment box. Following this the correct packaging can be ordered on the medication prescription sheet (e.g. no child-proof caps on bottles, or a dosette box).
- The patient completes the consent form with their team nurse. Teaching about their medication (e.g. what they take and why, what times they need to take it, and any side-effects to watch out for) will be given by the team nurse, who ensures that the patient understands the information. The information leaflet is handed out.
- The patient will ask his nurse for his medication within 1 hour of it being due. The team nurse will then administer that medication from the drug cabinet.

Phase 2
- The patient will receive his own supply of medication from the hospital pharmacy, labelled with instructions for his individual use. The drugs are kept in his own drug cabinet.
- The patient is responsible for asking his nurse at the correct time to unlock the drug cabinet. The patient selects and takes the correct medication, with supervision. This is recorded on the drug kardex.

Phase 3
- The patient is considered competent to take his medication unsupervised.
- The patient is given the key to his drug cabinet.
- The patient is responsible for:
  (a) taking his medication as prescribed
  (b) the safe-keeping of his medication
  (c) the safe-keeping of the drug cabinet key until discharge, when it is returned to the team nurse.
- The nurse will check, on each shift, that:
  (a) the patient has the key to his drug cabinet
  (b) the drug cabinet is locked, except when in use by the patient
  (c) there is sufficient medication.

■ **BOX 5.13 Procedure for individualised medication programme**

1. Hunters Moor Regional Rehabilitation Centre uses an individualised medication system.

2. Medication is kept locked in bedside drug cabinet.

3. All drug cabinets are locked, except when in use by the patient or nursing staff.

4. The drug cabinet has three master keys:
   (a) each team has a master key, which is handed on to the qualified nurse at each shift change
   (b) the third master key is kept in the general office.

5. The drug cabinets also have individual keys. There are two copies:
   (a) one copy is kept in a key cupboard located in the ward treatment room, and given to the patient at Phase 3 of the self-medication programme
   (b) the other copy is kept in the general office.

6. The key cupboard has three master keys:
   (a) each team has a master key, which is handed on to the qualified nurse at each shift change
   (b) the third master key is kept in the general office.

7. The key cupboard is locked, except when in use by nursing staff.

8. The patient's ability to self-medicate is discussed by the team at the key worker meetings.

See the procedure for the self-medication programme in Box 5.11.

REFERENCES

Abbott D 1992 Objective assessment ensures improved diagnosis. Professional Nurse 7(11):738–742
Addison R 1996 Faecal incontinence. Community Nurse 1(12):29
Alderman C 1989 Social stigma. Nursing Standard 3(16): 22–23
Anderson A 1995 Reducing bacterial contamination in enteral tube feeds. British Journal of Nursing 4(7):368–376
Arrowsmith H 1996 Nursing management of patients receiving gastrostomy feeding. British Journal of Nursing 5(5):268–273
Baille L 1993 A review of pain assessment tools. Nursing Standard 7(23):25–29
Braden B, Bergstrom N 1987 Clinical utility of the Braden scale for predicting pressure sore risk. Decubitus 2(3): 44–51
Chance R 1994 A problem we need not take for granted. Professional Nurse 9(7): 498–504
Clancey J, McVicar A 1992 Subjectivity of pain. British Journal of Nursing 1(1):8–10
Clos S J 1994 Pain in elderly patients: a neglected phenomenon. Journal of Advanced Nursing 19(6):1072–1081
Cohen A 1996 Delivery of total parenteral nutrition (TPN). Part II: Administration systems. Care of the Critically Ill 12 (Supp 1):S2–S3
Cornwell J 1994 How do nurses view their role in pain control? Nursing Times 90(5):11–12
Davis P 1994 Nursing the orthopaedic patient. Churchill Livingstone, Edinburgh
Davison C, Stable I 1996 Audit of nutrition screening in patients with acute illness. Nursing Times 92(8):35–37
Duxbury J 1994 Understanding the nature of sleep. Nursing Standard 9(9):25–28

East E 1992 How much does it hurt? Nursing Times 88(40):48–49

Fawcett H 1995 Nutritional support for hospital patients. Nursing Standard 9(48):25–28

Haynes S 1994 Intermittent catheterisation – the key facts. Professional Nurse 10(2):100–104

Hodgson L A 1991 Why do we need sleep? Relating theory to nursing practice. Journal of Advanced Nursing 16(12):1503–1510

Holden C, Brook G, Wills J 1996 Home parenteral nutrition: present management, future options. British Journal of Community Health 1(6):347–353

Holmes S 1996 Percutaneous endoscopic gastrostomy: a review. Nursing Times 92(17):34–35

Johnson J 1995 Achieving effective rehabilitation outcomes: does the nurse have a role. British Journal of Therapy and Rehabilitation 2(3): 113–118

Jones H 1994 Meeting personal care needs. Community Outlook 4(9):30–32

Kennedy J F 1997 Enteral feeding for the critically ill patient. Nursing Standard 33(11):39–43

Liddle K 1995 Making sense of percutaneous endoscopic gastrostomy. Nursing Times 91(18):32–33

Llewlyn S 1992 Attitude problems. Nursing Times 88(31):64–66

Lowthian P 1987 The classification and grading of pressure sores. Care Science and Practice 5(1):5–8

McGrother C W, Jagger C, Clarke M 1990 Handicaps associated with incontinence: implications for management. Journal of Epidemiology and Community Health 44(3):246–248

Melzack R 1975 The McGill pain questionnaire. In: Melzack R (ed) Pain measurement and assessment. Raven, New York pp 41–47

Norton C 1996 Faecal incontinence in adults. 1: Prevalence and causes. British Journal of Nursing 5(22):1366,1368,1370–1374

Norton D 1987 Norton revised scores. Nursing Times 83(41):6

Pomfret I J 1996 Catheters: design, selection and management. British Journal of Nursing 5(4):245–251

Pottle B 1992 Pulling together. Nursing Times 88(31):34–35

Robshaw V, Marbrow S 1995 Raising awareness of patients' nutritional state. Professional Nurse 11(1):41–42

Snelling J 1994 The effect of chronic pain on the family unit. Journal of Advanced Nursing 19(3):543–551

Southwell M T, Wistow G 1995 Sleep in hospitals at night: are patients' sleep needs being met? Journal of Advanced Nursing 21(6):1101–1109

Spiller J 1992 For who's sake – patient or nurse? Professional Nurse 7(7):431–434

Thomas G B 1987 Is anyone else out there? Nursing Times 83(21):31

Tierney A J 1996 Undernutrition and elderly hospital patients: a review. Journal of Advanced Nursing 23(2):228–236

US Department of Health and Human Services 1992 Pressure ulcers in adults: prediction and prevention. Maryland Agency for Healthcare Policy and Research, Washington

Walker J M, Akinsanya J, Davis B D 1990 The management of elderly patients with pain in the community: study and recommendations. Journal of Advanced Nursing 15(10):1154–1161

Waterlow J 1985 A risk assessment card. Nursing Times 81(48):49–55

Webb A 1994 Catheters and their care. Journal of Community Nursing 8(3):22–27

Willis J 1989 A good night's sleep. Nursing Times 85(47):29–31

Woodward S 1993 A checklist to meet longterm needs: continence assessment of neuroscience patients. Professional Nurse 8(4):222–230

Woodward S 1996 Nutritional support for head-injured patients. Professional Nurse 11(5):290–292

Development of the rehabilitation nurse as specialist

Greg Wain

Part A of this chapter explored the nurse as technical expert and provider of care, focusing predominantly on the normal remit of the practising rehabilitation nurse. It is now commonplace that this level of expertise is expanded beyond what is expected in the normal remit of the nurse. Clearly this is the case within the provision of rehabilitation as well as in other areas. The aim of this section is to examine the generic role of the clinical nurse specialist within the rehabilitation framework, exploring the development of this expanded practice, including that of 'specialist roles'. Coming from a tissue viability and plastic surgery background, I will discuss the clinical nurse specialist role amidst the struggles faced by nurses working in today's National Health Service (NHS), using examples from both personal experience and the literature. There has been a proliferation of clinical nurse specialist roles pertinent to rehabilitation (e.g. pain management specialist, urology nurse specialists, sexual health nurse practitioners, and nurse counsellors to name just a few) within the organisation in which I work. The NHS has undergone a period of rapid change in response to complex economic market forces, affecting provision of care and availability of resources. It is against this backdrop that the following discussion is offered. In examining the potential for such roles, examples within rehabilitation settings will be used to offer frameworks for both their development and the evaluation of their success.

THE CLINICAL NURSE SPECIALIST ROLE

The question has to be asked as to what the clinical nurse specialist does. The following essential functions of the clinical nurse specialist are identified by Castledine (1992):

- undertaking research
- providing clinical leadership, enhancing the development of nursing knowledge
- being an educator
- acting as a change agent.

Bale (1995) identifies that the concept of nurse specialism is far more advanced in other countries, especially the USA. In the UK, clinical nurse specialists are differentiated from generalist nurses by having a higher level of skills and knowledge within a specific area of nursing. McSharry (1995) states that the development of specialist nurses has been most prominent in those areas where the medical profession is least dominant. They often provide a service across a wide range of clinical areas within healthcare organisations, working constantly to enhance the quality of the service provided to the population. Unfortunately, clinical nurse specialists in the UK have, until recently, had no formal educational pathway to follow and no universally recognised qualification. Flanagan (1996) suggests that this has contributed to the haphazard development of such specialists and is reflected in, for instance, the large number of tissue viability specialists currently practising without relevant qualifications. In other countries clinical nurse specialists are expected to achieve a degree at master's level, but to date this has not been accepted in the UK, although this situation will change with the implementation of the United Kingdom Central Council of Nursing, Midwifery and Health Visiting's (UKCC's) standards for post-registration education (UKCC 1994). Such issues are discussed in more depth in Chapter 9, which focuses on the current and future opportunities available within education.

Some generalists have argued that, as nurse specialism becomes more developed, covering a greater number of nursing areas, care will become more fragmented (Bale 1995). However, this is not a view that appears to be commonplace, and not one this author would be keen to support, because of the potential benefits of specialism not only to the client but also to the professional credibility of nursing.

In my particular speciality of wound management, there have been many changes during the last decade, one of the most significant being the development of the clinical nurse specialist. The effectiveness of this role within a rehabilitation setting depends on how the specialist nurse functions and interacts within the multidisciplinary healthcare team. His interpersonal skills are likely to be an important factor in influencing the amount of cooperation obtained from professional colleagues. This concept of multidisciplinary and multi-agency working and the requirement for appropriate interpersonal skills to manage these often complex relationships are, I would propose, essential for all appointed to such nurse specialist posts.

The components of the clinical nurse specialist role can be divided into five subroles, as identified by Storr (1988):

- practitioner
- educator
- consultant
- researcher
- change agent.

In addition to the above, I would propose that the following subroles should be included:

- empowering agent
- coordinator
- monitoring and ensuring the quality of healthcare practices.

PRACTITIONER

The clinical nurse specialist acts as the role model for the nurse, being able to assess patients comprehensively and develop nursing care plans based on advanced clinical knowledge and expertise. Flanagan (1996) identifies that the amount of direct patient contact varies greatly between practising tissue viability nurse specialists, and is usually dependent on the allocation of time to indirect care activities such as research, education, or the formulation of clinical practice guidelines. This will obviously vary, depending not only on the particular expectations and client role within nurse specialist posts, but also on the organisation in which they are working.

EDUCATOR

The clinical nurse specialist can educate patients, families, nursing staff and other healthcare team members. This is particularly the case when there is a deficit between the theory taught in the colleges of nursing and the knowledge base of the ward nurses. In this situation, McSharry (1995) identifies the need for clinical nurse specialists to act as advocates for students, while supporting and educating the qualified ward nurse to rectify any deficits in theory or practice and to explore further the boundaries of existing clinical practice. Some clinical nurse specialists are joint appointments between academic institutions and the clinical speciality and are in a prime position to bridge the theory–practice gap, allowing education and practice to correspond with each other and be congruous in the aim of positively influencing the quality of nursing provided to the individual client.

CONSULTANT

This role can be formal or informal and is most effective when the clinical nurse specialist is readily available, or highly visible, to nursing staff. I would strongly suggest that this can only be achieved by being seen to be clinically credible at the 'sharp end' of nursing, and is important in implementing change. Nurses are more likely to learn from a tissue viability clinical nurse specialist seen performing wound-management procedures on complicated wounds, thereby role modelling advanced clinical practice based on current research. Conversely, learning and credibility are likely to be less where the clinical nurse specialist just theorises about a particular procedure.

RESEARCHER

Many consider that initiating and carrying out research is part of the specialist's role. In theory, the clinical nurse specialist is ideally placed to evaluate research findings for potential implementation in practice. In practice, McSharry (1995) identifies that the initiation of the research component of the clinical nurse specialist role is often very difficult to implement, as effort is generally directed at utilising and evaluating research. From a personal perspective the major influence on the ability to undertake this role is the limited resource of time. For example, the tissue viability clinical nurse specialist has to remain updated on the plethora of literature relating to pressure-relieving equipment and wound-care products, and sift out the paucity of research supporting its use and purchase. At the same time, the nurse must meet the excessive demand made by the role of patient-care provider. McSharry (1995) suggests that research is de-emphasised within the clinical nurse specialist role because of the lack of financial resources to fund nursing research and the inadequacy of support systems within the organisation available to the clinical nurse specialist undertaking research within the clinical environment.

CHANGE AGENT

The clinical nurse specialist is expected to act as the catalyst for change within the organisation to improve patient care, promote communication and improve nursing practice. The implementation of change is a complicated issue, but early change adoption is more likely if nurses feel a close affiliation with the particular change being implemented and with the clinical nurse specialist who acts as a primary change agent.

EMPOWERING AGENT

Clinical nurse specialists must not be protective of their special skills and knowledge, lacking in willingness to share with others. Nurses must be encouraged to reflect and grow both personally and professionally as a result of their new-found knowledge and expertise gained from the clinical nurse specialist. Every clinical nurse specialist should be aware of the potential danger of de-skilling less experienced colleagues if they become overly dependent on the clinical nurse specialist's clinical decision-making prowess.

COORDINATOR

The clinical nurse specialist coordinates and facilitates care for the individual patient using a system of formal and informal contacts, thereby working around bureaucratic obstacles for the benefit of the patient (Humphris 1994, cited in Bale 1995).

MONITORING AND ENSURING THE QUALITY OF HEALTHCARE PRACTICES

Quality assurance monitoring is an integral part of most clinical nurse specialist roles. Flanagan (1996) identifies that quality assurance and tissue viability became inextricably linked as a result of the 1994/1995 Priorities and Planning Guidelines, which set annual targets of at least 5% for the overall reduction of pressure sores and stipulated that contracts should record pressure sore prevalence based on the Department of Health's (1993) recommendations. The clinical nurse specialist is therefore closely involved in monitoring pressure sore incidence/prevalence using tools adapted to meet the demands of the organisation so that accurate and meaningful results can be obtained. The issues of measuring rehabilitation nursing are covered in detail in Chapter 7, and readers are encouraged to turn there for additional information.

DEVELOPMENT OF SPECIALIST ROLES: SCOPE OF PROFESSIONAL PRACTICE

The scope of professional practice (UKCC 1992a) could be perceived as one of the major developments in allowing nurses to expand their role. The impetus behind its development was concerns related to previous extended roles which nurses were undertaking. Within the UKCC document there is an acknowledgment that nursing practice must be sensitive and responsive to changes in the needs of clients, healthcare provision and society. Recognising the need for broad-based pre- and post registration education, it acknowledged the benefit of developing role beyond the traditional scope provided by this education. In practical terms, it is suggested that nursing should continue to change and there is a place for specialist roles to impact positively on meeting these client needs. The framework was designed to guide the development of new nursing roles, recognising the need for development of practice to be based upon personal experience, skill and education. The key principles on which adjustment of the normal scope of professional practice is made are outlined in Box 5.14.

■ **BOX 5.14 Principles for adjusting the scope of professional practice (UKCC 1992a)**

The registered nurse, midwife or health visitor:

1. Must be satisfied that each aspect of practice is directed to meeting the needs and serving the interests of the patient or client.

2. Must endeavour always to achieve, maintain and develop knowledge, skill and competence to respond to those needs and interests.

3. Must honestly acknowledge any limits of personal knowledge and skill and take steps to remedy any relevant deficits in order effectively and appropriately to meet the needs of patients and clients.

4. Must ensure any enlargement or adjustment of the scope of personal professional practice is achieved without compromising or fragmenting existing aspects of professional practice and care and that the requirements of the council's Code of Professional Conduct (UKCC 1992b) are satisfied throughout the whole area of practice.

5. Must recognise and honour the direct or indirect accountability borne for all aspects of professional practice.

6. Must, in serving the interests of patients and clients and the wider interests of society, avoid any inappropriate delegation to others which compromises those interests.

MEETING THE NEEDS AND INTERESTS OF THE CLIENT

Much has already been written in earlier chapters regarding the need for rehabilitation to be client centred. The first key principle in relation to the development of the scope of nursing practice follows the same primary aim. The key question must surely be how one can demonstrate that the development of a nursing role is actually based on better meeting client needs and interests.

A reasonable method that may fulfil this involves identifying the actual needs of clients or patients from a particular service. Again, reference has been made previously in this book to the validity of using 'the experts' (i.e. the clients themselves) to identify these needs. Through comparison of these identified needs against what is provided in practice, one can determine deficits, which could potentially be met through development of the scope of practice of a particular nurse's role.

COMPETENCE TO RESPOND TO THOSE NEEDS AND CLIENTS

Competence to meet the deficits in service provision by nursing will be based, as suggested by the UKCC (1992a), on personal experience, skill and education. Prior to implementation of any new role, there must be:

- a comprehensive person specification and job description
- an individual training needs analysis performed to determine what skills are required by the person who is to undertake the role
- a training programme that includes assessment criteria, developed to ensure competence in all the required skills.

ACKNOWLEDGMENT AND REMEDYING OF LIMITATIONS

There are clear links between this and the previous point, with regard to ensuring that adequate training is undertaken. It is likely that during the early days of a new post the individual nurse may encounter situations where it is clear that further training or supervision is required. During this period it is fundamental that the nurse must not attempt to move beyond the training given. Furthermore, the scope of the role must not be surpassed without further justification and support from the relevant organisation.

REQUIREMENTS OF THE CODE OF CONDUCT ARE MAINTAINED

It seems obvious to state that, in order to maintain the title and work as a registered nurse, one must not only fulfil the requirements for registration but also be active on that register. In doing this the nurse undertakes to adhere to the UKCC professional code of conduct (UKCC 1992b). Particularly important in relation to the development of nursing roles are the clauses relating to promoting and safeguarding the interests of individual patients and clients, accountability and, in those areas where the nurse is prescribing and delivering specific interventions, the issue of gaining consent. These are covered to some degree within other aspects of this framework for developing the scope of practice, but nevertheless merit emphasis.

RECOGNITION OF DIRECT AND INDIRECT ACCOUNTABILITY

Every nurse has three direct lines of accountability: professional accountability to the UKCC, contractual accountability to an employer, and accountability to the law.

Accountability to the UKCC (1996) is based on the principle that you have personal responsibility for what you do, that it is no defence to blame 'acting on orders'. Therefore the actions and decisions one makes must be entirely justifiable.

Contractual accountability to an employer determines the remit and scope of what the nurse is able and has a responsibility to perform on an day-to-day basis. Clearly the tool used to guide this is the job description. Any extended scope of practice should be recorded with the employer, and in those cases where expansion of role is tied with a 'specialist' job, as previously outlined, this should be reflected in the job description. In addition, the person specification for that particular post should reflect the educational requirements and experience that the nurse must possess.

AVOIDANCE OF INAPPROPRIATE DELEGATION

A nurse with an expanded scope of practice requires additional training and assumes a greater professional knowledge in the particular sphere of practice. It is fundamental in promoting the safety of clients that this is borne in mind when considering delegation or prescribing care for others to perform. This is not only vital in providing the client with safe care, but is also tied in with professional accountability (UKCC 1996). Clear lines of referral and written limitations of what is expected of a nurse who has not received additional training should be defined.

CONCLUSION

The role of the nurse specialist has provided, and should continue to provide, a positive contribution to the delivery of rehabilitation services. However, the role as outlined here should be clearly defined and supported in practice, through adventurous and forward-thinking management which will enable full use of the opportunities created through development of such roles. We have been clearly guided through the scope of professional practice document (UKCC 1992) as to how these roles should develop.

As with many other areas within the rehabilitation nursing remit outlined throughout this book, it is fundamental that we develop effective monitoring of the success of specialist roles, not only to demonstrate the positive aspects of the role, but also to guide future developments.

REFERENCES

Bale S 1995 The role of the clinical nurse specialist within the health care team. Journal of Wound Care 4(2):86–87
Castledine G 1992 The advanced practitioner. Nursing 5(7):14–15
Flanagan M 1996 The role of the clinical nurse specialist in tissue viability. British Journal of Nursing 5(11):676–681
McSharry M 1995 The evolving role of the clinical nurse specialist. British Journal of Nursing 4(11):641–646
Storr G 1988 The clinical nurse specialist from the outside looking in. Journal of Advanced Nursing 13:265–272
United Kingdom Central Council of Nursing, Midwifery and Health Visiting 1992a Scope of professional practice. UKCC, London
United Kingdom Central Council of Nursing, Midwifery and Health Visiting 1992b Professional code of conduct. UKCC, London
United Kingdom Central Council of Nursing, Midwifery and Health Visiting 1996 Guidelines for professional practice. UKCC, London

The rehabilitation nurse as team worker and coordinator

Team-working in rehabilitation nursing

Anne Seaman

INTRODUCTION

The aim of this chapter is to provide information relating to aspects of team-working in rehabilitation nursing and the organisation and personnel within those nursing teams. The principles of effective team-working are examined, and the general nature, roles and management of conflict within team-working are discussed. In addition, the concepts and processes involved in primary nursing are described, using examples from the rehabilitation environment in which the author works, enabling the reader to examine nursing teams in his own clinical setting.

Team work in rehabilitation has never been as important as it is today as, with advances in medicine, many more patients are surviving severe illness and traumatic injuries to live with severe impairments and their associated disabilities. In order to meet the needs of these patients, healthcare organisations have become complex; the emphasis has moved away from individuals providing care towards the use of teams (Blanchard et al 1990).

Commissioners, and previously purchasers, of rehabilitation programmes expect a service that delivers a comprehensive package of care, which should be both of a high quality and cost-effective. A complete care package for a patient who has suffered a cerebral vascular accident would include critical care, a rehabilitation programme, community liaison, and support and outpatient follow-up. Without doubt the number of agencies and disciplines, both hospital and community based, involved in the provision of such a package necessitates the use of effective team-working.

WHY USE TEAMS?

Team-working is recognised as being more effective than individuals working in isolation or as groups of workers. Groups can be mistaken for teams, but there are significant differences between the two. Groups can exist in name only, often referred to as 'work groups' or 'working parties'. The members are not always interactive and may not necessarily discuss or share information; this results in a lack of cohesiveness and productivity

(Hanks 1994). On the other hand, teams consist of members who are very interactive, working together as one, rather than in isolation; the members share information and ideas and work towards a common or shared goal.

Team members who work towards common goals form a highly cohesive body, make joint decisions rather than individual ones. In addition, when making decisions, the team can influence external forces, as a team decision is given more credibility than when only one team member speaks, reinforcing the notion that there is power in numbers (Zejdlik 1992).

PRINCIPLES OF EFFECTIVE TEAM-WORKING

TEAM COMMUNICATION

Communication is a priority for effective team-working. All members of the team must have an understanding of the roles of the team members. This refers to both the team role and the individual functional roles. Often there is potential for overlap; for example, both the physiotherapist and the occupational therapist may be able to assess seating and posture requirements. This may lead to each therapist assuming that the other will complete the assessment, and it is possible then that this aspect of care is missed. In these days when blurring of professional roles seems to be promoted for the benefit of clients (while recognising the specific areas of expertise of each discipline) the possibilities for confusion if responsibilities are unclear is obvious. Therefore, it is essential that each member is clear about their role in any aspect of care and responsibilities that they are expected to complete.

All members of the team must be familiar with the methods of communication that will be used. This may include the method of arranging a primary-care or goal-planning meeting, to ensure that all team members are aware of the meeting and can attend. Other methods may include the use of multidisciplinary care planning or case notes, team or ward meetings and dissemination of information relating to the particular organisation in which one works. Using the accepted methods of communication will ensure that everyone is kept informed of current and future events, thus preventing confusion.

TEAM ROLES

The effectiveness of the team is reflected in its members. Individuals demonstrate behaviours which, when clustered together, are given the term 'team role'. The team roles are influential and a balance is necessary if the team is to be successful.

Belbin (1993) identified nine team roles, each of which makes a particular contribution to the team as a whole (Table 6.1). An effective team incorporates members who are capable of fulfilling all the roles identified, which often proves difficult in practice. It is also important to find a balance of roles in a team. Selecting or inviting team members who function in the same or in a similar manner may result in an ineffective

Table 6.1 Team roles (Belbin 1993)

Role	Behaviours
Plant	Demonstrates creativity, is imaginative, may be unorthodox and has problem-solving abilities
Coordinator	Is a mature, confident chair-person, who clarifies goals, promotes decision-making and delegates well
Shaper	Is dynamic and challenging, has both the courage and drive to overcome obstacles and thrives on pressure
Resource investigator	An extrovert who is enthusiastic and explores opportunities, a good communicator who makes useful contacts
Specialist	Is dedicated and experienced, possessing rare knowledge and skills and is single minded
Implementer	Is disciplined, reliable and efficient, has the ability to put ideas into practice
Team worker	Is cooperative, perceptive and diplomatic, has good listening skills, mediates and avoids friction
Completer	Is conscientious, anxious and thorough, meets time-scales
Monitor/evaluator	Uses strategies, sees all the options and has the ability to judge accurately

team. A team that consists of several members who are 'coordinators' may result in all of them trying to organise the team, which could result in the team not having a clear coordinator and lead to confusion and lack of cohesiveness. Not all willing team members may have developed their skills well enough to be fully effective within a team role; however, they should not be ruled out. A compromise may produce favourable results, when their strengths are used and their weaknesses are managed (Belbin 1993). An imaginative approach may be used, such as providing the experience to develop skills, where support and supervision are available or by arranging a place on a specific training course. For example, an E grade nurse who is often in charge of the ward for a shift may need to develop management skills; this could be achieved by the ward sister supervising the nurse taking charge of the ward for a shift or, alternatively, the nurse may attend a 'skills for management' course. Some weaknesses may be tolerated and, indeed, expected if other team members are able to make up the shortfall through their contribution. This in essence highlights one of the key benefits of a team approach.

TEAM CONFLICTS

Even cohesive teams experience disagreements between members from time to time, which may be due to professional, cultural or, sometimes, personal reasons. Disagreements or disputes can escalate into conflicts, which are described as clashes between hostile or opposing members (Gillies 1994). Team members are very dependent on one another if they are to provide effective quality patient care, and disputes are said to be normal within multidisciplinary teams planning patient care (Kaluzny 1989, cited Gillies 1994). Walton 1984 suggests that there are five areas that give rise to disputes.

- Facts – when information received is different or incomplete or when it is interpreted differently.
- Goals/objectives – these may be interpreted differently.
- Methods – how to proceed with the task or problem encountered.
- Values/ethics – includes issues of power, morality, patient rights or confidentiality.
- Resources – availability of funds, equipment or time to achieve the goal or objective.

Ideally, disputes or conflicts should be resolved within the team. This may be facilitated either by another team member or by the individual disputants. If the dispute develops into conflict and the team is unable to resolve it themselves, the members may seek a mediator, such as their manager.

A conflict mediator, whether from within the team or not, needs to understand the cause of or the reason for the individuals' motivation for conflict and how willing each disputant is for negotiation. Resolution is only possible if at least one disputant is willing to negotiate. Neutral ground is often beneficial and the mediator may suggest an acceptable time and venue for a meeting. The mediator aims to equalise the power between the disputants; this may be achieved by the mediator intervening to ensure that each has an equal say (Gillies 1994).

Usually disputes are resolved through compromise, which may have been suggested by the mediator or by a disputant. It is important to note that this level of intervention is rarely required and disputes are usually resolved fairly easily, either directly by the disputants or within the team environment.

NURSES AS TEAM WORKERS

The nurse's role within a team is influenced by how nurses organise themselves. Understanding nursing hierarchy and methods of team-working enables nurses of all levels to understand their role and how they fit into the team.

THE ORGANISATION OF NURSING

Team work is essential to providing effective nursing care, and within a National Health Service (NHS) Trust there is a network of nurses all working towards the promotion of quality nursing care. Leading this network is the nurse director, who may also be a member of the Trust's executive board. This post may not be incorporated within a direct line of management, but acts as a liaison between the nursing teams and the management teams within the Trust. Throughout the UK the posts vary, although there are five main elements of responsibility (Box 6.1).

■ BOX 6.1 The responsibilities of the nurse executive director

There are five main elements of nurse executive responsibility:

- Nursing leadership
- Development and leadership of nursing practice
- Direct/organisational management
- Contribution to corporate management
- Human resource management

(NHSME 1992)

The first element is nursing leadership, which is considered central to the job. Development and leadership of nursing practice includes manpower and skill mix reviews and restructuring. The third element involves direct/operational management. This role does vary between Trusts; some have significant general management responsibilities, while others do not. Nurse executive directors also have a responsibility to contribute to corporate leadership and management in areas other than nursing; this may include corporate decision-making involved in strategic and organisational development. The fifth element is human resource management; this is the most common role, the nurse director acting as an advisor to the director of human resources (NHSME 1992). Nurse directors are often supported by a deputy or assistant nurse director who represents the director in situations when the director is unable to be present. The deputy also has other responsibilities, which are usually based on a particular aspect of nursing management such as nurse education (Townsend 1994).

Senior nurses are given many different titles, such as senior clinical nurse, nurse manager and unit manager. Most will have similar responsibilities, having direct management of the nursing workforce within a specified unit within a directorate. Often this is a department or a group of wards that provides a specific aspect of care, for example a group of surgical wards that may include urology and cardiothoracic surgery. Ultimately, the senior nurse is responsible for the quality of the nursing care within the unit.

Within the ward or unit environment there is also a hierarchy. This relates mainly to the clinical grading structure introduced in 1988. Some Trusts have moved away from clinical grading and have developed a unique system. Nurses' roles relate directly to their clinical grade, although titles may be different. This is very evident for F grade nurses, who are called either junior sisters or senior staff nurses. There are also the healthcare support workers who may have a higher grade than auxiliary nurses.

At ward level, just as at the organisation level, team work is essential to providing effective nursing care. Rehabilitation nurses work in at least two teams: they work as a member of a ward-based nursing team, and as part of the rehabilitation team.

The use of shift patterns to cover nursing care over the 24-hour period influences the team-working of nurses. The team of nurses working an early shift on one day is unlikely to be the same the following day, and therefore nurses need to be adaptable if they are to work effectively during each shift.

Nurses are also members of the ward team as a whole. Each nurse will have a clearly defined role, with specific responsibilities outlined within his job description (e.g. ward sister, primary nurse or team leader, associate nurse and auxiliary nurse).

THE ORGANISATION OF NURSING CARE

Over time, four methods of organising nursing teams have emerged:

- patient allocation
- task orientation
- team nursing
- primary nursing.

Nursing is continually developing with the aim of promoting professionalism and cohesiveness of working, with the desired result being a client-centred, high standard of care through the provision of a service that is continuous and consistent over the 24-hour period. Therefore, task orientation has largely become obsolete, as the approach described above is preferred to the more fragmented nursing care which task allocation may produce. The major means through which nursing is delivered and organised seem to be primary nursing and team nursing. The choice may depend on the perceived advantages or disadvantages of possible approaches and the type of client group with which the nursing team is dealing. In addition, commonplace in rehabilitation is the concept of using a key worker or case manager who may be from any discipline. For the purposes of this chapter the concept of primary nursing will be the focus. Most nurses will be less familiar with primary nursing, and therefore it merits this deeper exploration. Key workers and case managers have been discussed briefly in Chapter 1. In addition to the information already given there, these roles are examined further in Part B of this chapter.

PRIMARY NURSING

Primary nursing has been slow to take off in the UK. In 1989 the Department of Health recommended that 'the development of primary nursing should be encouraged.' Today it is a popular method of managing patient care. Its use has been described in many settings, such as medical wards (Chilton 1991), intensive care units (Manley 1989) and the community hospital setting (Pearson 1988), and in the author's experience it is particularly beneficial for patients undergoing rehabilitation.

Many definitions of the concept of primary nursing have been offered. While the definitions differ, there is some agreement that it is a philosophy, an organisational method of delivering nursing care, or both. The quality of nursing care is dependent on the performance of the nurses within the system.

In their analysis of the definitions of primary nursing, Ersser & Tutton (1991) suggest that there are four key elements:

- particular patterns of responsibility, authority, autonomy and accountability
- continuity of care
- the care planner is also the care giver
- direct communication with the patient and family.

These relate closely to Manthey's (1992) four elements:

- allocation and acceptance of individual responsibility for decision-making to one nurse
- assignment of daily care by case method
- direct person-to-person communication
- one person is responsible for the quality of the care given to patients on a ward or unit, 24 hours a day, 7 days a week.

It is important that primary nurses understand the implications of their role, which can be applied to all primary nurses, no matter what their additional organisational role may be. For example the ward sister's organisational role includes overall ward management, while the E grade nurse may be responsible for the management of a span of duty. Primary nurses are supported and supervised by the primary nurse coordinator, who is ultimately accountable for the quality of nursing care (Bartels et al 1977, Ersser & Tutton 1991). The minimum requirements for the role of primary nurse could include:

- employed full time, with internal rotation
- relevant specialist course and over 2 years within speciality
- ENB 998 or equivalent
- skills for management course.

This is to ensure that the primary nurse is competent to practise (Ersser & Tutton 1991). Using the four elements described by Ersser & Tutton (1991) it is worth exploring the primary nursing role in more detail. These elements can be used as the basis for the development of primary nursing in any clinical area.

Element 1: Responsibility, authority, autonomy and accountability

This first element is at the heart of primary nursing. Primary nurses accept the responsibility for making decisions about the nursing care of patients. This begins at the time of the patient's admission and continues with 24-hour responsibility through to the patient's discharge (Manthey 1992).

The primary nurse is expected to plan and be involved in providing direct nursing care. This ensures that the nurse is in the best position to decide how nursing care is to be given, and also allows the nurse to take on a proactive approach rather than a reactive one. This assumes that the primary nurse is suitably qualified to fulfil the role in a competent, safe and effective manner. As primary nurses are responsible and accountable for the care provided over the 24-hour period, which of course they are unable to provide themselves, the proactive approach enables them to direct the nursing care in the form of a patient care plan. This plan is discussed with the patient and other nurses who provide care in the primary nurse's absence. If a patient's condition requires a change in the nursing care planned by the primary nurse, the care can be altered, but any changes must be justified and discussed with the primary nurse on his return to duty. Even then, the primary nurse has both the authority and the autonomy to change the care plan, and thus retains accountability for the nursing care. Without the above it is impossible for primary nurses to be accountable (Ersser & Tutton 1991).

Element 2: Continuity of care

The primary nurse has continuous responsibility for a named group of patients, and, while it is accepted that there is 24-hour responsibility, as discussed earlier, it is also suggested that this responsibility extends beyond the inpatient stay. This might involve primary nurses taking continued responsibility for patient re-admissions and clinic visits (Anderson & Choi 1980). The former notion may not be as difficult as it first seems; primary nurses often continue to be responsible for episodes of patient re-admission, this being dependent on the same nurse being available. With outpatient clinic visits, it is likely that this will not be possible, as managing the nurse's time and duty rota to facilitate this could prove to be very difficult. While it could be said that it would promote continuity of care, in fact it could have just the opposite effect. The continuity of care for inpatients would be interrupted due to the absence of the primary nurse. Therefore, it may well be more practical if a case manager or community liaison nurse takes over such responsibility at the time of discharge.

Element 3: Care planner as care giver

As primary nurses are also the providers of care, there is the expectation that each primary nurse will care for his 'primary patients' when he is on duty. However, this does not address how much time the primary nurse needs to spend with his patients in order to enable him to make decisions and plan the care required effectively.

The number of hours that a primary nurse works will influence the time he has to plan and provide care for his patients. It has been suggested that primary nurses should work full time in acute areas, where the rate of admission is high and the length of stay short. In areas where changes in the patient's condition occur at a slower rate, primary nurses could work part time (Ersser & Tutton 1991). This is debatable. While change is perceived to be slow in rehabilitation, this is not always the case, and re-assessment is often necessary on a daily basis. Therefore, it is preferable that primary nurses are employed on a full-time basis.

Element 4: Direct communication

First of all, primary nurses use their contact time with their patients to gain knowledge of their needs and problems. This information can then be passed on to nurses taking over the patients' care on the next shift. Primary nurses also function as the key communicators within the team, and convey information to other healthcare workers involved in the patients' care (Black 1992). In the rehabilitation setting this would indicate communication within the primary rehabilitation team. Communication is essential to the continuity and quality of the patients' care.

ROLE STRUCTURE

The success of primary nursing depends on the roles played by all members of the ward and/or unit team. The role and functioning of the primary nurses has been described above. Clearly there are other key members of the nursing team who are essential for the successful implementation of primary nursing. Such team members include the primary nurse co-ordinator, who is usually the ward sister or charge nurse, the associate nurses (qualified nurse), the care assistants or auxiliary nurses, and the ward clerk (Mead 1990).

Primary nurse coordinators

Primary nurse coordinators are essentially the ward managers. Overall responsibility involves enabling the nursing team to provide the optimum standard of nursing, through good leadership, advocacy and acting as a clinical expert. Minimum requirements for such a post could include:

- employed full time, with internal rotation as necessary
- relevant specialist course
- considerable experience in nursing within that client group
- ENB 998 or equivalent
- managerial training.

The associate nurse

The associate nurse is a trained nurse who is responsible for supporting the primary nurse. When the primary nurse is off duty the associate nurse takes over the patient care (Wright 1990). Primary nurses may also ask associate nurses to contribute to patient care when they are on duty. Typical examples of this may arise when a patient requires some intervention such as a dressing change or, possibly, a period of teaching. This may allow the primary nurse to attend to another of his 'primary patients'. Generally associate nurses are more junior registered nurses. Initial experience following appointment will vary from the newly qualified to those with experience in other fields of nursing who have changed their nursing speciality. Induction to the clinical area and in-service training is provided shortly after appointment.

The care assistant

The care assistant role, often referred to as the auxiliary nurse, has been discussed with some uncertainty in the literature. While few fulfil the role of associate nurse (Easton 1989, Fox 1988), generally two roles have been identified: one of support and one of facilitator.

The supportive role involves the care assistant acting as an associate to the primary nurse, but within limits; she is not able to replace the primary nurse in his absence but can provide care under the supervision of either the primary or associate nurse. The role of facilitator involves the care assistant helping the primary nurse perform aspects of care that require two people, such as manual handling tasks. Domestic duties are often considered part of the role and care assistants may be employed as a ward/unit 'housekeepers', in which case they are not linked to a particular primary nursing team (Armitage et al 1991). Whatever the case, care assistants perform an important role. Initially, experience in either nursing care or in rehabilitation specialities is not essential, although obviously it is advantageous. An in-service training programme is vital, and a record of competency should be kept. These issues are covered in more depth in Chapter 8.

ORGANISATION OF THE TEAM USING PRIMARY NURSING

Organising the team to ensure that the skill mix is at an optimum for each shift may often be a difficult task. There must be a balance of primary nurses, associate nurses and auxiliary nurses. In addition, in the absence of a primary nurse coordinator/ward manager, there may be a need for a suitably trained member of staff to assume overall responsibility for the management of the clinical area for the shift.

In the clinical area with which the author is most familiar, a 6-week duty rota is used. Nurses are grouped into 'lines', which consist of a primary nurse, two associate nurses and two auxiliary nurses. The rota consists of 4 weeks day duty, working 7 days at a time, one week of night duty (7 nights) followed by 7 days off. This ensures that all 'line' members have the same days off, and therefore they work on the same days, but not necessarily the same shift. The result is that three 'lines' are on day duty at all times, and one 'line' is on night duty. This pattern reinforces team work. There are a few nurses who are prepared to work flexi-time to ensure a good skill mix on some shifts as required. An example of the skill mix on each shift is given in Table 6.2.

THE PROCESSES WITHIN PRIMARY NURSING

PRIMARY NURSE PATIENT ASSIGNMENT

Again referring to the clinical area in which the author works, the expectation is that the primary nurse will have a maximum of five primary patients, at least one of whom would be a short-stay re-admission patient.

Table 6.2 Shift patterns and skill mix in primary nursing

Early shift		Late shift		Night shift	
Role	Line	Role	Line	Role	Line
PN	2	PNC		PN	5
PN	4	PN	3	AN	5
AN	3	AN	2	AN	5
AN	4	CA	4	CA	5
CA	2	CA	2	CA	5
CA	3				
CA	4				
CA	3				

PNC, primary nurse coordinator; PN, primary nurse; AN, associate nurse; CA, care assistant/auxiliary nurse.
Other nurses belonging to lines 2, 3 and 4 may be away due to annual leave or training. Staff on lines 1 and 6 are on days off.

The aim is to share the workload. Patient dependency (in the long term) is taken into consideration when the primary nurse is assigned a new patient. Clearly this may differ depending on the dependency and case mix of the particular clinical area.

- *Planned patient admission.* The primary nurse is assigned prior to admission; the primary nurse should be on duty to welcome and assess the patient.
- *Emergency admission.* The primary nurse is assigned within 24 hours, but may not be on duty at the time of admission.

The admitting nurse should explain the primary care system to the patient and family as soon after admission as appropriate, usually within 24 hours. The primary or admitting nurse will be present during the medical examination, and will conduct an assessment within the first few hours of admission. The multidisciplinary team is informed of the patient's admission and condition, so that they can begin their plan of action. Ideally, in those areas in which it is possible, the primary nurse should be involved as soon after injury as possible. During the acute phase of injury or illness, even if the patient is being managed in a different area, the primary nurse should arrange contact and begin the planning process prior to transfer to the rehabilitation area. In those areas that have patients at acute and rehabilitation stages this is clearly not a problem. Indeed, the continuity this facilitates may be a major factor in this actually becoming the standard means of organising the package of care in the healthcare services described earlier.

Primary care meetings will be arranged by the primary nurse, who will invite all members of the multidisciplinary team assigned to the patient and his family. Central to the team is the patient and his family (if the patient wishes), who attend all the meetings. During the first meeting, discharge planning is discussed. Figure 6.1 demonstrates the communication pathways involved in primary nursing and the multidisciplinary team.

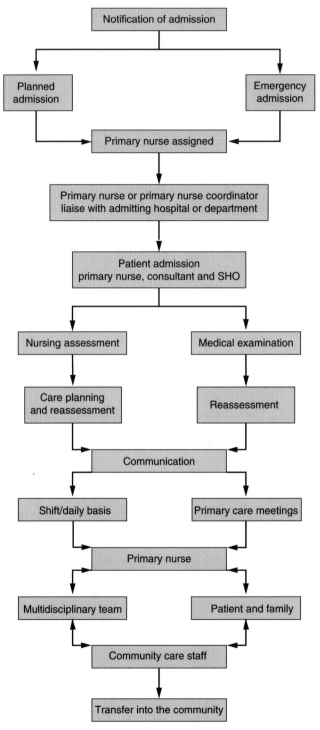

Figure 6.1 A system of primary nursing and multidisciplinary team-working.

In the event of a primary nurse leaving the unit, a replacement should be agreed with the patient and a handover period arranged between the two primary nurses, to ensure continuity of care.

ADVANTAGES AND DISADVANTAGES OF PRIMARY NURSING

As with all methods of working, there are both advantages and disadvantages of primary nursing. The lists below identify these. They will help you to understand some of the benefits and some of the difficulties that need be overcome when utilising primary nursing in practice.

Advantages

- Nursing roles are clearly defined.
- Patients receive individualised care.
- Joint care planning with the patient promotes patient autonomy and empowerment (Black 1992).
- Continuity of care and patient satisfaction are increased (Roberts 1980, cited Black 1992).
- Communication between the nurse, patient and family is improved (Kemp & Richardson 1994).
- Discharge planning is more effective.
- The patient has an advocate if one is needed (Kemp & Richardson 1994).
- There is an increased rapport between the patient and the three or four nurses who care for him, with increased security and trust (Kemp & Richardson 1994).
- The primary nurse develops his managerial skills in relation to providing patient care, especially in providing rehabilitation nursing.
- There is enhancement of multidisciplinary teamwork; team members know to approach the primary nurse who has a greater knowledge of the patient (Kemp & Richardson 1994).
- Patient education is improved if there is a named person responsible (e.g. primary nurse).

Disadvantages

- Requires full cooperation of all members of staff.
- The primary nurse may have a heavy workload if he has several primary patients, especially if several are high-dependency patients.
- There may be problems if there is a clash of personalities between the patient and the primary nurse.
- There is a risk of the primary nurse becoming overinvolved and overprotective of his patients.
- The primary nurse may become overwhelmed by the 24-hour accountability.

- Primary nurse autonomy may result in an overconfident nurse who fails to seek advice (Kemp & Richardson 1994).
- Those nurses who are on permanent night duty and some part-time nurses are unable to be primary nurses. This may result in bad feeling within the nursing team, proving a source of conflict.
- The ward sister may not communicate with patients (Kemp & Richardson 1994).
- The members of a multidisciplinary team have to communicate with a number of nurses to obtain information, rather than approaching the ward sister or nurse in charge of the shift.
- Caring for the same group of patients on every shift may mean not getting to know other patients very well.
- Primary nurses may feel unsupported if one of their patients is unpopular.
- Some primary nurses perceive 24-hour accountability as a disadvantage.
- Patients may be allocated without the primary nurse's knowledge if he is on leave (long-term patients).
- Allocating short-stay patients can be difficult.
- Primary nursing requires an appropriate skill mix.
- Off duty can be difficult to write.

INTRODUCING PRIMARY NURSING

Introducing primary nursing to your ward or unit is a complex task that requires team work if the transition is to be successful. Prior to considering any in-depth work, it is essential to talk to your colleagues to gain support for your proposal. In particular, you should approach your senior nurse and ward sister/charge nurse for support, preferably with an outline of any initial plans (Box 6.2).

Your manager may supply you with some useful resources to enable you to develop your proposal, such as giving you time away from the clinical area to hold meetings, and to plan and research primary nursing.

At some point you will need to meet and discuss your proposal with the other members of the multidisciplinary team. Without their support

---

■ **BOX 6.2 Seeking support from your manager**

When you approach your manager for support, it will be useful if you have some initial plans prepared. The following could be included:

- an outline of how primary nursing will benefit both the patients and staff
- first impressions of staff support for the change
- an outline of the research into primary nursing required, and how you may achieve this
- preliminary ideas for how you could put primary nursing into practice.

primary nursing will not be successful, and communication in particular may break down. This meeting should only be arranged when the nurses are knowledgeable about primary nursing. Questions are bound to be asked and you will need to demonstrate your knowledge in order to gain the support of other team members (Black 1992).

THE PROJECT TEAM

Selecting members of your project team is an important task. You need to bear in mind the specific tasks involved in researching and planning and the team role behaviours described earlier. You need a team that is committed to introducing primary nursing and willing and able to contribute. It is important to recognise that, although you may have been the initial driving force, you may decide that you are not the best person to lead the project team. Therefore, it may prove useful to invite others who may have experience of working in project teams and who may fulfil specific roles within the team, including the team leader. If staff are willing, all grades of nurses should be included. Promoting ownership in this way will help in implementation of the project and, ultimately, in primary nursing in practice.

The size of the team is important. It should be kept small (5–8 members maximum). Too few will result in members becoming overburdened, while too many can result in a less cohesive team.

There should be regular and frequent meetings of the project team to discuss research, development and implementation of primary nursing. The meetings will promote continued enthusiasm, particularly when everything seems to be coming together.

Take care to set a realistic time frame. Undertaking a project such as this, where all staff will require training, is a lengthy process. Setting deadlines, which are subsequently missed, may result in low morale. Assessing progress at regular intervals will allow you to set realistic dates, particularly for implementation and review.

THE PROCESS OF INTRODUCING PRIMARY NURSING

Each clinical area is different, and therefore how you implement primary nursing in your clinical area will be unique and designed to meet the needs of your speciality, patients, staff and environment.

The project team members will need to consider how they intend to manage the development and implementation process. Dividing the main tasks into stages may be helpful. The stages given in Box 6.3 and described below are based on Black's (1992) suggestions and are guidelines. You will need to adapt these to include your own ideas.

Stage 1: Understanding primary nursing

1. Conduct a literature search; there are numerous articles and books so do not attempt to read everything that you find. Be selective, while

> ■ **BOX 6.3 The process of introducing primary nursing**
>
> There are five stages:
>
> - understanding primary nursing
> - sharing primary nursing
> - preparation for implementation
> - implementing primary nursing
> - evaluation of primary nursing in practice.

at the same time ensuring that you read a broad selection of relevant information.

2. In the light of the information gained, review your current working methods. Identify elements that work well and that you think you should retain. For example, begin with your nursing mission statement. Does it reflect what you are doing? Does it need to be renewed? Will primary nursing help you to meet your mission statement? Another element that you may wish to consider is the nursing model you are using. Is it the most appropriate?

3. Attending conferences and study days about primary nursing may be useful, especially to hear how others have put it into practice.

4. Make contact with staff within your trust who are using primary nursing. Visit their clinical areas and discuss their difficulties and achievements

Stage 2: Sharing primary nursing

- Encourage other staff to read about primary nursing.
- Leave relevant articles in a suitable place for staff to use.
- Arrange study days and visits for staff.
- Hold a meeting for all members of the multidisciplinary team to explain primary nursing and to seek support and promote understanding.
- Use a display board to highlight aspects of primary nursing.
- Publish minutes of the project team meetings to promote feedback.
- You could write an information sheet on primary nursing for all staff.

Stage 3: Preparation for implementation

- Use feedback from discussions with all staff to enable you to address areas of difficulty (e.g. primary nurse assignment, the decision-making process, responsibility and accountability).
- Write clear role profiles for all nurses involved.
- Identify the involvement of the multidisciplinary team.
- Agree communication methods between nurses and the multidisciplinary team.

- Identify any additional resources required (e.g. training needs, off-duty rota, documentation).
- Consider how you will evaluate the effects of primary nursing for patients and staff.

Stage 4: Implementing primary nursing

- Agree and set an implementation date.
- Ensure that the project team members are available in the first few days to support staff.
- Expect some difficulties.
- Encourage each other.

Stage 5: Evaluation of primary nursing in practice

Now that you have primary nursing running in your clinical area, you will need to address some of the difficulties and the successes.

- Project team meetings should continue.
- Continue to support the ward staff while primary nursing is new to them.
- Evaluate primary nursing; this will identify the achievements and some aspects that may require further work.
- Enjoy your project and ward team's successes.

WORKING WITH OTHER DISCIPLINES AND AGENCIES IN REHABILITATION

As stated earlier, any section of the NHS has a complex network of care providers. This is particularly pertinent in rehabilitation, where patient issues may be many and complex (Ryan 1994). Professionals working in rehabilitation aim to provide client centred care. Team work using the skills of all of these disciplines is essential if rehabilitation is to be successful; it is unlikely that a single profession is capable of providing client-centred care on its own (Barnitt & Pomeroy 1995). Therefore, the rehabilitation provided can only be considered to be completely client centred if the skills of all the disciplines are present. The nature of this team-working within the whole rehabilitation team is covered in Part B of this chapter, but it is worth noting here that nurses do not work in isolation, but as part of this multidisciplinary team. This quite simply emphasises the fact that any reorganisation of nursing will impact on the other disciplines within rehabilitation. It seems reasonable, therefore, to ensure that other team members not only understand the benefits and processes within any nursing system used, but are actually consulted during the planning and implementation stages. The benefit of this is that it may help in reducing conflicts between nursing and other disciplines, and therefore facilitate successful implementation generally.

EVALUATION OF TEAM COMMUNICATION

As identified earlier, communication is vital for effective team-working. Evaluation of team communication can be achieved through clinical audit. Although audit and measuring of rehabilitation nursing is the focus of Part A of Chapter 7, it is worth demonstrating here how the process may be used to improve team-working. Auditing how well communication takes place between the team members will not only promote team development, but will also provide information that can be used as a basis for planning and developing communication tools and procedures.

THE AUDIT CYCLE

The audit cycle consists of three phases: the setting phase, the monitoring phase and the action phase. During each phase there are tasks to be completed before moving on to the next phase. This is explored further in Part A of Chapter 7.

The setting phase

The audit will involve assessing and evaluating the team's communication based on standards that have been predetermined (Vaughan & Pillmoor 1989). Examples of standards might include the following.

- Primary care team meetings will take place every 6 weeks as a minimum.
- Primary care team meeting summary sheets are completed and distributed within 48 hours of the meeting.

You will have identified these standards when you decided on your methods of communication within primary nursing with the multidisciplinary team. The audit will allow a continuous assessment and evaluation of such standards relating to team-working, to ensure that they are reasonable and achievable (Vaughan & Pillmoor 1989). You can audit several standards at once, although you will find it easier to share the load with the members of your project team, and audit a standard each.

Next you need to select your indicators, devise a data collection method and complete a design sheet and indicator sheet (Boxes 6.4 and 6.5).

■ **BOX 6.4 Communication audit design sheet**

Topic:	Primary Care Team communication
Topic coordinator:	Staff Nurse Smith
Departments involved:	Orthopaedic Unit and secretariat
Pilot sample:	4 Primary Care Team meetings
Main sample:	3 months, approx. 20 meetings
Pilot collection dates:	1.5.98–31.5.98
Main collection dates:	1.7.98–1.10.98
Collected from:	Secretary

■ **BOX 6.5 Communication audit indicator sheet**

Topic: Primary Care Team communication
Objective: To ensure that Primary Care Team meeting summary sheets are available 48 hours following the meeting

Aspect of care	Standard	Exception	Definition
Turnaround time for completion and distribution of summary sheets to be no more than 48 hours following the meeting	100%	Meetings that take place on a Thursday or Friday, these should be available on Monday	Turnaround = time from meeting to distribution

■ **BOX 6.6 Example of a communication audit data collection sheet**

No of meetings	Date of meeting	Date of summary sheet distribution	Indicator – distributed within 48 hours	Reason indicator not met
1	12.7.98	14.7.98	Y	
2	14.7.98	19.7.98	N	Secretary off sick
3	18.7.98	19.7.98	Y	
4	22.7.98	25.7.98	N	Photocopier not working

The monitoring phase

A data collection form needs to be designed (Box 6.6). The secretary who photocopies and distributes the summary sheet is the ideal person to record the data. You would of course need to obtain the secretary's agreement. Following data collection, the data are analysed and evaluated against the standard.

The action phase

Following evaluation of the data, you will identify any action that needs to be taken in order to improve on performance and meet the standard set. The audit can be repeated to assess the results of the action taken. Meeting the standards set will ensure quality care for the patient and his family.

SUMMARY

In discussing general issues relating to team-working and focusing on the issues on team work related to nursing, the author has attempted to promote in the reader a desire to critically evaluate the organisation of nursing team work within his particular nursing environment. The focus has been on primary nursing, as opposed to other forms of nursing team work, simply because this is a less familiar way of working in most rehabilitation areas and because the author's experiences of primary nursing have been particularly positive. It is clear, however, that there is no absolute hard methodology through which primary or team nursing should be operationalised. The prime aims of developing a system that not only facilitates client centred care but also enables nurses to perform their work effectively and efficiently should be paramount. Any system merits adaption according to the specific nature and needs of the particular clinical area. Whichever system is implemented there is an indisputable need for effective communication. A key principle which every reader should take away is the need to facilitate this through formalised audit of the communication processes that occur in your nursing team.

REFERENCES

Anderson M, Choi T 1980 Primary nursing in an organisational context. Journal of Nursing Administration 10:26–31

Armitage P, Champney-Smith J, Andrews K 1991 Primary nursing and the role of the nurse preceptor in changing long-term mental health care: an evaluation. Journal of Advanced Nursing 16:413–422

Barnitt R, Pomeroy V 1995 An holistic approach to rehabilitation. British Journal of Therapy and Rehabilitation 2(2):87–92

Bartels D, Good V, Lampe S 1977 The role of the head nurse in primary nursing. Canadian Nurse 26–30

Belbin M 1993 Team roles at work. Butterworth-Heinemann, Oxford

Black F 1992 Primary nursing: an introductory guide. King's Fund Centre, London

Blanchard K, Carew D, Parisi-Carew E 1990 The one minute manager builds higher performance teams. Fontana, London

Chilton S 1991 A change for the better – primary nursing in a medical ward. In: Ersser S, Tutton E (eds) Primary nursing in perspective. Scutari, London

Department of Health 1989 A strategy for nursing – a report of the steering committee. Department of Health, Nursing Division, London

Easton N 1989 Educating auxiliaries. Primary Nursing News 11(3):2

Ersser S, Tutton E (eds) 1991 Primary nursing in perspective. Scutari, London

Fox T 1988 Feel the quality. Geriatric Nursing and Home Care 8(7):12–13

Gillies D A 1994 Nursing management: a systems approach, 3rd edn. W B Saunders, Philadelphia

Hanks D 1994 Teamwork in rehabilitation: learning from sports. Journal of Rehabilitation 60(1): 12–16

Kemp N, Richardson K 1994 The nursing process & quality care. Edward Arnold, London

Manley K 1989 Primary nursing in intensive care unit. Scutari, London

Manthey M 1992 The practice of primary nursing. King's Fund Centre, London

Mead D 1990 Research report: collegial relationships among primary and associate nurses. Nursing Times 86(42):68

NHSME 1992 One year on. The nurse executive director post: report on the role and function of the nurse executive director post in first wave NHS Trusts. NHSME

Pearson A 1988 Primary nursing in the Burford and Oxford Nursing Development Units. Chapman & Hall, USA

Ryan T 1994 All for one and one for all: team building and nursing. Journal of Nursing Management 2:129–134

Townsend R 1994 Organizational structure. In: Gillies D A (ed) Nursing management: a systems approach, 3rd edn. W B Saunders, Philadelphia

Vaughan B, Pillmoor M (eds) 1989 Managing nursing work. Scutari, London

Walton M 1984 Management and managing: a dynamic approach. Harper & Row, Cambridge.

Wright S 1990 My patient – my nurse. Scutari, London

Zejdlik C 1992 Management of spinal cord injury, 2nd edn. Jones & Bartlett, Boston

The coordinating role of nursing within rehabilitation

Amanda Pearson

INTRODUCTION

This section moves on from the previous discussions regarding nursing teams, and attempts to address more specifically the role of nursing within the rehabilitation team. Through exploring the coordination role within nursing in rehabilitation, this role is examined on both a general level within the clinical environment, and at a specialist level looking at this particular role which nursing is ideally suited to undertake. The key aspects covered in this section are:

- why, what and how nursing should coordinate
- the nature and processes involved within the specialist nursing rehabilitation coordinator role
- case management
- a framework for discharge planning, including the need for the development of relationships with community professionals.

THE REHABILITATION NURSE AND COORDINATION

Traditions within rehabilitation are being challenged and must change. Rehabilitation has traditionally been seen as a therapy, the majority of which was physiotherapy, occupational therapy and social work driven. Nursing, has often been perceived as somewhat supplemental to rehabilitation, the 24-hour caring service which ensured that during the recovery period the patient did not develop any untoward complications, such as pressure sores or urinary tract infections (Wood 1993). Clearly there is more to rehabilitation nursing than this, and this concept is promoted and explored throughout this book. However, this perception of the nurse's role being less 'important' may lead some to suggest that nurses could not or should not coordinate rehabilitation. Quite clearly, as a rehabilitation coordinator and a nurse, these are views that the author would oppose. Conversely, the author would argue that as a profession we are in an unique position to undertake such a role. Because of our close contact with the client, we are in the best position to identify the patient's needs and to ensure that each patient has an individual plan of rehabilitation, which is reflected across the 24-hour period. We can also provide the ultimate communication link between all professionals involved in the process (Johnson 1995, Wolf 1989).

In a clinical position the need for a nurse in this role is clear. Within the rehabilitation process the involvement of many professionals and agencies can appear most confusing to patients and their significant others.

The one constant within it all and whom they all recognise is the nurse. This universal identity places the nurse ideally when communication, clarification and advice is required. Uniquely, nurses are available 24 hours a day, 7 days a week.

More than in any other discipline, nurses are expected to be 'generic' in their working, not only providing nurse-prescribed intervention and evaluation but also interventions prescribed by other disciplines. This aspect has been covered extensively Chapter 6 Part A, and so requires no further exploration here. However, it does suggest that nursing is best placed not only to coordinate the day-to-day activities within the rehabilitation environment, but also to provide the overview required to coordinate the rehabilitation process as a whole. Key to this is effective and objective evaluation. To give an example, we have all had patients who perform wonderfully in the gym or the assessment kitchen, but on return to the ward are completely different; it is nurses who will be able to identify this. Thorough and objective evaluation of the rehabilitation provided for any individual is paramount in achieving the optimum level of independence. It is the nurse who is able to provide this. In addition, due to this more 'generic' style of working, it follows that nurses have a greater awareness of the role of other disciplines and agencies than perhaps any other health workers. Again this is fundamental if appropriate referral and effective collaboration are to be achieved, both of which are vital elements of coordination.

In the nursing role we often act as the centre for communication, and this is probably the key to both the need for and success of the coordinating role (Booth & Waters 1995, Brillhart & Sills 1984). If we were to identify areas of weakness within our rehabilitation environments, often the reasons could be traced to ineffective communication (Henderson et al 1990, Strasser et al 1994). If we were then to highlight the key skill we require to ensure maximum efficiency, we would also say communication. The coordination role, which generally nursing provides as a pivotal point in health care, must therefore hinge on the need to facilitate communication. Again this is the case at a ward level or unit level, through the use of a specified specialist rehabilitation coordinator.

THE NURSE COORDINATOR IN REHABILITATION

At a time when our patients are living longer and have more complicated medical problems, where in-patient and discharge resources are limited, despite the barriers to be overcome, successful and meaningful rehabilitation must remain the goal. More than ever this changing health-care situation suggests the need for effective team-working facilitated by a coordinated approach. The coordination of this process should aim to develop a team the performance of which is greater than the sum of the individual contributions. Many authors have promoted interdisciplinary team-working rather than a traditional multidisciplinary approach (Davies et al 1992, McGrath & Davies 1992, Wood 1993). The key differences between the two approaches are briefly outlined in Box 6.7.

■ BOX 6.7 Comparison of interdisciplinary and multidisciplinary team approaches to rehabilitation

Interdisciplinary team-working	Multidisciplinary team-working
• Recognises and uses skills of many disciplines	• Recognises and uses skills of many disciplines
• Roles more blurred, often joint working	• Clear and defined discipline roles
• Client-orientated goals	• Professional goals (e.g. physiotherapy, nursing, occupational therapy goals)
• Often utilises collaborative patient notes	• Usually utilises individual discipline notes
• General move towards rehabilitation models that are socially orientated, focusing on handicap	• Focus tends to be on impairment or physiological functioning

In examining what the achievement of this involves, it is worth first defining what one needs to be able to undertake in order to perform the role of specialist rehabilitation coordinator. To be able to coordinate effectively:

- you must have a professional background which contributes to an understanding the process
- you must be prepared to become generic in nature
- you must be an advocate for all other professions involved in the process
- you must have an open/collaborative leadership style
- you need to understand the society to which your patients belong.

The establishment and maintenance of interdisciplinary working within the process is paramount to effectiveness. The coordinator is key, in that he is able to evaluate objectively discipline-based activities, team-working and the effects of both of these on patient outcome.

The development of such a role involves research, piloting and implementation of projects and evaluation, and needs a consistently rigorous approach and enthusiasm, not only for the role, but also towards the aims and success of the service itself. In order to carry this out effectively there is a need to identify the needs of the patient group, the needs of all professionals involved in that process, and the quality or outcomes expected.

For example, in the early stages of the introduction of a rehabilitation process to the orthopaedic/trauma area in which the author works, two key projects were implemented to facilitate rehabilitation team-working between disciplines, thereby contributing to improved rehabilitation services. These were:

- collaborative patient notes
- the establishment of regular patient-focused interdisciplinary meetings.

These demonstrate well how the coordinator is able to facilitate the process through centralising communication systems and identifying clear channels of communication. These two projects alone were the main focus for the first 3 months of the project. As a nurse, the overview the author had of the other disciplines enabled her to investigate current practices, absorb new information and skills, and establish an effective relationship with significant personnel, in order to drive forward such collaborative ideas.

In the case of the collaborative notes it was not about implementing a new idea, but rather introducing a new concept, and enabling colleagues to unravel their individual needs and wants to create a working document. The role of the coordinator was to ensure that the team members met regularly, agreed some time-scales, shared responsibility, and kept a patient focus at all times.

The role of coordinator is not confined to leading interdisciplinary working, but also includes investigating and challenging existing practices and leading the development of new practice. In the redesigning of rehabilitation services roles such as key workers and case managers have been developed. Their role is, in essence, to coordinate the effective and efficient rehabilitation and timely discharge of their individual patients.

This ability to challenge, suggest, question and predict freely based on case-related incidents exposes the core objectives for a project plan and for establishing performance measures. The rehabilitation co-ordinator, being exposed to vast amounts of information related to all aspects of rehabilitation, can then proceed to coordinate innovative changes, research, clinical practice, the sharing of management/leadership tools, and objectively evaluate as the needs of the process and the changing health service demands. For example, again from actual clinical practice, a standard that the average length of stay for a fractured neck of the femur should be 15 days was examined. This statement provided a tool to explore current practice, identify key activities to track performance, set targets based on achieving best practice (where we want to be) and establish the baseline (where we are now). Outline results of the activities that were identified as being required to meet this standard more effectively are given in Box 6.8. This demonstrates not only the value of interdisciplinary working, but also the need for effective leadership. Furthermore, it shows that, even though all those involved are managed independently, they all work within a process that aims towards common goals. The author suggests, therefore, that a coaching and facilitation style of leadership is preferable.

In order to see the true effects of change, all those involved, however great or small their contribution, need to see the progress being achieved. As a team it is essential that the members agree common ground for the sharing and displaying of data, especially if it is to be seen or used process-wide. In the initial stages individuals are protective of their own data; later, they will see that the data are an evaluation tool, and that their primary use will inevitably be to identify the deficit between need and the resources available. In the beginning, agreeing common ground may be difficult; however, if there is a joint written mission statement and goals, together with ground rules agreed by all involved, a point to evaluate

■ **BOX 6.8 Coordinating improvements in meeting standards**

Performance measure:
Average length of patient stay for a fractured neck of the femur

Baseline: average length of stay 21 days		Target: 100% within 15 days	
Discussion	Action	By whom	By when
1. Assessment of patients on admission for PT and OT within 24 hours	• To remove referral form, all patients will be discussed each morning to establish the need for PT input • OT still need referral forms as they are centrally managed. To monitor effectiveness of system and suggest adopting system used for PT	Senior II physiotherapist Head III occupational therapist	1 January
2. All disciplines need to make assessment material available in the collaborative patient notes	• All staff within the process to receive teaching regarding effective use of the notes. • OT and PT at present need to keep patient notes centrally, a summary of input will be documented in the collaborative notes	Rehabilitation coordinator Senior II physiotherapist and head III occupational therapist to inform all staff and to monitor increase in administration time	1 month 1 month
3. There is a need for weekly multidisciplinary meetings. All disciplines must attend. Aim for collaborative discharge planning with team responsibility for effectiveness	• Form a list of 'good' times for the meetings from each discipline. • Format for meetings to be universal, rehabilitation coordinator to chair	Rehabilitation coordinator, senior II physiotherapist, head III occupational therapist and link social workers	2 weeks

■ **BOX 6.8 (contd)**

Discussion	Action	By whom	By when
4. It was felt that we were not effectively using the patient's day, i.e. when OT came to do washing and dressing with patients, they may have been already washed by nursing staff. The social worker would visit to complete an assessment and find the patient had gone to the PT gym	• To schedule the patient's day. All staff involved in the process to receive information.	Rehabilitation coordinator	2 weeks
	• Both rehabilitation wards to obtain and set up scheduling boards	Ward-based keyworkers	2 weeks
	• Scheduling to be the framework for the working day	Rehabilitation coordinator, senior II physiotherapist, head III occupational therapist, social worker, keyworkers	3 weeks

OT, occupational therapy; PT, physiotherapy.

from and work towards is established. Such a mission statement could be as follows:

As a team we will provide an interdisciplinary approach to rehabilitation in order to effect a safe and timely discharge. We will involve all significant others within this process, relatives, carers, specialists, and community professionals. We will regularly monitor and evaluate our process to ensure that we maintain high standards.

From this goals are identified, which enable the achievement of the mission. These may include, for example:

1. We will hold interdisciplinary meetings weekly, ensuring that all relevant professionals are present.
2. We will set a discharge date for all our patients within 24 hours of admission.
3. We will make referrals to all other relevant professionals within 24 hours of assessment of need.
4. We will involve relatives/carers in all discharge plans.
5. We will monitor and review our set performance measures monthly, and develop an action plan to address any issues arising.

Here we see the need for performance monitoring as one of the main goals, a topic which often tends to be a delicate one, especially when the monitoring crosses discipline boundaries (Strasser et al 1994). Team members may perceive a threat through concern that it will indicate poor individual performance, potentially resulting in the true data not being shared. It is essential that agreement is reached regarding to whom and in what format this information will be given. The need is for an approach that is sensitive to the 'threat' which some may perceive, while also being firm.

In the author's experience the most effective way to use data from performance tracking is to display it positively or predictively. If you show what you are able to achieve, the target set, the reasons for the deficit and proposals for improvement, you are in an excellent position to obtain resources. If a target was set that 75% of patients referred to a social worker would be seen within 2 days of referral, knowing that the establishment of social workers for the number of patients was insufficient, the performance measure would actively support this if achievement was consistently well below target. However, the workers involved would initially be apprehensive, aware that the data could reflect personal effects on their case load. There is a great need for consistent education/support to ensure that regular review of performance does not become demoralising. In the author's experience, for example, simply choosing in the beginning to display the number of neck of femur fracture data allowed everyone to incorporate data collection in their daily workload and reinforced that this was not a threat but a valuable basis upon which to build cases of need.

Having monitored this performance measure for several months, it was soon apparent that a lot of effort was going into data collection, but it was unclear what use it was. The team discussed what they needed to demonstrate. A core theme was the essence of a 7-day service from all professionals. It was therefore agreed to monitor the percentage of patients discharged within 15 days, inclusive of the weekend, even though there was no physiotherapy, occupational therapy or social work input. This would enable the team to identify quickly what could be possible and make a judgment about the extra resources that would be required. The new data proved to be more powerful, especially the collated quantitative data, which enabled us to define clearly the reasons for high or low performance (Fig. 6.2).

CASE MANAGEMENT AND DISCHARGE PLANNING

Case management has core aims that are well documented (Gerber 1994, Hale 1995, Waterman et al 1996) and include:

- management and coordination of the acute, rehabilitation and reintegration process for individual clients
- to increase liaison and collaboration with community professionals
- to increase rehabilitation knowledge within the community
- to decrease the dependency of community professionals on acute NHS provisions
- to empower patients and their relatives and promote independence, self-reliance and self-esteem.

	February	March	April	May	June	July
% of #NOFs discharged within 15 days	46	48	50	55	60	70
Target	100	100	100	100	100	100

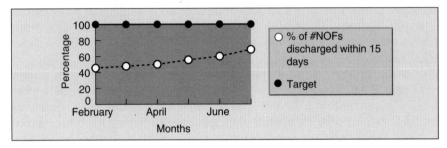

Figure 6.2 The percentage of patients with neck of femur fracture discharged within the target period of 15 days.

Case management allows an individualised, multiprofessional, yet co-ordinated approach to rehabilitation, which takes into account the needs of everyone involved in the process. It involves providing the patient with a constant person during what can be a complex experience, someone who holds an overview of the case, who is able to address specific needs and has a trusting relationship with the patient and his relatives/carers.

The essence of case management is a framework for efficient and effective rehabilitation and discharge planning. There are seven key points in effective discharge planning:

- assessment of social circumstances on admission
- early diagnosis and medical plan
- early setting of a multidisciplinary agreed discharge date
- early establishment of communication with relatives/carers
- appropriate referral to community professionals
- clear patient-focused rehabilitation and discharge plan
- a method of evaluating the effectiveness and efficiency of the processes in place.

For a rehabilitation process to have clear direction, specifically related to the clinical process of rehabilitation and discharge, it is essential to develop a project plan. The plan should include all relevant project work, internally derived from the process, and also external work that directly influences the working of the process (Fig. 6.3).

Alongside the plan there must be a clear framework for discharge planning within the process. The key to a successful discharge framework is the production of a clear, concise document which is user-friendly at clinical level. Most NHS trusts have well-established local discharge frameworks, their main strength being that they are jointly developed with the Department of Social Services. However, the common criticism is that, as working documents, they are jargonistic, complex and contain ill-

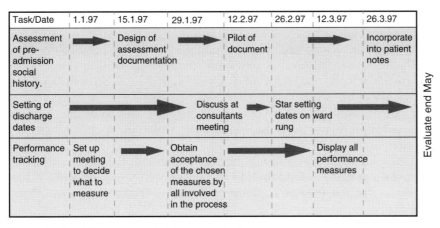

Task/Date	1.1.97	15.1.97	29.1.97	12.2.97	26.2.97	12.3.97	26.3.97	
Assessment of pre-admission social history.		Design of assessment documentation		Pilot of document			Incorporate into patient notes	Evaluate end May
Setting of discharge dates				Discuss at consultants meeting	Star setting dates on ward rung			
Performance tracking	Set up meeting to decide what to measure		Obtain acceptance of the chosen measures by all involved in the process			Display all performance measures		

Figure 6.3 Rehabilitation and discharge project plan.

defined criteria. The rehabilitation coordinator is fundamentally important in ensuring that the specific framework designed for his client group is in line with local policy, but compensates for its weaknesses. On investigation of the use and relevance of such a framework, it is clear that breaking down the terminology and choosing an appropriate way to demonstrate it are essential in its transferable use to clinical practitioners.

An example of such a framework could be in the form of a planner. If a discharge planner was incorporated into collaborative patient notes it would provide instant access by anyone to information from any relevant discipline. The key sections of the planner would include:

- planned discharge date
- actual discharge date (this allows for automatic auditing of reasons for delay)
- list of equipment provided, from where it was ordered, when and where it is to be delivered, or by whom it is to be collected
- list of items to leave the ward with the patient
- the tablets prescribed to take home, the supply sent, and information given to the patient and relative/carer
- the date and time of the follow-up appointment if required, and by whom it was arranged
- the amount of social care arranged (i.e. the number of visits and their purpose)
- name and address of the general practitioner to which the discharge summary was sent
- list of referrals to community professionals, reason for referral, supplies provided and contact numbers
- mode of transport arranged, and date and time
- name of relative/carer informed of the discharge
- a section for the discharging professional to sign on the day of discharge.

This planner should be a working document, incorporated in the interdisciplinary meetings and the daily evaluation of care. It will facilitate effective collaborative communication of the plan with the patient, relatives and fellow professionals. It is common for the majority of relatives to visit out of hours and at weekends when not all professionals are available. This document, if efficiently maintained, will enable anyone to provide information, relevant to all disciplines, based on their assessments. This type of planner also enables new or less experienced staff to understand the discharge process, have instant evidence of the standard expected from them and, most importantly, a place to document relevant information.

A copy of the planner should be sent home with the patient, as again it provides valuable information to all who are involved with a individual at home, whether they be community-based professionals or family and friends.

The role of community professionals in the success of hospital discharge cannot be emphasised enough. Discharge planning must incorporate early and appropriate referral so that a smooth transition from hospital back to the client's community can be achieved. As with all services, resources are limited, and therefore it is often such forward planning of their allocation which is needed to effect a timely discharge. There is a need for both an understanding and an appreciation of how community services are funded and managed to ensure that we refer appropriately. In rehabilitation environments it is important to include in the process:

- opportunities for regular sharing of knowledge and skills
- the building of relationships
- problem-solving
- a forum to evaluate effectiveness.

It is not unreasonable to suggest that any conflict between hospital and community-based professionals is perhaps due to the lack of the above. For example, it is not uncommon for hospital discharges to occur on a Friday or a weekend. However, if a patient requires complex district nurse input, this will be an inappropriate day for discharge, as the staff available is limited. Awareness of service provision out of hours and at weekends will ensure that such cases do not occur. As professionals, generally we are not very accommodating of criticism or complaints. However, the most effective way to manage such situations would be to turn them into needs. If the resources of the community were not properly evaluated prior to discharge and a problem occurs, it would be valuable to invite that professional to an interdisciplinary forum in which he can share the problems/ issues he faces and jointly decide on how to prevent their reccurrence.

The forum that provides the best environment for joint planning is the home visit. This provides the hospital-based professionals with the real picture, and enables precise assessment of abilities within the patient's own environment and of limitations placed on community professionals which would not have been seen if the assessment had been hospital based. A problem arises that in most environments we are only able to arrange such visits for complicated cases, which limits the opportunities to network. From the author's experience with complex discharges, early involvement of community professionals not only enables identification of problems, access to local resources, and an added perspective, but also a more efficient discharge, where going home becomes a part of the process instead of the end of hospitalisation and the beginning of care in the community.

SUMMARY

To end this section you should consider the following key points as essential within the development of a coordinator's role:

- Identification of key performance measures related to your process, which the role would affect.
- An evaluation of current rehabilitation and discharge, from which goals are jointly set.
- The establishment of effective and efficient interdisciplinary team-working.
- The reduction of barriers and improved communication with community professionals.
- The ability to affect the efficiency and quality of rehabilitation and discharge.
- To develop and implement innovative ideas/concepts, move the role forward and maintain a focus on changing patient needs.

Although there has been a focus on the development of this specialist role, one would emphasise that all nurses in the rehabilitation environment have coordination as one of their key roles. Often it is this day-to-day coordination outlined earlier in the chapter which is fundamental to the success or otherwise of the whole rehabilitation process.

REFERENCES

Booth J, Waters K R 1995 The multifaceted role of the nurse in the day hospital. Journal of Advanced Nursing 22:700–706
Brillhart B, Sills F 1984 Analysis of the roles and responsibilities of rehabilitation staff. Rehabilitation Nurse 19(3):145–150
Davies A, Davis S, Moss N et al 1992 First steps towards an interdisciplinary approach to rehabilitation. Clinical Rehabilitation 6:237–244
Gerber L S 1994 Case management models: geriatric nursing prototypes for growth. Journal of Gerontological Nursing 20(7):18–24
Hale C 1995 Case management and case managed care. Nursing Standard 9(19):33–35
Henderson E S, Morrison J A, Young E A, Portland B 1990 The nurse in rehabilitation after severe brain injury. Clinical Rehabilitation 4:167–172
Johnson J 1995 Achieving effective rehabilitation outcomes: does the nurse have a role? British Journal of Therapy and Rehabilitation 2(3):113–118
McGrath J R, Davies A M 1992 Rehabilitation – where do we go and how do we get there? Clinical Rehabilitation 6:225–235
Strasser C, Falconer J A, Saltzmann D 1994 The rehabilitation team: staff perceptions of the hospital environment, the interdisciplinary team environment, and interprofessional relations. Archives of Medical and Physical Rehabilitation 75:177–182
Waterman H, Waters K, Awenat Y 1996 The introduction of case management on a rehabilitation floor. Journal of Advanced Nursing 24(5):960–967
Waters K R, Luker K A 1996 Staff perceptions on the role of the nurse in rehabilitation wards for elderly people. Journal of Clinical Nursing 5:105–114
Wolf Z R 1989 Uncovering the hidden work of nursing. Nursing and Health Care 10:463–467
Wood R 1993 The rehabilitation team. In: Greenwood R, Barnes M P, McMillan T M, Ward C D (eds) Neurological rehabilitation. Churchill Livingstone, Edinburgh, p 41–49

The rehabilitation nurse as auditor and researcher

7

The rehabilitation nurse as auditor

Mike Smith

INTRODUCTION

The aim of this chapter is to explore the principles relating to the measurement of rehabilitation nursing. The concept of evaluation and measurement is introduced, including an examination of the reasons why we need to evaluate rehabilitation nursing. A brief discussion of the types and characteristics of measurement tools is given, before looking in more detail at the practical aspects of measuring what we are doing in rehabilitation nursing practice.

Two basic principles form the basis of measuring nursing. These are the need for objectivity (i.e. that something is indeed measurable), and the need to test whether a service or intervention has achieved a particular goal or standard (St Leger et al 1992).

Objectivity is vital if results from evaluation or measurement are to be considered useful. It suggests a freedom from any potential bias in the person undertaking the measurement and, therefore, reasonable accuracy. It is the combination of these two factors that enables the use of the results in the clinical setting. In simple terms, for something to be objective it must have a particular unit of measurement attached to it (e.g. a time-scale, a weight or a distance).

The second factor is that of the requirement to measure against a particular goal or standard. The principles of goals were covered in Chapter 1. In essence, goals are usually in the form of a stated aim (e.g. 85% of patients will return to work following myocardial infarction, or the client will be able to inject his own insulin independently).

COMPONENTS OF THE EVALUATION PROCESS

As with any activity related to the delivery of health care, effective planning is the key to successful implementation of any measurement. The key factors that must be taken into account prior to undertaking any type of formal measurement (Agency for Health Care Policy and Research 1992) are listed in Box 7.1, and form the basis of this chapter.

■ **BOX 7.1 Key factors in measurement**

- Who wants it? (This will often indicate what and why it is to be done.)
- Which measuring tool is to be used?
- How is measurement to be done?
- Are the people responsible able to do it?
- How is it to be used?

- Identification of the persons or agencies requiring evaluation will often determine what exactly is to be measured and how detailed or complex the evaluation needs to be.
- Identification of which measuring tool(s) is to be used will be discussed in detail later in this chapter.
- When deciding how the evaluation process will be implemented, one must identify the person(s) responsible for undertaking the evaluation (e.g. individual or team), the actual process to be used and how results will be disseminated.
- The personnel involved may need training in order to undertake the required evaluation.
- How the information gained will be used and any relationship between this information and other evaluations performed need to be identified. The often complex nature of rehabilitation may mean that different measurement tools are being used at the same time. It may be that the results of a particular measurement will impact on the interpretation of other results.

WHY MEASURE REHABILITATION NURSING?

The persons requiring or demanding the evaluation or measurement must be identified, so that the content and extent of information detail required can be determined. It is worth stressing that evaluation of what we do within rehabilitation nursing is not an optional exercise, it is demanded by all parties involved in the delivery of rehabilitation services. Although some of these issues are covered in greater detail later in this chapter, it is worth emphasising them here, and they are briefly outlined below.

THE CLIENT

Clearly the major interested party is the individual on the receiving end of the service. The patient or client is entitled to receive the optimum service available and, rightly, expects and desires meaningful outcomes. In Chapter 1 much importance was placed on rehabilitation services being client centred. If we are to demonstrate that we have done a good job, this underpinning philosophy of identifying client needs and goals (rather than professional goals) will prove essential. With developments in technology there are increased expectations of health care generally, including in the field of rehabilitation, and much has been made of the rights of patients, notably within documents such as *The Patient's Charter*.

NURSING PROFESSION

By indicating the success or otherwise of what we do within rehabilitation nursing, measurement or evaluation is at the very foundation of decision-making in the continuous nature of the nursing process within clinical practice. As well as it being ethically correct to aim for optimum effectiveness within our work for the client, and to provide evidence of such, it is also vital in maintaining professional credibility. The low profile that rehabilitation nursing has had in comparison with other rehabilitation disciplines may have been due in part to this lack of professional credibility with regard to nursing 'making a difference'. Anecdotally, public opinion of nursing and what it does still appears very favourable. This will undoubtedly be reinforced and indeed strengthened if we can demonstrate our effectiveness formally.

OTHER REHABILITATION PROFESSIONALS

As outlined in earlier chapters with reference to the role of the nurse as team worker, the intervention of other team members will often be dependent on information provided by nurses. This is obviously particularly apparent in rehabilitation, where interdisciplinary team-working is often a fundamental principle as a means of delivering services. Therefore, through their unique 24-hour system of work, nurses are not only well placed to evaluate prescribed 'nursing care', but also to contribute to the evaluation of the prescribed interventions of other disciplines.

PURCHASERS OR COMMISSIONERS OF REHABILITATION

The introduction of the White Paper *Working for Patients* (Secretary of State for Health 1989) and the resulting purchaser–provider relationship has had a substantial influence on rehabilitation units. The exact implications of the recently announced changes to the structure of the National Health Service (NHS) are not yet entirely clear. However, it is certain that the commissioning bodies will be determining what services rehabilitation clients are to be offered. As with any 'buyer', the bottom line remains whether or not such a system delivers value for money. Purchasers of rehabilitation services do have a right to know that they are paying for an effective and efficient service. It would be a mistake not to emphasise this fact. It cannot be ignored, as the very viability of rehabilitation services may be threatened without evidence of this. Clearly, without continuing purchaser support, and therefore financial security, some healthcare services will not survive.

THE ORGANISATION

The organisation within which rehabilitation services are provided is responsible for the accurate allocation of resources to particular units. A major part of this is the issue of manpower planning. Measurement of the influence of nursing is vital in order to minimise the potential for inappropriate skill mix or inadequate levels of staffing.

GOVERNMENT

There is currently a government-led demand to deliver evidence-based practice, and the motives behind this may be viewed with suspicion (e.g. cost cutting to health services). Despite such concerns one must continue to stress that it is professionally and ethically correct to prove that what we do is worthwhile. To emphasise this desire for evidence-based health care, the Department of Health (NHS Executive 1994) has suggested that evidence may potentially determine future priorities for funding within health care.

MEASUREMENT TOOLS

WHAT ARE WE TO MEASURE: STRUCTURE, PROCESS, OUTCOME?

In view of the above agencies requiring measurement of the success or otherwise in meeting goals or standards, it is reasonable to surmise that the emphasis is focused ultimately on outcome (i.e. the impact or result of a service). However, it is also important to measure structure (represented essentially by a service's fixed costs, e.g. staff, equipment and environment) and process (i.e. the processes through which a service is delivered). These three variables, originating from the work of Donabedian (1980), provide a framework within which to measure all aspects of rehabilitation. Clearly this is important because, to reach any end-point could involve both effective and ineffective processes, and both good and poor use of resources.

CLASSIFICATION OF MEASUREMENT TOOLS

Measurement tools can be classified into one of four distinct categories: nominal, ordinal, interval or ratio. A brief discussion of each is given below. However, the reader is encouraged to refer to other texts for more detail.

Nominal measures

Nominal measures categorise items into groups, allowing frequencies to be measured. No particular order is measured. For example, nominal measures include classifying subjects as male or female or into particular diagnostic or impairment groups (e.g. traumatic brain injury, Parkinson's disease or lower limb amputees).

Ordinal scales

Ordinal scales are used to put sets of data into some form of rank order, often using some form of 'scoring'. It is important to emphasise that a difference in score is not an indication of absolute mathematical difference, but a rank order only. An obvious commonly used example is pain scales. In this case, although one may get an indication of the intensity of pain on a scale of 0 to 5, the difference between a score of 1 and a score of 2 does not indicate that the pain is twice as severe or that the difference in pain severity is the same as if the score had risen from 3 to 4. Other ordinal scales used in rehabilitation include many of the functional measures related to disability (e.g. Barthel and FIM) based on grading levels of independence.

Interval measures

The distinct difference between an ordinal and an interval scale, as the name suggests, is that in the latter an identical interval exists between scores (i.e. the difference between a score of 2 and a score of 3 is the same as the difference between 4 and 5). An important point to note is that interval measures do not rely on an absolute zero being present in the measurement tool. Such tools are less commonly used in rehabilitation than are nominal and ordinal measures.

Ratio measures

As with interval measures, in a ratio measure the interval between scores is identical. The major difference is that a ratio measure involves the presence of an absolute zero. Examples include measuring time, distance or weight.

CHARACTERISTICS OF MEASUREMENT TOOLS

Once the type of scale to be used has been determined, the next stage is to assess the appropriateness of particular measuring tools. There are six key characteristics to consider when choosing a measuring tool (Wade 1992):

- relevance
- validity
- reliability
- sensitivity
- simplicity
- communicability.

The development of measuring tools can often be difficult, and it is undoubtedly worth considering the use of a previously validated tool that will serve the purpose.

Relevance

Relevance is concerned with focusing exclusively on the key issues to be measured. Collection of data is often expensive in terms of resources, both financial and in terms of that most valuable resource, the rehabilitation nurse's time. Therefore, it is essential that the measure is specific to what is needed in a particular situation and does not collect too much or too little information.

Validity

A valid tool can be defined as one that measures what it is designed to measure. This involves removal of variables that may adversely affect the accuracy of the result. There are many aspects to validity (e.g. environmental, the presence of other impairments, and time-scale (particularly in retrospective studies)), which again the reader is encouraged to investigate further.

Reliability

Reliability refers to how repeatable the test is with regard to obtaining the same 'score'. One could examine this from two standpoints. First, would the same score be obtained by the same observer on another occasion; and, second, would the same score be obtained by two or more different observers. Factors influencing reliability include the provision of adequate training for observers and the complexity of the measure being used.

Sensitivity

In some cases the ability of the measuring tool to detect change (i.e. its sensitivity) may be questioned. Using again the example of pain scores, a scale that offers three alternatives would not be as sensitive as one that offers ten points when measuring the same variable. A scale that is insufficiently sensitive may not produce meaningful results, whereas a scale that is complex and contains many points may affect reliability due to its recording errors of the investigator.

Simplicity

Simplicity refers to how user-friendly the measurement tool is. A tool that is simple in design and easy to complete will aid both compliance and accuracy of response.

Communicability

Communicability refers to the ease with which the results can be reported and understood by others. If the results of any measurement are designed to affect the practice of rehabilitation nursing, this is obviously vital.

EVALUATION OF REHABILITATION NURSING OUTCOME

Evaluation within the nursing process is continuous, involving both the nurse and the patient. Progress against set goals should be measured, either by the nurse exclusively or, commonly in rehabilitation, by the inter-disciplinary team. Such evaluation may occur on a continual basis during care delivery, or on a 'snap-shot' basis (often at the end of shift).

There are four possible broad results of evaluation:

- the expected result has been achieved
- some aspects have been achieved
- new or different priorities have been identified, and therefore the goal is no longer valid
- the expected result has not been achieved.

After the evaluation has been performed, planned interventions can be maintained as currently prescribed, adapted, reprioritised or abandoned if the intervention is completely ineffective. If client goals related to nursing activity have been only partially achieved or not achieved at all, the evaluating nurse must question why this is (e.g. were the goals set realistic in terms of time or resources; did the client want to meet or have the capability of meeting the goal?) The care plan must also be examined to ensure full implementation, from both the nursing and the client perspective.

In the case of goals set with the whole team, there should be inter-disciplinary measures of outcome (Freeman et al 1996). Formal outcome measures can and often are used within rehabilitation environments. The use of measures of disability (e.g. FIM (Hamilton et al 1987) and the Barthel index (Mahoney & Barthel 1965)) and, more recently, those of handicap (e.g. the Craig handicap assessment and recording technique, i.e. CHART (Whiteneck et al 1992)) and quality-of-life, is becoming increasingly common. Although these measures are usually performed on an inter-disciplinary basis, it is important that the nursing contribution to outcome can be determined in both the rehabilitation practice and process. This is the key means by which we can evaluate nursing performance, and so justify the specialism of rehabilitation nursing.

EVALUATING REHABILITATION NURSING PROCESSES

Generally speaking, processes are the way in which the service is organised and performed. Although it is important to determine the success of the processes used in service delivery, because there is commonly involvement and interaction of many agencies in rehabilitation, it can be difficult to extract the information relating specifically to nursing. Despite this, it could be suggested that the established interdisciplinary team approach that rehabilitation commonly adopts contributes well to the evaluation of process, in comparison to other areas. Three potential approaches are described here: peer review, nursing audit and integrated care pathways.

PEER REVIEW

Peer review is the process through which one's performance is critically evaluated by others. There is little evidence in the recent literature of this being used in many practice areas, however guidelines have been offered by some authors (Burnard 1987) for its implementation. If peer review is to be used, a key first stage is to create an environment that facilitates this. Without the level of trust necessary to enable the rehabilitation nurse to pass judgment on and accept judgment from a colleague, it is a system clearly doomed to failure. All participants must accept the process before implementation, which may require a significant amount of persuasion, education and support.

A less threatening practical approach to implementing peer review, and therefore one that may prove to be more acceptable, is one where the nurse presents, using the processes of reflection, a case study or critical incident in which he was involved. The relevant peer could then contribute suggestions on how the intervention could have been improved.

An undoubted advantage of peer review is that it promotes the idea that quality of performance is the responsibility of the practitioners, rather than exclusively a responsibility of nursing management. In addition, it promotes ownership of developments and improvements in nursing practice.

NURSING AUDIT

By definition, nursing audit is a quality assurance mechanism for monitoring and evaluating the quality of interventions provided by nursing. The audit process has distinct stages that can be used to evaluate any practice within the rehabilitation setting. Formal nursing audit can be complex or relatively simple, depending on the particular issue being measured. Regardless of the degree of complexity of the audit, the stages in the process are the same and can be artificially separated into three broad categories: development of the audit tool, the preparation required, and implementation of the audit process. Each stage is explored below, using as an example a relatively small area of nursing practice.

Development of the audit tool

There are three stages in this category. These are listed in Box 7.2, and illustrated using the example of recording fluid balance.

Preparation for the audit

This comprises two stages. First, it must be ensured that the auditors are trained in the use of the tool, so that the reliability of the audit is maximised. In the above example the auditors must be familiar with the fluid balance chart and with the audit tool. Not only would a pilot scheme of using the tool be of benefit in assessing its usability, but this could also prove an effective means of training staff in its use. Secondly, once training

■ BOX 7.2 The development of an audit tool

Stage	Example
1. Identification of the practice/ intervention to be evaluated	Recording fluid balance
2. Development of standard which the audit team believe is acceptable	A comprehensive and accurate record of fluid intake and urinary output should be kept on all patients who are using an intermittent catheter for bladder management
3. Development of the criteria necessary to achieve the standard	• The patient has a fluid balance chart for the previous day • The patient's target intake is specified at the top of the chart • There is an entry in the intake column for every hour, either stating the volume of fluid taken or that fluid was refused by the patient • The intermittent catheter times are specified at the top of the chart • There is an entry in the output column against each of the specified times • The intake column has been totalled • The output column has been totalled • There is an entry in the kardex relating to fluid balance

is complete, a formal date should be set for the audit to take place. Results obtained prove to be more valid if this date is not known to the clinical staff, as in this way a 'real' picture is obtained.

Implementation of the audit process

The audit process itself is cyclical in nature and comprises four stages.

1. The auditors perform the audit, using the criteria and 'rules' for assessment as identified above.

2. The results from the audit are analysed, often in the form of frequencies or percentages (e.g. 80% of charts audited had intake totals recorded). This will serve to indicate 'problem areas' in the defined area of practice.

3. An action plan is developed using a standard objective-setting format

with the nursing team to address the identified problem areas. Often such actions are educational in nature (e.g. the importance of monitoring fluid balance may need to be reinforced, or it may be that the area of practice is not clearly defined and procedures or policies need revision).

4. A data for re-audit is agreed, allowing sufficient time for actions to be implemented. The process begins again.

Audit and research

Although research in rehabilitation nursing is not within the remit of this section, it is worth briefly outlining the similarities and the definite differences between audit and research (Table 7.1).

INTEGRATED CARE PATHWAYS

Commonly originating from acute services within the USA, clinical care pathways (or integrated care pathways) are a tool that has been used to guide the multidisciplinary team process and activity involved in providing health care. They act as an audit tool which potentially highlights improvements that can be made to the service delivery. Hotchkiss (1997) suggested six features which are inherent in an integrated pathway.

1. It is the only record of patient care used by the whole multidisciplinary team.

2. It is located near or actually with the patient. Although currently

Table 7.1 Comparison of audit and research

	Audit	Research
Purpose	Evaluate and improve nursing practice at a local level	Provide additional nursing knowledge, which can be generalised to populations or clinical groups, on which to base clinical practice
Process	Analysis of quality (cyclical process)	Scientific inquiry (linear process)
Methods	Utilises data that already exist as a result of current nursing practice	Utilises data that often require the use of additional measuring tools
Sample	Measurement against a standard with one or more clients	Statistical significance is required. Strict inclusion criteria are necessary and, often, large groups of patients
Reporting of findings	Primarily nursing staff working in area. The standard and audit tool may be disseminated to other similar centres	Responsibility to disseminate results widely so results can be applied on a global scale
Time-scale	Changes are immediate and ongoing as part of the audit cycle	Changes may take a significant period of time

most seem to be paper based, it is likely that such pathways will become computerised on a network system, allowing team members to input information in their own department. This will also facilitate the speed with which the information can be analysed.

3. It provides information relating to the sequence and types of intervention, time-scales and person(s) responsible. An advantage of this is the ease with which nursing interventions can be identified.

4. Variances from the pathway plan are recorded. These are often recorded on a separate variance sheet (Baldry & Rossiter 1995), which would include the reason for the variance. This would allow easier analysis and action planning to address any deficits or difficulties.

5. A plan or practice may be adjusted following audit of the variances.

6. As they are often pre-printed, there is minimum free text.

Feedback from rehabilitation areas that have implemented integrated care plans has been almost entirely positive in nature (Metcalf 1991, Rossiter & Thompson 1995). Improvements that have been cited include:

- better cross-discipline communication
- a reduction in duplication of information within documentation
- facilitating staff training and orientation/induction programmes
- through the audit process, it impacts positively on the care provision, process and outcome of care.

Although the author is enthusiastic about investigating the use of integrated care pathways, further work is needed to determine if such benefits are actually commonplace. However, we must take care to ensure that such pathways do focus on systems only (e.g. goal-planning every 2 weeks, the need for referral and involvement of appropriate disciplines, and formal patient education). It seems essential that the pathways do not entirely dictate what we do. If client needs are indeed related to the individual and his interaction with his society, as promoted throughout this book, then interventions will be specific to those needs. Therefore, to be real to that person, there must be a built-in flexibility in the pathways that allows for this individuality. Without this we are inadvertently promoting a professional-orientated process of rehabilitation.

EVALUATING STRUCTURE: RESOURCES FOR REHABILITATION NURSING

The resources for rehabilitation (the structure) incorporate the relatively stable characteristics of the service, such as staff distribution, qualifications and structure. As rehabilitation nursing skills and experience are part of the resources, the evaluation and development of the individual nurse has obvious importance. This is covered in detail in Chapter 9. Other aspects of structure include the physical environment in which rehabilitation takes place, including available equipment. Overall, it could be fairly stated that the structure related to rehabilitation nursing should facilitate rather than inhibit the processes involved.

EVALUATION OF THE REHABILITATION NURSING ENVIRONMENT

There appears to be little in the literature that gives clear specific practical guidance on measuring the appropriateness of the environment in which rehabilitation nursing takes place. In examining the environment, one could divide the issues into those that impact on the client and those that may affect the ability of the nurse to facilitate rehabilitation. These obviously will differ depending on the needs of the particular client group. There are undoubtedly many issues involved, and some are appropriate to both perspectives. A few suggestions of issues that could form the basis of an audit tool are given in Tables 7.2 and 7.3.

NURSING-SKILL MIX IN REHABILITATION

Earlier in the chapter, when discussing the need for evaluation, one of the agencies mentioned was the organisation that determines the staff resources. Unless the contribution of nursing within rehabilitation is clear, the assessment of the appropriate nursing staff numbers, grades and experience is surely at best simply guesswork. One attempt to evaluate the need for nursing staffing levels could be through a patient dependency score. If there is an objective measure of client dependency, and the number of nurses needed for varying levels of dependency is defined, it may be

Table 7.2 Environmental issues from the client's perspective

Issue	Example
Has the client full access to all necessary areas within the rehabilitation environment? (This would include aspects which minimise the impact of disability)	Clear signs suitable for clients with visual impairments. Doors wide enough and open in a way that allows wheelchair use. Does the client have access to all relevant equipment to be self-caring?
Appropriate floor coverings	Is there a non-slip surface facilitating the safety of a client using a walking aid? Does the surface facilitate wheelchair use?
Temperature of the environment	An environment that is too cold may result in physical discomfort, affecting the client's desire to participate, or even causing physical harm to those who have altered ability to control body temperature
Availability of recreational/relaxation facilities	Is there an area where the client can socialise with others? Often re-engaging in social activities is an important part of the rehabilitation (e.g. in gaining peer support) of those with altered body image
Access to areas that allow privacy	Is there a quiet area where a client can discuss issues with his partner?

Table 7.3 Environmental issues from a nursing perspective

Issue	Example
The physical space available to perform prescribed interventions	Sufficient space to assist with mobility without endangering the nurse's back
Areas for meetings and educational activities	Defined area on the ward where in-service training can be provided to increase the knowledge base for rehabilitation
Sufficient storage space	Are there defined and organised areas for storage of equipment which facilitate easy and quick access?
If computerised systems are to be used, are there sufficient terminals and keyboards?	Are there occasions when nursing time is wasted waiting for access?
Appropriate client-to-nurse, and nurse-to-nurse communication systems	Do the nurse call systems work for every patient?
Appropriate systems and facilities for the safe disposal of clinical waste and general rubbish	Are linen skips and rubbish bins overflowing because they have not been removed?
Support from domestic, portering and cleaning services within the rehabilitation area	Are client's appointments delayed due to unavailability of portering?
Sufficient supplies	Are there occasions when nurses must insert an in-dwelling catheter because no intermittent catheters are available?

possible that changes in staffing levels could be made as appropriate. Clearly there is a requirement for duty rosters to have a constant degree of flexibility to facilitate this, otherwise it may only be useful in establishing changes year on year.

Assuming this is a possibility, the next stage is to use a score that can indicate levels of experience or skill mix required. More complex dependency scoring tools may allow this to some degree. One such tool that is under development (Brown & Idiols 1995) allocates a particular score to each specific nurse intervention; if one can relate each intervention to a grade of nurse, the skill mix required can be determined. However, although by totalling of scores an overall dependency score for each patient can be ascertained, this stage has not yet been attempted.

SUMMARY

With the exception of the evaluation performed as part of the day-to-day nursing process, other forms of evaluation have appeared to be less frequently used to date. However, it is clear from the increasing demands from many agencies to demonstrate effectiveness in rehabilitation nursing, that nurses must now view these other methods of evaluation as essential. Not only will they promote the continuation of rehabilitation nursing, they will also enable the desire to improve rehabilitation nursing practice, through guiding areas of development, to be met. Systems must be developed to limit the impact on the time available for practical hands-on nursing (e.g. through the provision of time and resources to undertake this). This is vital, not only for the benefit of the client, but also for nursing itself, which needs to be able to stand proud among other healthcare professions and objectively state the difference it makes. The reader is encouraged to look at his own practice area, to determine to what extent the nursing practice is objectively measured, to define which measurements are possible and beneficial, and to seek out the training and managerial support and resources needed to undertake these measurements.

REFERENCES

Agency for Health Care Policy and Research 1992 Using clinical practice guidelines to evaluate quality of care. US Department of Health and Human Resource Services, Rockville, MD
Baldry J A, Rossiter D 1995 Introduction of integrated care pathways to a neurorehabilitation unit. Physiotherapy 81(8):432–434
Brown S, Idiols J 1995 The London Spinal Unit dependency score. Royal National Orthopaedic Hospital Trust, Stanmore (unpublished).
Burnard P 1987 Self and peer assessment. Senior Nurse 6(5):16–17
Donabedian A 1980 Explorations in quality assessment and monitoring. Vol. 1: The definition of quality and approaches to its assessment. Health Administration Press, Ann Arbor, MI
Freeman J A, Hobart J C, Thompson A J 1996 Outcomes-based research in neurorehabilitation: the need for multidisciplinary team involvement. Disability and Rehabilitation 18(2):106–110
Hamilton B, Granger C V, Sherwin F S, Zielezny M, Tashman T S 1987 A uniform national data system for medical rehabilitation. In: Fuhrer M J (ed) Rehabilitation outcomes analysis and measurement. Brooks, Baltimore
Hotchkiss R 1997 Integrated care pathways. NTResearch 2(1):30–37
McGrath J R, Davies AM 1992 Rehabilitation – where are we going and how do we get there. Clinical Rehabilitation 6:225–235
Mahoney F, Barthel D W 1965 Functional evaluation – the Barthel index. Maryland State Medical Journal 14:342–346
Metcalf E M 1991 The orthopaedic critical path. Orthopaedic Nursing 10(6):25–31
NHS Executive 1994 Priorities and planning guidance for the NHS 1995/96. NHS Executive, Leeds, (EL(94)) 55
Rossiter D, Thompson A J 1995 Introduction of integrated pathways for patients with multiple sclerosis in an inpatient neurorehabilitation setting. Disability and Rehabilitation 17(8):443–448
St Leger A S, Schnieden H, Walsworth-Bell J P 1992 Evaluating health services' effectiveness. Open University Press, Milton Keynes
Secretary of State for Health 1989 Working for patients. HMSO, London
Wade D T 1992 Measurement in neurological rehabilitation. Oxford University Press, Oxford
Whiteneck G, Charlifue S, Gerhart K, Overholser J, Richardson G 1992 Quantifying handicap. A new measure of long term outcomes. Archives of Physical and Medical Rehabilitation 73:519–526

FURTHER READING

Parsley K, Corrigan P 1994 Quality improvement in nursing and healthcare. Chapman & Hall, London
Pilling D, Watson G 1995 Evaluating quality in services for disabled and older people. Jessica Kingsley, London

The nurse as rehabilitation researcher

Sylvie Thorn

INTRODUCTION

A number of challenges face the nursing profession in its attempt to provide high-quality nursing care. In particular, research and its utilisation in practice are thought to be major factors in the provision of high-quality nursing care. Research-based clinical practice has long been recognised as an essential element for the growth of the National Health Service (NHS) and the nursing profession. Indeed, the NHS Research and Development Strategy requires that the care delivered by healthcare personnel be firmly based on research (Department of Health 1991). Nurses, like other healthcare professionals, need to address their responsibilities in the area of research by using, initiating and conducting research that will allow them to deliver the best possible care. However, there is much evidence to suggest that the nursing profession as a whole is still poorly developed in the area of research. Much research conducted by nurses remains limited both in quantity and quality, and their findings are generally poorly disseminated and utilised (Gould 1986, Hunt 1981, Vaughan & Edwards 1995).

The speciality of rehabilitation nursing is also poorly developed in the area of research. Although as rehabilitation nurses we have achieved much in the last decade to raise our profile, we are still failing to act as equal members of the multidisciplinary team in the amount of research we generate. Within the area of rehabilitation, the literature shows that, unlike nurses, other healthcare professionals, in particular doctors, have been very productive in generating research. Although there has been a growth in research conducted by rehabilitation nurses in other countries, particularly the USA, the number of studies initiated and conducted by British nurses is limited in comparison. Results from American studies can provide some useful information, but the differences in culture and healthcare provision make it difficult for British rehabilitation nurses to generalise these findings to their own setting. To be credible the studies would often need to be replicated in this country, and this does not appear to be happening.

The lack of nursing research conducted by rehabilitation nurses is not the only factor inhibiting research-based practice in this field. Other factors, such as the size and quality of those studies conducted and the dissemination of the results, also have an important influence. Much of the research conducted by British rehabilitation nurses (with the exception of a few well-known studies, e.g. Waters & Luker (1996)) have been small-scale, one-off studies. The size and quality of these projects and their non-replication means their findings cannot be considered significant. Furthermore, because many of these studies are conducted for academic reasons and are presented in the form of unpublished dissertations, they are not readily available to nurses, and their potential utilisation in practice is limited. If the speciality of rehabilitation nursing is to develop further in this country, nurses need to overcome these problems, becoming more actively involved in initiating and conducting research. Failure to address the lack of nursing-generated research in this area will place rehabilitation nurses in an disadvantageous position (Wahlquist 1982).

The purpose of this section is to introduce the concept of research-based practice and to outline the advantages of adopting a research-based culture in the field of rehabilitation nursing. Using research in practice does not require postregistration diplomas or degrees, nor does one need to be an experienced researcher. However, a basic understanding of the processes involved is important to all nurses, whether directly conducting research or simply applying existing research findings. For this reason, a large part of this section provides an overview of the steps involved in using and conducting research.

In order to ensure that our research knowledge base advances in a systematic way and in a way that has maximum impact on improving the nursing care of rehabilitation clients, we need to set research priorities for this speciality. This section therefore concludes with a discussion of how nurses might identify research priorities for their field and for the rehabilitation nursing speciality as a whole.

RESEARCH-BASED PRACTICE

Evidence-based practice, or 'research-based practice as it is most commonly known in nursing (Hek 1996), appears to have been derived from the concept of evidence-based medicine (White 1997). Research-based practice is a process which uses the best available research evidence to guide clinical decisions (Appleby et al 1995, Hek 1996, Sackett et al 1996). The widespread use of this approach in health care has been encouraged by national initiatives, such as the research and development strategy for the NHS launched in 1991. The major aim of this strategy was to create a knowledge-based health service where decisions were based on sound research findings (Department of Health 1991).

So what is research? The literature contains numerous definitions of this term. One of the best and most concise examples is that provided by Hockey (1996) who defines research as a 'process of systematic enquiry undertaken according to certain scientific rules: the research process'. McLeod Clark & Hockey (1989) added that it was a process that attempted to add to the body of knowledge by the discovery of new facts or relationships. Therefore, research is an activity concerned with investigating a problem or question, according to certain rules, and research-based practice is about evaluating and utilising the results of this activity.

THE BENEFITS OF RESEARCH-BASED PRACTICE

Research can strengthen the practice of rehabilitation nursing in a number of areas, including clinical practice, management and the further development of the speciality.

Benefit to clinical practice

All rehabilitation nurses want to deliver care that is up to date, is of the highest quality and produces the best possible outcome for patients and families. A meta-analysis of nursing intervention studies found that patients who receive research-based nursing interventions can expect a 28% better outcome than patients who receive non-research-based care (Heafer et al 1988). Research will also strengthen the knowledge base of rehabilitation nursing and will make available a wider range of rehabilitation nursing practice options. It can provide evidence of weaknesses and strengths in rehabilitation nursing, and can help nurses to recognise which practices have a sound basis and which are based purely on experience and tradition (Cormack 1996). Finally, it can help us define good practice and can provide a basis for standard setting (Crow 1981) and audit.

Benefits to managing rehabilitation nursing

Research findings can enable nurses to make managerial decisions based on a clear and sound rationale. For example, research can help to identify those interventions that are cost-effective and those which are not. Research on wound cleaning has questioned the use of sterile saline for some types of wound, and has suggested that the cheaper option of tap water is equally effective (Angeras et al 1992). In a climate of limited resources, this finding has particular significance. Conversely, research findings could be used to provide evidence to demand additional resources. An example of this is research that has illustrated that families experience extreme stress after brain injury in a family member (Lezak 1978, Livingston 1986, Livingston et al 1985, Maus-Clum & Ryan 1981, Oddy et al 1978). Since family involvement is recognised as an important factor in the success of the rehabilitation of these individuals (Johnson & Higgins 1987), such research might be used to argue for additional healthcare personnel to work with families in the rehabilitation setting.

Development of the speciality

As professionals we are accountable for our actions. Practice that is based on sound research findings will increase our credibility and accountability by establishing scientifically defensible reasons for rehabilitation nursing activities. Research into the impact of nursing interventions may help to highlight the contribution of nurses to the rehabilitation process. This will aid in raising the profile of rehabilitation nursing both nationally, within nursing itself, and within the multidisciplinary team, by making it more visible and valued.

USING RESEARCH IN PRACTICE

When utilising and conducting research there is a series of distinct steps that need to be undertaken. Both processes require the formulation of an answerable research question from a chosen clinical problem, a search of the literature surrounding the topic, and evaluation of the research evidence. In research-based practice these initial steps conclude with a decision as to whether or not to implement the findings (Sackett et al 1996).

When conducting research there are a number of further steps that need to be undertaken: the writing of a proposal, selecting a research design, choosing data collection tools, deciding on method of data analysis, deciding how to present the data, and finally how to disseminate the findings (Cormack 1996). These steps, from the formulation of the research question to the dissemination of findings, are known collectively as the research process (Fig. 7.1). Each step in this process is now described in sequence.

IDENTIFYING THE RESEARCH QUESTION OR TOPIC

Whether planning to conduct your own research or just looking to use research findings, the first and most important step is to identify your research question (Sayner 1987). Research questions in rehabilitation nursing can be identified from a number of sources, the main ones being clinical experience and the literature.

Clinical practice is the source of many research questions in nursing (Grant & Davies 1995). A wealth of potential research questions can be identified by any nurse practising rehabilitation who applies a questioning and reflective approach to his practice. Furthermore, the fact that rehabilitation nursing practice has received limited research interest means that there are many untouched areas for research investigation. The rehabilita-

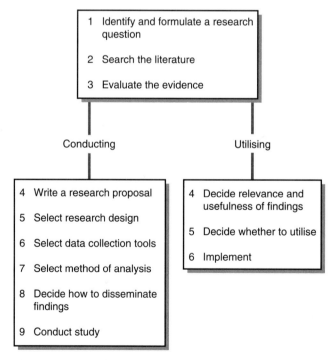

Figure 7.1 The research process: steps involved in conducting and utilising research.

tion nurse should therefore readily be able to identify many potential research questions from his observations and experiences during his everyday activities. A recent research report by Bennett (1996) provides an example of how research topics can arise from clinical work. As a staff nurse in a stroke rehabilitation unit, Bennett became aware that nurses felt unable to help stroke patients with the emotional and psychological impact of sudden disability, and tended to refer such patients to the social worker or chaplain. She wondered why nurses felt this way, and these obser- vations and thoughts led her to identify the research topic for her study. Following a search of the literature this idea was formalised into answer- able research questions: What was it that nurses felt unable to do and what could improve the situation?

The literature can also provide ideas for research topics and questions. A search of the literature may identify a gap in the knowledge base that needs addressing or may uncover previous research and existing theory that may raise further questions and issues for investigation.

Critical care pathways and standards are other potential sources for research ideas. The process of writing critical care pathways and setting standards may highlight clinical practices or procedures that are unsup- ported by empirical knowledge, thus indicating potential research topics. Likewise, local policies and national initiatives can also provide ideas for research, by highlighting areas that need to be researched (Fig. 7.2).

Before proceeding to develop a research idea further, the researcher should consider a number of factors including:

- The relevance of the topic to practice.
- The potential of the idea to improve patient care.

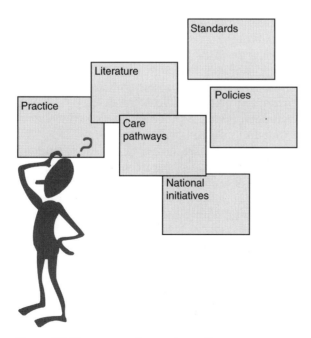

Figure 7.2 The sources of research questions.

- The usefulness of the idea to nurses and the extent to which it can contribute to existing nursing knowledge.
- Whether there are any potential practical or ethical constraints that may prevent the topic from being researched.
- The feasibility of the project must be considered. The research topic may be too ambitious in terms of the researcher's own skills and experience, or it may be too expensive to undertake due to the time and resources required.

SEARCHING AND EVALUATING THE LITERATURE

Once you have selected your research topic your next step is to review the literature. A literature review is 'the process of systematically identifying published materials which meet set pre-determined criteria' (Cormack 1996, p. 69). It is a crucial part of research-based practice and should be initiated at the beginning of any research project and continued throughout its development (Burns & Grove 1987). A search of the literature has a number of purposes. First, it will verify the knowledge base related to the research question by identifying areas that have been studied and those that have not. Second, it will identify the strengths and weaknesses of any previous research (Burns & Grove 1987). Finally, it serves to refine a research problem which was initially broad and general (Grant & Davies 1995).

Literature searches can either be conducted manually (using printed indexes such as *The Cumulative Index to Nursing and Allied Health Literature* (CINAHL), *The International Nursing Index* and the *Index Medicus*) or by using a computer and specially designed databases. Whichever method you choose, your first step must be to determine your search terms and the parameters you wish to set.

To set your search terms you need to brainstorm around your chosen subject, noting every word or phase that could be used to describe your area of interest. For example, if your area of interest is patient participation your key words might include 'patient control', 'patient education' and 'patient empowerment'. Many articles now identify key words at the beginning of the document, and therefore articles located on the subject could be used to help to identify further key terms.

In order to prevent your search being too wide and unmanageable, your next step should be to set parameters. Parameters might include the diagnosis and age of your study population, the language of the article, the country or date of publication. Date of publication is of particular importance, since the age of the study often affects its relevance to current practice. Many authors on this subject suggest that the last 3–5 years of the literature should be considered current. However, one exception to this rule is classic studies that have formed the theoretical basis for much of the recent research (Schira 1992). For example, in the author's own study of the information needs of families in the rehabilitation setting (Swift 1992) the current literature referred to the classic work of family theorists. Since these represented significant works in the author's area of interest, it was important that she reviewed these articles, even though they were published 20 years ago. Finally, it is important to focus on research reports rather than descriptive or anecdotal articles, and primary rather than secondary sources (Schira 1992).

Once the literature search has been completed and the relevant articles collected, the process of evaluation begins. Since publication is no guarantee of the quality or reliability of an individual piece of research (Hek 1996), all nurses need to be able to make a systematic, logical and balanced examination of the studies they read. This will enable them to come to an independent decision about the quality and significance of the research. Any review should start by determining whether the report is an original piece of research rather than a literature review or descriptive article (Hek 1996). This should be followed by a detailed examination of each part of the report. The reviewer should examine:

- the research problem and the purpose of the study
- the literature review
- conceptual background to the work
- research questions and hypotheses
- the location
- size of sample and method of sampling
- data-collection technique
- data analysis
- results
- limitations and recommendations.

An examination of these areas should enable the reviewer to identify the strengths and weaknesses of the study, and therefore its overall value to practice.

UTILISING RESEARCH FINDINGS

The main purpose of research-based practice is to utilise the findings of research. In order that you implement findings which are relevant and appropriate to your practice, the review and evaluation of the literature should be followed by a consideration of several other criteria. The rehabilitation nurse must:

1. Determine whether the research base is sufficient to justify a change in practice. Horseley et al (1983) suggest that the research base must include more than one study in order for the scientific merit of the work to be established.

2. Consider the extent to which the findings are transferable to another setting or client group. For example, the transferability of the findings of a research study conducted in the USA to another country may be limited due to cultural differences, even though it may involve a similar patient group.

3. Be certain that the findings would bring about an improvement in nursing care, and that these benefits of the intervention outweigh any risks involved (Horseley et al 1983).

4. Determine how feasible it is to implement the findings (Horseley et

al 1983). Although the intervention may meet all the above criteria, it may be too expensive or impractical to implement.

PREPARING A RESEARCH PROPOSAL

If you are conducting your own research, your next step is to write a proposal. A research proposal is a 'written summary of what the researcher intends to do, how and why' (Seaman & Verhonick 1982). It is an important exercise for three main reasons.

- It assists the initial planning of the research (Parahoo & Reid 1988).
- It provides detailed information on the project that can be used to convince the relevant authorities that the proposed study has practical and theoretical significance, is of acceptable quality and is ethically sound (Cormack 1996, Parahoo & Reid 1988).
- Funding bodies will expect to see a research proposal when considering applications for financial support.

In general, although individual proposals may vary in the level of detail required, all research proposals need to provide certain basic information about the study and the researcher undertaking the work (Cormack 1996, Parahoo & Reid 1988). A list of the main areas that need to be addressed in a proposal is given in Box 7.3. For more detailed guidelines on writing a research proposal, see Cormack (1996).

SELECTING A RESEARCH DESIGN

The research design refers to how and when the subjects will be studied (Jacox & Prescott 1978). There are three main types of research design: experimental, quasi-experimental and descriptive (Jacox & Prescott 1978).

■ BOX 7.3 Areas that need to be addressed in a research proposal

- Abstract
- Background and purpose of study
- Specific research question or hypotheses
- Definition of terms
- Methods and procedures
- Sample and setting
- Data collection
- Data analysis
- Ethical considerations
- Limitations
- Timetable of project
- Communication of findings
- Personal experience and qualifications of the researcher

Experimental designs are used to test cause and effect. In this type of research the researcher has control over the introduction of an independent variable and over the assignment of subjects to an experimental or control group. A second type of design is the quasi-experiment. This approach is very similar to an experimental design, but has one major difference in that subjects are not randomly assigned to an experimental or control group. This design is usually used where the researcher wishes to use an experimental design but practical or ethical considerations prevent this (Jacox & Prescott 1978). The third type of design is the descriptive approach, which is used by researchers who wish to describe the characteristics of a person, situation or group. The most frequently used descriptive designs are the case study and the survey (Jacox & Prescott 1978).

Although different health professional groups appear to favour particular research designs (e.g. doctors tend to use experimental approaches and nurses descriptive designs), no single approach is necessarily better than another (Jacox & Prescott 1978). However, according to Brink & Wood (1988), there are a number of factors which need to be considered in selecting an appropriate design. As the aim and purpose of the proposed research has a major influence on the choice of design, this must be the first consideration. For example, if the researcher is particularly interested in the views of patients or families, the most appropriate design would be one that would enable their viewpoints to be presented. Therefore, a descriptive design would be the best choice in this case. Conversely, if the researcher wishes to explore relationships or differences, then an experimental approach would be the most appropriate choice.

Another factor influencing the choice of design is the current level of knowledge available on the topic. If the literature search reveals that little is known about the topic, a descriptive approach should be used. The use of an experimental design in this situation would not be possible, as the knowledge base would not be sufficiently developed to allow the testing of relationships. This initial descriptive approach may then yield the knowledge base, and the relationships could then be tested using an experimental design in the future.

Other factors may also limit the choice of design. For example, for ethical reasons it may not be possible to randomly assign subjects to intervention and control groups, thus making use of an experimental design impossible; or the resources available, including the experience of the researcher, may limit the size of the study and thus the approach.

DATA-COLLECTION TOOLS AND METHOD OF ANALYSIS

There are many tools available for collecting data. The most common include observation, questionnaires, attitude scales, interviews and records such as nursing or medical notes. For nurses new to research it is advisable to consult an expert in this field before selecting a data-collection tool. However, there are some general factors that should guide this decision. These include the type of data that one wishes to collect and practical factors such as cost and time (Jacox & Prescott 1978). For example, if the researcher wishes to gain in-depth information about the patient's point of view, interviews as a method of collecting data might be chosen. However, the use of interviews can be very time-consuming and costly; therefore, time and resource constraints may lead the researcher to choose a tool that is quicker and cheaper to administer, such as a questionnaire. In the author's own study (Swift 1992) a questionnaire was chosen in preference to interviewing as a method of collecting data from nurses because of time and resource constraints, and because questionnaires had the additional advantage of permitting wider contact and avoiding interviewer bias.

Once the data have been collected, they will need to be analysed. There are a number approaches to data analysis, which fall into two main categories: descriptive and inferential statistics (Jacox & Prescott 1978). Descriptive statistics are appropriate to descriptive research designs, where the researcher describes a sample such as case studies or surveys. Inferential statistics are designed to identify differences between groups, and are therefore appropriate for use in experimental approaches.

The collection of data and their analysis is a large subject and entire textbooks have been devoted to it. The above description provides a very basic outline of the approaches available. Those nurses contemplating undertaking research will need a greater understanding of the subject and will therefore need to read around the subject in more detail. They should consult a general nursing research textbook (e.g. Burns & Grove 1987, Cormack 1996) and an introductory guide to statistics (e.g. Knapp 1985, Rowntree 1991). This also may be achieved through using experienced researchers or statisticians to whom one may have access, and who have a responsibility to guide the inexperienced researcher through the process.

DISSEMINATION OF FINDINGS

Even before your study is complete you need to consider how best to disseminate your research findings. Failure to publicise your results will mean that your efforts will have little impact on clinical practice. There are several ways in which you could disseminate your research. You could present your work at seminars or workshops, either locally or nationally, but this will only reach the group present. The most effective way of disseminating findings is publication of the report in a journal. This might be a general nursing publication or a journal read by those nurses practising in the area of your research. Many nurses are nervous about submitting work to national journals, feeling that their work is not good enough. Hicks (1995) found that only 10% of nurses who had conducted research had submitted it for publication. The main reasons given for this were a lack of confidence and time. However, the findings also suggested that there was little foundation for this lack of confidence. It was found that most nurses who had submitted research for publication had been successful in getting it accepted. This suggests that nurses should not be put off by their own feelings, and should always attempt to have their work published.

PRIORITIES FOR RESEARCH IN REHABILITATION NURSING PRACTICE

At a national level there is increasing recognition that research in the health service has developed in an unsystematic fashion. This has resulted in a wide range of one-off studies with small samples and a lack of replication work (Mulhall 1995, Simms et al 1994). Consequently, many areas of clinical practice have not been examined in sufficient depth to allow the development of a sound evidence base (Simms et al 1994). This is particularly true in the nursing profession, where many specialities (including rehabilitation) have a poorly developed research knowledge base. The field of rehabilitation nursing, like many other areas of nursing, urgently needs to address this problem. We need to direct research efforts so that a knowledge base of sufficient depth is accumulated quickly and efficiently.

So how do we go about identifying and setting research priorities for rehabilitation nursing? Research priorities can be identified from a number of sources. We have seen that the literature can be used to identify areas that need investigation or further development, or that the literature may highlight an interest or urgency in the profession to address a particular issue or problem. The views of nursing colleagues can also be used in identifying priorities for nursing research: for example, Gordon et al (1996) described a study in which rehabilitation nurses' views were used to help identify research priorities for this speciality in the USA.

Consumers of health care might also be consulted in any research-setting exercise. In fact their involvement is widely supported in the literature. Mulhall (1995) argues that: 'for research to contribute to policies which are truly beneficial to the health of the nation, then both policy and research must be underwritten by consumer needs.' Rehabilitation nurses in setting a research agenda relevant to the needs of rehabilitation clients should involve client groups as much as possible in the process. However, Mulhall (1995) offers a word of caution, commenting that it is important to remember that such groups may frequently reflect the views of only a small percentage of the population. It is important that any research priority-setting exercise is not focused entirely on personal or local interest, but is also congruous with national initiatives which identify research priorities in health care, not least because this may facilitate funding. For example, the NHS Research and Development Initiative (Department of Health 1991) identified a wide range of healthcare priorities for research. Those particularly relevant to rehabilitation nurses included:

- measurement and evaluation of rehabilitation outcome for stroke patients
- rehabilitation after acute myocardial infarction
- equipment for people with physical and complex disabilities
- effectiveness of current therapies for physical and complex disability
- consumers' views of rehabilitation services.

The nursing profession has also started to identify research priorities to enable the profession to focus its research efforts. Kitson et al (1997)

■ **BOX 7.4 Research priorities for nursing as determined by the Royal College of Nursing and the Centre for Policy in Nursing Research National Initiative**

- Patient perspectives of care and how they are assessed
- The role of informal carers and how health and social care are/will be integrated
- Nursing interventions and nurse-led services
- Access to and exit from health services and nurses' role in this process
- Chronicity and how to facilitate coping with chronic illness
- Evaluating the effect on nursing practice of new technologies

---

·described a project set up by the Royal College of Nursing and the Centre for Policy in Nursing Research, which aimed to identify research priorities for the nursing profession. Although not specific to rehabilitation nursing, many of the topics identified have relevance to all types of nursing, including rehabilitation (Box 7.4).

However, the setting of national priorities has been criticised by some who feel that the process limits individual creativity and initiative (Marvin et al 1991) and does not necessarily take into account the views of those in clinical practice (Sleep et al 1995). To avoid any such limitations, we need to involve ourselves in the process and allow our voice to be heard. It is clear that rehabilitation nursing, as well as the rest of the profession, would benefit substantially from a programme that guides research development in a way that best achieves an improvement in the quality of patient care. It is worth strong emphasis that concerns related to any limitations on setting a research agenda are insignificant compared with the problems that may arise from maintaining the status quo.

CONCLUSION

The advantages of becoming a research-based speciality are clear. However, these will only be achieved if rehabilitation nurses become more involved in research activity at all levels. Rehabilitation nurses must incorporate research into their practice by reading and utilising findings. More rehabilitation nurses need to initiate and conduct research relevant to rehabilitation practice in order to develop the research knowledge base of this speciality. Furthermore, they need to raise their profile in this area by leading or co-authoring multidisciplinary research projects in their field. To achieve this we need to ensure that the speciality develops a culture that supports and fosters research-based practice.

Research should not be the sole remit of professional researchers and academics; it is clinically based nurses who are in the optimum position to be able to identify relevant clinical nursing research problems. It should be the role of those with research experience to facilitate the less experienced clinically based nurses to find the answers to problems themselves.

Research activity must be seen as an integral part of everyday rehabilitation nursing practice, rather than an additional task to undertake if time is available. Investment in nursing research must be given a high priority and more research opportunities for nurses need to be developed as a matter of urgency. Failure to address any deficiencies in this area will have disastrous results for rehabilitation nursing, and indeed may lead to the death of this nursing speciality (Wahlquist 1982).

REFERENCES

Angeras M H, Brandberg A, Falk A, Seeman T 1992 Comparison between sterile saline and tap water for the cleaning of acute traumatic soft tissue wounds. European Journal of Surgery 158(33):347–350

Appleby J, Walshe K, Ham C 1995 Acting on the evidence. A review of clinical effectiveness; sources of information, dissemination and implementation. NAHAT, Birmingham, research paper 17

Bennett B 1996 How nurses in a stroke rehabilitation unit attempt to meet the psychological needs of patients who become depressed following stroke. Journal of Advanced Nursing 23:314–321

Brink P, Wood M 1988 Basic steps in planning nursing research: from question to proposal, 3rd edn. Jones & Bartlett, Boston

Burns N, Grove S K 1987 The practice of nursing research: conduct, critique and utilisation. W B Saunders, Philadelphia

Cormack D (ed) 1996 The research process in nursing, 3rd edn. Blackwell Science, London

Crow R 1981 Research and the standards of nursing care: what is the relationship? Journal of Advanced Nursing 6:491–496

Department of Health 1991 Research for health: an R&D strategy for the NHS. HMSO, London

Gordon D L, Sawin K J, Basta S M 1996 Developing research priorities for rehabilitation nursing. Rehabilitation Nursing 5(2):60–66

Gould D 1986 Pressure sore prevention and treatment: an example of nurses' failure to implement research findings. Journal of Advanced Nursing 11:389–394

Grant J S, Davies L L 1995 Using the literature to design a study in the rehabilitation setting: an example with stroke patients. Rehabilitation Nursing 20(3):144–148

Heafer B, Becker A, Oloon R 1988 Nursing interventions and patient outcomes: a meta-analysis of studies. Nursing Research 37(5):303–307

Hek M A 1996 Guidelines on conducting a critical research evaluation. Nursing Standard 11(6):40–43

Hicks C 1995 The shortfall in published research: a study of nurses' research and publication activities. Journal of Advanced Nursing 21:594–604

Hockey L 1996 The nature and purpose of research. In: Cormack D (ed) The research process in nursing, 3rd edn. Blackwell Science, London, ch 1

Horseley J A, Crane J, Crabtre M K, Wood D J 1983 Using research to improve nursing practice: a guide (CURN project). W B Saunders, Philadelphia

Hunt J 1981 Indicators for nursing practice: the use of research findings. Journal of Advanced Nursing 6:189–194

Jacox A, Prescott P 1978 Determining a study's relevance for clinical practice. American Journal of Nursing 1882–1889

Johnson J R, Higgins L 1987 Integration of family dynamics into the rehabilitation of the brain-injured patient. Rehabilitation Nursing 12(6):320–322

Kitson A, McMahon A, Rafferty A, Scott E 1997 High priority. Nursing Times 93(42):26–30

Knapp B G 1985 Basic statistics for nurses, 2nd edn. Wiley, New York

Lezak M D 1978 Living with the characterologically altered brain-injured patient. Journal of Clinical Psychiatry 39:592–598

Livingston M G 1986 Assessment of need for coordinated approach in families with victims of head injury. British Medical Journal 293:742–744

Livingston M G, Brooks D N, Bond M R 1985 Three months after severe head injury: psychiatric and social impact on patients' relatives. Journal of Neurology, Neurosurgery and Psychiatry 48:876–81

McLeod Clark J, Hockey L 1989 Further research for nursing. Scutari, London

Marvin J A, Carrougher G, Bayley B, Weber B, Knighton J, Rutan R 1991 Burn nursing: Delphi study. Nursing Forum 12:190–197

Maus-Clum N, Ryan M 1981 Brain-injury and the family. Journal of Neurosurgical Nursing 13(4):165–169

Mulhall A 1995 Nursing research: what difference does it make? Journal of Advanced Nursing 21:576–583

Oddy M, Humphrey M, Utterley D 1978 Stresses upon the relatives of head-injured patients. British Journal of Psychiatry 133:507–513

Parahoo K, Reid N 1988 Research skills: writing a research proposal. Nursing Times 84(41):49–52

Rowntree D 1991 Statistics without tears: a primer for non-mathematicians. Penguin, Harmondsworth

Sackett D L, Rosenberg W M C, Gray J A M et al 1996 Evidence-based medicine. What it is and what it isn't. British Medical Journal 312:71–72

Sayner N C 1987 Conceptualising researchable neuroscience nursing problems in the clinical setting. Journal of Neuroscience Nursing 19(1):49–52

Schira M G 1992 Conducting the literature review. Journal of Neuroscience Nursing 24(1):54–57

Scofield J 1990 Practical standards. Nursing Times 86(8):31–33

Seaman C C, Verhonick P J 1982 Research methods for undergraduate students in nursing. Appleton-Century Crofts, New York

Simms C, McHaffie H, Renfrew M J, Ashurst H 1994 The midwifery research database, MIRIAD. Books for Midwives Press, Hale

Sleep J, Renfrew M J, Dunn A, Bowler U, Garcia J 1995 Establishing priorities for research: report of a Delphi survey. British Journal of Midwifery 3(6):323–331

Swift S A 1992 The information needs of families of traumatically brain-injured individuals – perceptions of nurses and families. Kings College, London, thesis (unpublished)

Vaughan B, Edwards M 1995 Interface between research and practice. Kings Fund, London

Wahlquist G I 1982 Promoting research in rehabilitation nursing. Rehabilitation Nursing 20:19–20

Waters K, Luker K 1996 Staff perspectives on the role of the nurse in rehabilitation wards for elderly people. Journal of Clinical Nursing 5:105–114

White S J 1997 Evidence-based practice and nursing: the new panacea. British Journal of Nursing 6(3):175–178

Support for rehabilitation in adult nursing: the role of the healthcare assistant

8

Mike Smith

INTRODUCTION

This chapter explores the use of support workers in rehabilitation and focuses specifically on the development of the healthcare assistant (HCA) role. It will describe and attempt to examine constructively some of the concerns raised by nursing, arguing that the HCA role may provide a means by which nursing has the opportunity to develop to its full potential. Guidelines for support roles produced by the United Kingdom Central Council for Nursing, Midwifery and Health Visiting (UKCC 1992) are outlined and discussed. The impact on nursing at ward level is examined, providing practically orientated guidelines for support and supervision of the HCA role.

It is worth pointing out that little formal work appears to have been done on the role of the HCA, most of the related literature being 'opinion' articles rather than based on hard evidence. In addition, many of these articles are either unjustifiably provocative or lack clarity or conclusion, and so contribute little to a balanced or objective debate. Consequently, this chapter aims to provide a balanced view, acknowledging concerns but also suggesting practical solutions and ways forward in an area which for many ward-based nurses often appears to create major anxiety.

Healthcare assistants, or nursing auxiliaries as they were formally known, have been a part of healthcare provision for many years. It is recognised by some that their contribution to nursing has been invaluable, and indeed as an integral part of the nursing team their impact has been considerable (Barrett 1994, Dickson & Cole 1987, Stubbs 1987). Many readers will have no doubt heard, or indeed perhaps have said themselves, that 'a good HCA is worth her weight in gold'. Despite this, in recent times some authors have highlighted concerns regarding the role of HCAs (Redfern 1994). Some perceive the HCA as a threat to nursing today, as many are trained to undertake the tasks which were, in the not too distant past, solely within the remit of the qualified nurse (Friend 1991, Nicholson 1996). Examples of some of the tasks which are often are carried out by the HCA are outlined by Rowden (1992), and the author's personal experience is outlined in Box 8.1.

The list given in Box 8.1 is by no means exhaustive and the reader will be able to identify other tasks that the HCA regularly undertakes in their own clinical area. Differences, not only from organisation to organisation,

■ **BOX 8.1 Tasks currently performed by HCAs**

- Assisting patients with hygiene requirements
- Bowel care
- Intermittent catheterisation
- Taking temperature, blood pressure and pulse
- Recording fluid and dietary intake
- Assisting in prevention of pressure sore development
- Assisting in mobilisation of patients (e.g. supervision of walking and transfers)
- General 'tidying' within clinical area
- Positioning patients in wheelchairs
- Identifying client distress or anxieties
- Performing last offices

but also within an organisation, do little to contribute to the clarity of the HCA role. Although the range of tasks that HCAs undertake may depend to a degree on the way in which the nursing team operates (e.g. primary or team nursing) (Thomas 1993), clearly this situation is far from acceptable.

A major concern expressed is that the employment and development of the HCA is simply a cost-cutting exercise. The regular skill-mix reviews, which many readers will have been subjected to in recent times, seem, with few exceptions to result in diminishing qualified staff levels. This is exacerbated by the apparent lack of objective measurement against the effect on client outcome. Often the rather less acceptable measures of throughput and volume seem to have been used as the sole measures of the effect of such changes (Wynne 1995). Although this may be a difficult issue to discuss objectively when feeling under 'threat', the following four points are a reality in today's climate and are worth the reader's consideration.

COSTS OF HEALTH CARE

Due to changes in the demographics of the population, increased public expectations and increased use of technology, the costs of health care continue to rise.

USE OF FINANCIAL RESOURCES

There is a finite amount of money for healthcare available within the system. Although there are few within the health service who would doubt the need for substantial increases in health service spending, this must be combined with financial responsibility regarding the resources that are provided.

DELEGATION OF TASKS TO THE HCA

Nurses are performing tasks within the scope of current HCA role, and on occasion, tasks performed by other ancillary workers. Each reader will be able to think of many examples which are particular to his clinical area (e.g. giving out meals, pushing a patient to a therapy department, or the many fairly basic administrative tasks that the qualified nurse traditionally seems to get involved with on a regular basis). Nurses must question whether this is an appropriate use of their skills and qualifications, which they have undoubtedly worked hard to gain during training and post-qualification work. In addition, referring to Box 8.1, there are aspects of care which nurses are doing that could be delegated to suitably trained HCAs. Although one would not suggest that the qualified nurse should never do these tasks, it is surely right to consider delegation when the other skills that he may have (or may want to develop), which the HCA does not generally possess (e.g. educating, psychological care or the other roles of the rehabilitation nurse described in this book) are needed by clients within his care.

It cannot be emphasised enough that, if the HCA is to undertake such tasks, appropriate training and supervision must be available, and the HCA must continue to work under the direction of the registered nurse (Rhodes 1994, UKCC 1992).

Another point to note when discussing the tasks performed by un-qualified workers, is what we expect of partners and family members in the community when taking their loved one home. Lack of training and support for them is surely a real travesty. They may often be expected to carry out all the tasks in Box 8.1 along with many more, particularly if they are caring for a person with multiple health problems or major disability.

FULFILLING THE POTENTIAL OF QUALIFIED NURSES

When nurses perform the tasks that are within the HCA role, the ability of nursing practice to make full use of the potential of the qualified nurse is diminished. Such tasks do take time, thereby inhibiting this potential. In addition, and perhaps somewhat ironically, this may also impact adversely on the provision of proper supervision of the HCA. Some critics may be concerned about the potential effect of delegation appearing to be the removal of the qualified nurse from the bedside, and will complain that the hands-on aspects of nursing are what nursing is all about. The author suggests that this is at best short sighted, and at worst to the detriment of nursing and the patient.

In reality, the aspects of care that nurses will be able to provide when they delegate these other tasks to HCAs will take them closer to the patient. We should be able to create the time to sit by the patient and allow him quality time to discuss his fears and anxieties regarding the impact of his injury or illness. We should be able formally to provide the education patients require in order to manage effectively their own change in health status. Nursing has a history of developing its role according to the needs of society. Barrett (1994), in discussing the changes in nursing, suggested that the more traditional measures of what makes a good nurse (e.g. how quickly or well you can make beds or give out meals) are no longer valid. Looking further back in time at what nursing was doing as a profession, we no longer dust and clean the sick room as we did in the 1940s; now we employ domestic staff to release our time to perform tasks appropriate to our training. Surely this must be positive; there must be few who would actually like to be judged using such dated performance criteria. In looking forward Barrett proposed that 'nursing must define specific roles, relinquishing previous job responsibilities in exchange for new ones'.

If one could highlight a mistake in the example above, it is that we lost control of these essential members of the ward team through the creation of domestic or 'hotel' service departments within particular organisations. More recently, the situation appears to have worsened through contracting out such services, and with the inflexibility imposed by service level agreements. We must ensure that this does not happen with the HCA.

Put simply, the emerging role of the HCA may indeed be vital in enabling the qualified nurse to undertake the roles for which he is (or should be) specifically trained (Dewar 1992, Redfern 1994). Not to undertake these roles is not only potentially to the detriment of the client, but also to the profession, and inhibits the development of nursing overall.

If we look at, for example, the nurse's role as first-line psychological support as outlined Chapter 4, there will be few readers who believe they are able to undertake this particular aspect of their role effectively in their current way of working. Colleagues are frequently heard saying, 'We don't have the time.' Yet when we have the opportunity to delegate to the HCA some of the daily tasks we perform, and actually spend some quality time with the client or patient addressing some of their psychological needs and concerns, we become protective in the extreme regarding what we perceive as our traditional role. This is despite the obvious fact that nursing has and will continue to change its role. The same argument could obviously be extended to other roles identified within this book.

It is really worth questioning what the basis of our fears is regarding the developing role of the HCA. The author is convinced that there are multiple causes for any concerns we may have, and would encourage the reader to consider the points outlined in Box 8.2 as possible factors that have contributed to current concerns. The points raised may be worth formal exploration in future research, in order to define strategies to overcome them. Some of these issues are addressed later in this chapter.

Although supporting the structured and clearly defined use of HCAs, and the development of the HCA role to facilitate the development and scope of the qualified nurse, the author is not directly advocating in any way the replacement of qualified nurses by HCAs. If a suitable opportunity does arise, any such changes in skill mix must only be made when and if measures of patient outcome are in place. Formal studies should be undertaken as a pilot project to determine the effectiveness of such changes, and any savings should be invested back into that clinical area. Despite the concerns of almost the entire profession, until recently there has been an apparent lack of willingness by both the United Kingdom Central Council

■ **BOX 8.2 The origin of concerns regarding the HCA role**

- There have been difficulties in defining the role of the qualified nurse. If we are not clear about our role it is no surprise that we have difficulty in clarifying the role of the HCA. This has been exacerbated by the lack of direction from professional nursing bodies. Such role ambiguity can be nothing but unproductive and, with few exceptions, has been referred to by all authors discussing the HCA (Ahmed & Kitson 1993, Rhodes 1994).

- The HCA role may often have evolved not according to a definite structure or plan, but as a result of 'firefighting' responses to nursing shortages nationally. This has enforced the need to use increased numbers of agency staff, who are often familiar with neither the clinical area nor the speciality. The HCA may often have been trained, and relied on, to cover for the deficits created by this the lack of skilled nurses. There is a clear need for a structural framework which should facilitate clarity of roles and direction for nursing and support workers such as the HCA (Ahmed & Kitson 1993).

- Has the lack of formal training for qualified nurses in some of their roles, particularly in the psychological and educational aspects of care, resulted in a discomfort in performing these roles, meaning that some nurses are less willing to delegate tasks that they do feel comfortable with to others?

- Has the lack of formal training for the HCA, including failing to outline the limitations of their role, created practical problems that have threatened standards of care?

- Has the lack of this training, and what we are asking the HCA to do in actual clinical practice, also resulted in abuse of the HCA?

- Does the absence of regulation by nursing professional bodies create the impression, or the reality, that nursing has little control over the development of the HCA?

- Has the apparent lack of research related to the HCA role contributed to this role ambiguity, not only of the qualified nurse but also of the HCA?

for Nursing, Midwifery and Health Visiting (UKCC) and the Royal College of Nursing (RCN) to address bringing the HCA formally into the nursing fold, despite encouragement to do so (Chudley 1988, MacAlister 1997), a move which would enable a degree of control and regulation. Anecdotally this seems to be what nursing is keen to obtain, and not to do so seems to be counterproductive in allaying the fears of nursing. One would hope that the UKCC will take a lead in the formal debate about the role of the HCA announced in March 1997, and that this debate will prove fruitful.

In view of all of the above, one would conclude and propose that the development of the HCA role is worthwhile on two counts. First, it is beneficial in terms of the optimum use of resources, and therefore in exercising financial responsibility and so enabling more patients to be treated. Second, it is essential in enabling qualified nurses to attain their full potential to provide care, and the nursing profession to develop.

UKCC GUIDELINES

Despite the above concerns and the criticism of our professional bodies, in the *Scope of Professional Practice* document (1992), the UKCC has commendably recognised the requirement for support for professional clinical nursing practice. Although they acknowledge that they have no responsibility for the training of support workers, the UKCC has demonstrated a long overdue awareness that support roles will have an impact on the provision of standards of nursing practice. As a response to this awareness, guidance in the form of seven key principles was outlined in the same document (Box 8.3).

These guidelines are potentially invaluable in clarifying the scope of the HCA role. In addition, the guidelines may act as an initial framework that the nurse in the rehabilitation environment can use to guide and justify the need for training, both of the appropriate support workers and of those who will undertake the supervision role. Not only will this assist in ensuring that standards of care are maintained, but it will also allow the qualified nurse to be assured that he will be able to fulfil the roles of nursing to their full potential while these standards are maintained. However, it is worth emphasising that these guidelines are just a start. Further work and direction is needed from the UKCC and RCN to facilitate this further. Nevertheless, it is worth exploring each of the UKCC guidelines in more detail.

SUPERVISION OF THE HCA BY REGISTERED NURSES

The requirement for supervision of the HCA by a registered nurse could not be stated more clearly. The registered nurse has a key responsibility to prescribe new nursing interventions for the client. Certainly there is scope for the HCA to contribute or assist in the assessment and evaluation of that prescribed care. Often the HCA's observations will undoubtedly be valid; however the onus rests with the qualified registered nurse to carry out or to supervise any action that is taken following a judgment being made of the situation. Clearly, then, there is a need for appropriate guidelines for the HCAs, given at the commencement of their employment, regarding the limitations of their role, and these guidelines must also be made clear to qualified nursing staff.

ACCOUNTABILITY OF THE HCA

The accountability of the HCA is related to the need for appropriate delegation by the qualified nurse. A key point emphasised throughout the whole *Scope of Professional Practice* document is that registered nurses are accountable for their own actions, and that part of this is to ensure that

■ **BOX 8.3 The Scope of Professional Practice and support roles (UKCC 1992)**

The UKCC's position in relation to support roles is as follows:

- HCAs to registered nurses, midwives and health visitors must work under the direction and supervision of those registered practitioners.
- Registered nurses, midwives and health visitors must remain accountable for assessment, planning, and standards of care and for determining the activity of their support staff.
- HCAs must not be allowed to work beyond their level of competence.
- Continuity of care and appropriate skill/staff mix is important, so HCAs should be integral members of the caring team.
- Standards of care must be safeguarded, and the need for patients and clients across the spectrum of health care to receive skilled professional nursing, midwifery and health visiting assessment must be recognised as of primary importance
- HCAs with the desire and ability to progress to professional education should be encouraged to obtain vocational qualifications, some of which may be approved by the UKCC as acceptable entry criteria into programmes of professional education.
- Registered nurses, midwives and health visitors should be involved in these developments so that the support role can be designed to ensure that professional skills are used most appropriately for the benefit of patients and clients.

subordinates have the correct skills and knowledge to undertake a particular intervention. This emphasises the need for a record of competence to be maintained for each HCA. In other words, it is right that the HCA should be allowed to develop, as this supplements the nursing provision within the clinical environment, enabling qualified nurses to utilise their skills fully. However, this development must be under an umbrella of formalised education and supervision, in order to avoid potentially disastrous consequences, not only for the client but also for the delegating nurse.

WORKING WITHIN LEVELS OF COMPETENCE

Clearly linked to the above point is the need to demonstrate competence prior to undertaking a task. A standard framework and system for recording and developing competence should be developed and maintained within each ward area. Such systems should be organisation wide, and indeed one could argue that they should be regulated nationally by the nursing profession. The vehicle of the competence based National Vocational Qualification (NVQ) can and should be tied in with existing or developing orientation and on going training packages, the essence of which are described in Part B of Chapter 9. However, without regulation, or at least clear guidance from the UKCC and RCN, how can we possibly expect to develop systems that work in tandem with, rather than in competition with, nursing, and to ease the concerns of individual nurses (Healy 1996). It remains a concern that reports regarding lack of formal training continue. Rhodes (1994) indicated that most learning appears to be through informal observation rather than formal instruction. It is not surprising, therefore, that there is a lack of clarity regarding the limits of the role of the HCA.

THE HCA AS AN INTEGRAL TEAM MEMBER

The *Scope* document recognises unequivocally that HCAs are a valid and valuable part of the team providing nursing. Surely this is yet another justification for bringing the HCA more directly under the control of the nursing profession.

MAINTAINING STANDARDS OF CARE

It is only through adhering to the above points that the standard of care we desire for the clients for whom we have responsibility will be upheld. If formalised training ensuring competence, clear guidance and regulation of the HCA role, and a recognition that the HCA does have a valid contribution to make, is absent the result will surely be a threat to the quality of service. When these are in place the effects can only be beneficial for all, and the ability to develop further the qualified nursing role using the guidelines laid down in the *Scope of Professional Practice* document is facilitated.

VOCATIONAL AND PROFESSIONAL TRAINING AND EDUCATION

Clearly, many HCAs will develop skills through experience within the nursing practice environment that may indicate their potential to undertake further training. The contribution of the NVQ in developing and recording competence has previously been mentioned, and it is probably a valuable tool (Chapman 1990, Rhodes 1994) despite the ongoing problems in its implementation. In this section, the *Scope* document suggests, and quite correctly in the author's opinion, that some HCAs may reach a stage when the opportunity to undertake a formal nurse training programme may be considered. It is a responsibility of nursing not only to facilitate this, but also actively to promote it, particularly in the current climate of the UK national shortages of qualified nursing staff.

REGISTERED NURSES IN THE DEVELOPMENT OF THE HCA ROLE

In the recent nursing literature some authors have expressed concerns regarding the lack of nursing involvement in the developing role of the

HCA. However, it is worth bearing in mind that the HCA is an integral part of nursing provision, and if the desire to maintain high standards of care is to be met, we as a profession must stop burying our heads in the sand regarding this issue. It is our responsibility to be proactive in the development of the HCA, through reasoned debate and a degree of regulation. To do otherwise will be to the detriment of nursing generally, and lead to further abuse of the role of the HCA.

DEVELOPING AN HCA PROGRAMME WITHIN THE CLINICAL AREA

In view of the above there appear to be several key aspects of the HCA role that could be put into place within the clinical rehabilitation environment. The overall aims of such action would be to ensure that the guidelines are adhered to and, equally essential, to clarify the situation for the qualified nurse, the HCA and, importantly, the client. The eight-stage framework outlined below is designed to provide practical advice for the clinical nursing team in meeting these aims. The framework is designed to be used in its entirety, as a staged qualified nurse/HCA development programme. However, it is recognised that some clinical areas may choose to focus on points 6–8 initially as a base from which to reflect on the current situation, addressing other issues at a later stage when further development of the HCA and qualified nursing roles is planned. Possible methods for achieving each of the stages are suggested. This is by no means a definitive list, and readers may have alternative methods more suited to their particular situation.

Eight-stage qualified nurse/HCA development programme

Stage 1

Identify any deficits in current nursing ability to provide what is part of their fundamental role as a nurse in the rehabilitation of clients in their care.

Potential methods. Use the roles defined in Chapter 2 in nursing the client undergoing any sort of rehabilitation programme as a basis, i.e:

- educator
- team worker
- first-line psychological support
- researcher/auditor
- coordinator
- technical expert and provider of care.

Compare current perceptions of the clinical nursing team regarding what they believe they should be doing under each of the roles above with what they are actually able to do in practice. It will also be useful to ascertain the reason behind any deficits identified (e.g. lack of training, time or resources). This could be done using a survey, a focus-group or through a formal ward meeting using a brainstorming technique.

Results from this will not only highlight the deficits in provision, but may also assist in clarifying role boundaries and emphasising areas and opportunities for development. The results should be fed back to all qualified nursing staff.

Stage 2

Identify which aspects of current nursing practice could be safely delegated to the HCA, provided that:

- appropriate training is undertaken
- supervision of the HCA practice is maintained.

Potential methods. Identify current nursing activities by using a survey or by interviewing a selection of qualified nurses across all grades. Using a different sample of nurses and stressing the criteria above, perform a simple survey using the activities identified previously (e.g. see Fig. 8.1). It is worth emphasising that, to be productive, this must be seen in context with the opportunities identified in Stage 1.

Stage 3

Identify which of the deficits demonstrated in Stage 1 could be overcome if the HCA was able to perform the activities identified in Stage 2.

Potential methods. Bearing in mind the training needs of the qualified staff, the results from Stages 1 and 2 viewed together should indicate actual possibilities for development. These should be outlined to all staff members. Resource implications must obviously be considered and planned for, and a formal action plan developed accordingly (see Stages 4–8), highlighting the responsibilities of all concerned. Again, to gain a degree of ownership and to facilitate compliance a multigrade group of staff should be involved.

Do you think the following activities could be delegated to the HCA provided that

- appropriate training is undertaken
- supervision of HCA practice is maintained?

Activity	Yes	No	Comments
Activity A			
Activity B			
Activity C			

Figure 8.1 HCA activity survey.

Stage 4

Identify audit methods that could be used to demonstrate that standards of care are maintained.

Potential methods. The first consideration in this stage is to ensure that standards exist for all aspects of care. This area is covered extensively in Chapter 7, where guidance for auditing against standards is provided.

Stage 5

Identify methods by which the positive effects of HCAs fulfilling their potential roles could be demonstrated.

Potential methods. There are many ways in which the impact of implementing the above could be demonstrated, and the author suggests that it is through a combination of such methods that a complete picture will be obtained. These should be referenced in the action plan developed as described above. The following are a few suggestions:

- staff clarity and satisfaction with role
- client satisfaction with care provided
- measuring client outcome
- recording nursing developments
- recording nursing research activity and results of audit of clinical practice
- retention of qualified nursing staff and HCAs.

It is worth stressing that a true reflection of the impact will only be gained by measuring any of the above both prior to and after implementation of the action plan.

Stage 6

Document the current HCA role and the potential role that she could have following training. For both the current and the potential role, identify the limitations of the role, and lines of responsibility for reporting adverse occurrences. These should be distributed to the entire ward team, and a named person allocated to answer queries.

Potential methods. To facilitate role clarity for both qualified nurses and HCAs, clear guidance must be available to all. The use of comprehensive job descriptions, policies and standards, which should include responsibilities, be used properly and be available to all, seems the most logical means by which this can be achieved. The development of these features should be inherent in any action plan.

Stage 7

Develop an orientation programme to ensure that the needs of the current HCA and qualified nurse roles are met. Include within this a method of recording the successful completion of the orientation programme.

Potential methods. Again detailed information is provided in other chapters related to this aspect of an action plan. Chapter 9 Part B gives an in-depth description of orientation programme development. It is worth emphasising that many of the principles outlined are transferable between development programmes, whether for qualified nurses or HCAs.

Stage 8

Develop a staged, competence-based training programme to meet the potential HCA and qualified nurse roles. This would include clear guidelines relating to educational content, assessment of competence for each aspect of the role, and a means of recording successful completion of the programme.

Potential methods. Again this is discussed in depth in Chapter 9, and the reader is referred to that section of the book.

As the reader may have recognised, there are three common threads running through all the stages outlined above which will facilitate both the development and the implementation of the HCA role.

1. All the above stages should form the basis of the action plan referred to in Stage 1. This ensures that the focus remains on the opportunities for the qualified nurse and the ultimate benefits for the provision of client care, rather than on the potential threat to nursing of HCAs.

2. Consultation with and involvement of qualified staff of all grades should be an inherent part of every stage within the process. As the major concerns and practical problems appear predominantly to originate with and affect nurses at grades D to F, a top–down approach which neglects to use the resources and opinions of this group is more likely to fail.

3. There is a significant amount of work involved in undertaking such a project. Clearly, appropriate facilitation and guidance (possibly through the use of external parties), realistic time-scales, definition of responsibilities, formally booked time invested away from the clinical area and other resource support (e.g. administration of data collection, replacement of staff involved) are all fundamental to the success of the venture.

SUMMARY

This chapter has been based on the premise that the HCA is a valuable part of the provision of nursing in the rehabilitation of any client. The concerns that exist, although in some cases justifiable, have been contributed to by a lack of clarity regarding the roles of the qualified nurse and the HCA. The lack of clear guidance from the professional bodies has been detrimental to the situation, and must be resolved if nursing is to be proactive in the development of the HCA role. Such clear guidance is also important with regard to the development of nursing as a profession generally, and the ability of nurses to fulfil their potential role may well be dependent on developing the role of the HCA. We must remember that changing the role of nursing is not new, but has a historical basis. The guidelines regarding support roles produced within the *Scope of*

Professional Practice are a valuable start in providing us with some indication as to how we should both implement and limit the development of the HCA role. In addition, the framework proposed in this chapter should be facilitatory in such developments, provided that the three key principles outlined are adhered to.

Any developments should be in the best interests of the client and standards must be maintained. One could argue that, if nursing is able to develop its key roles fully, the development of the HCA role will not only improve standards and the contribution of nursing, but will also enable the return of the qualified nurse to the 'bedside', something which some would suggest has been increasingly absent in recent times.

Nurses can no longer afford to resist such change, digging in our heels, without (if we are honest) the evidence to back up our fears and our claims of a threat to nursing. If we want the best for nursing and for the patient, we must be proactive in such developments. The alternative is that changes may be imposed on us by others, and the opportunities to develop and implement new nursing roles will be quashed forever.

REFERENCES

Ahmed L B, Kitson A 1993 Complementary roles of nurse and health care assistant. Journal of Clinical Nursing 2(5):287–297
Barrett A 1994 Bendable or expendable? Nursing Standard 8(18):44
Chapman P 1990 In need of qualification. Nursing Times 86(17):46–47
Chudley P 1988 Levelling down. Nursing Times 84(20):59–60
Dewar B 1992 Skill muddle? Nursing Times 88(33):24–27
Dickson N, Cole A 1987 Nurse's little helper? Nursing Times 83(10):24–26
Friend B 1991 Sliding away. Nursing Times 87(6):22–23
Healy P 1996 Protecting the weakest. Nursing Standard 10(51):24–25
MacAlister L I 1997 Health care assistants need to be regulated. British Journal of Nursing 6(6):302.
Nicholson T 1996 Are we giving away nursing? Accident and Emergency Nursing 4(4):205–207
Redfern L 1994 Health care assistants – the challenge for nursing staff. Nursing Times 90(48):31–33
Rhodes L 1994 What can HCA's be asked to do? Nursing Times 90(48):33–35
Rowden R 1992 More input required. Nursing Times 88(33):27–28
Stubbs J 1987 The auxiliaries' tale. Nursing Times 83(10):27.
Thomas L 1993 Comparing qualified nurse and auxiliary roles. Nursing Times 89(38):45–48
United Kingdom Central Council for Nursing, Midwifery and Health Visiting 1992 Scope of professional practice. UKCC, London
Wynne T 1995 Skill mix in nursing: efficiency and quality? Journal of Nursing Management 4(3):189–191

Educating rehabilitation nurses

9

Curriculum issues for rehabilitation nursing

Peter Davis

INTRODUCTION

Nurses, midwives and health visitors practice in an environment of constant change. There are new and expanding roles for health professionals, increasing technological advances in treatment and care, and continuing reorganisation of resources. It is, therefore, essential to continue to develop knowledge and competence throughout a career to be able to respond to these demands and the complexities of professional practice (United Kingdom Central Council for Nurses 1995). These issues and concepts apply to any profession, and are predominantly addressed through education. In recent years there has been a paradigm shift in the education of many healthcare professionals, in that it is now the responsibility of the individual to seek to ensure their competence in order to maintain registration with their professional body. For nurses this professional body is obviously the United Kingdom Central Council for Nurses, Midwives and Health Visitors (UKCC). This chapter focuses on some of the opportunities created through the current educational climate. In doing this, reference is made to some issues addressed within other chapters, and these are reinforced through provision of information regarding the educational context within which they fit.

LIFE-LONG LEARNING AND PREP

It has never been realistic or logical to expect any profession's initial few years of preparation to equip its students to work for forty years, or more, with no further compulsory education or development during their careers. However, this is the situation that has existed until relatively recently. Fortunately, most professions, including those concerned with healthcare, have realised the need to insist on updating knowledge and the development of the individual through mandatory requirements for professional recognition, usually through the registration process.

Since the early 1990s, nursing in the UK has been preparing and implementing a process for Post-Registration Education and Practice (PREP). It defines what nurses must do in order to maintain an effective registration on the different parts of the UKCC register. The details are set out in the UKCC's document on the future of professional practice (UKCC 1994). Fundamentally, nurses are responsible for seeking opportunities to learn and to improve their level of competence in the interests of patient and client care. The UKCC provide only a few stipulations for learning related to PREP.

- The learning must be appropriate to the practitioner's current area of practice.
- Learning outcomes should be set and be appropriate to the practitioner's individual needs.
- The process should be recorded in a professional profile.

The UKCC have also established five broad categories to help individuals to plan their studies. These are designed to be flexible, to ensure that individuals can meet their own needs in the context of their practice. The categories are:

- patient, client and colleague support
- care enhancement
- practice development
- reducing risk
- education development.

The essence of all of these categories is the requirement for the individual continually to address personal development needs, which are not necessarily directly related to patient and client care, for example developing the skills and knowledge to become increasingly reflective and critical as an individual.

The principle of continuity of education throughout the span of one's professional practice is encompassed in the concept of life-long learning (English National Board for Nursing, Midwifery and Health Visiting 1994).

If rehabilitation nursing is to develop for the benefit of patient and client care, then its destiny is in the hands of nurses themselves. This is easy to expound, but more difficult to follow. Many nurses still find it difficult to be proactive and take the lead with other healthcare colleagues as their equals.

SELF-EMPOWERMENT

By promoting health and providing quality nursing care, the rehabilitation nurse should aim to empower the patient and client. This may be difficult to achieve in environments as varied as the hospital and community, and in individuals with a span of acute and/or chronic healthcare problems. To be able to empower others, one must be capable of self-empowerment. Personal development of this nature is primarily achieved through education.

Self-empowerment is a means by which individuals can draw on their inner strengths and resources. Everyone can become more self-empowered; care professionals, patients or clients, and families. The more selfempowered an individual becomes the more he will be able to help bring about this process in others. Self-empowerment may be considered as 'a process of becoming increasingly more in control of oneself and one's life, and thus increasingly more independent' (Fenton & Hughes 1989). To facilitate self-empowerment, the rehabilitation nurse would need to develop appropriate beliefs and attitudes, such as the following (Fenton & Hughes 1989).

- Each individual is unique, valuable and worthy of respect.
- Education, therapy and self-empowerment are value based.
- The more self-empowered a person becomes, the more they will be able to help others to be the same.
- Once people have learned to respect, love and value themselves, they will be able to respect, love and value others.
- It is helpful to differentiate between the behaviours that encourage the developing parts of a person, and those that serve to anchor them in states of depression, hostility, fear and/or insecurity.
- Taking risks and learning from mistakes is effective and valuable.
- Everyone has something to teach and something to learn.

Box 9.1 lists characteristics of the more or less self-empowered individual

---

■ **BOX 9.1 Characteristics of more or less self-empowered individuals**

More self-empowered	Less self-empowered
• Proactive	• Reactive
• Open to change	• Closed to change
• Considers others in situations of change	• Considers only self in situations of change
• Assertive	• Non-assertive or aggressive
• Self-accountable	• Blames others
• Self-directed	• Led by others
• Uses feelings	• Overwhelmed by or fails to recognise feelings
• Learns from mistakes	• Debilitated by mistakes
• Confronts	• Avoids
• Realistic	• Urealistic
• Seeks alternatives	• Tunnel vision
• Likes self	• Dislikes self
• Values others	• Negates others
• Considers others' needs	• Selfish
• Interested in the world	• Self-centred
• Enhances other people's lives	• Restricts the lives of others
• Can say no	• Difficulty in saying no

and provides goals and directions for those seeking to promote self-empowerment.

Rehabilitation nurses' perspectives of patients and clients are rapidly developing and reshaping. To understand and utilise these changes requires education. As nurses, our own attitudes, beliefs and knowledge directly affect the way we care. Furthermore, these ideas are relevant and valid for both patients and nurses and other healthcare professionals. That is, in seeking to understand their own attitudes and beliefs nurses are encompassing exactly the same knowledge base as is essential to their patients and clients. Two important examples of this, which are related to the concept of empowerment, are locus of control and health beliefs.

Rotter (1966) described individuals who believe they have a lot of personal control over events as having an internal locus of control. Alternatively, those who believe that they have little control over events and situations, who believe instead in luck or fate, are defined as having an external locus of control. A rehabilitation nurse with an external locus of control is poorly prepared to act as an advocate for a client or to drive forward necessary changes within rehabilitation.

In literature reviews by Bailey (1992) and Smith & Draper (1994) it was shown that, in the past, patients were seen as passive recipients of care. However, due to changes in society and nursing, there is a move towards increasing the control of health care of patients themselves. These changes must be understood and accepted by nurses and other healthcare professionals. Equally, rehabilitation nurses *must not* become or remain passive recipients of changes within health care.

The role of a health promoter is to remove obstacles to empowerment (Robertson & Minkler 1994). Feelings of well-being can enhance one's ability to cope with ill health, and Downie et al (1990) suggest that well-being can be achieved by empowerment. Cohen (1997) relates the concepts of empowerment and well-being to health belief models. Health belief models, such as the one described by Rosenstock et al (1998), incorporate concepts of self-efficacy. Self-efficacy refers to the amount of control one perceives one has over one's own health. A rehabilitation nurse, with low self-efficacy, would find it difficult or incompatible to try to persuade a client to take more control of their health when they themselves feel they have little control over their own health.

SPECIALIST PRACTICE

The International Council of Nurses (1992) believes that the development of nursing specialities is critical in stimulating the growth of nursing knowledge and expertise. Increasingly, evidence is being cited of the benefits of the specialisation trend: quality of care is enhanced and there is greater job satisfaction resulting from the mastery of knowledge and skills achieved and the increased recognition accorded to specialist status. To rehabilitation nurses world-wide the benefits of specialisation may appear obvious and indisputable, but this view is not held by all those who have an influence on healthcare provision.

There is a fundamental difference between a nurse working in a speciality and a nurse who is a specialist. Dicks (1996) suggests that nurses working in a speciality provide everyday care to patients in practice-based positions with limited in-depth knowledge and experience. They will draw on the experience and support of specialist nurses who have successfully completed higher and advanced level educational programmes.

The need to acquire further academic qualifications is a contentious but essential element of speciality status. Academic qualifications, however, are not the only factor by which to judge. Many rehabilitation nurses could rightly consider themselves to be specialising as they use a common language, have common interests at an advanced level and develop specialised nursing skills.

At present there is a profusion and confusion of titles, such as specialist practitioner and clinical nurse specialist. There is also a need to identify clearly the differences between advanced and specialist practice. In overcoming this confusion the nursing profession has a challenging and interesting future to embrace.

SPECIALIST AND ADVANCED PRACTICE

The development of specialist and advanced nurse practitioners in the UK has stimulated debate within nursing itself and outside the profession. It has been suggested that the statutory bodies have been deliberate in choosing not to offer a succinct definition of advanced practice because they are waiting for the profession itself to develop its own parameters (Castledine 1996). However, the UKCC (1996a) has published transitional arrangements for specialist and advanced nurses, with the promise of firmer arrangements in the near future. The UKCC (1994) defines specialist practitioners as 'practitioners who are able to demonstrate higher levels of clinical decision making and develop practice through research, teaching and support of professional colleagues.' Also, to qualify as a specialist practitioner, the individual will be required to undertake additional preparation and education. Educational programmes should be to first degree level and contain 50% theory and 50% practice (UKCC 1994).

Advanced nursing practice has not been so clearly characterised by the professional bodies. The transitional arrangements, published in September 1996, state that the title of 'nurse consultant' has been suggested as more accurate and appropriate than the term 'advanced practice'. During the ensuing deliberations, it was agreed that advanced practitioners are expected to be grounded in practice, but to have research, education and consultancy functions as well. The interim report also recommended that preparation for advanced practice should be via individually tailored pathways at masters or doctoral level.

Patterson & Haddad (1992) defined advanced nurse practitioners as those nurses who 'will push beyond the known boundaries of their profession, are willing to take the risks and face the challenges associated with breaking new ground and have the ability to articulate their thoughts clearly as they move ahead and develop new nursing knowledge and skills thus leading their profession forward to meet the needs and demands of society.' Advanced nursing practice is concerned with personal attributes and qualities associated with exploring as yet uncovered professional territory and developing new domains as well as 'advancing clinical practice, research and education to enrich professional practice as a whole' (UKCC 1994).

Jester (1997) identifies several concerns about advanced nursing practice.

- Is the advanced nurse practitioner a mini-doctor or maxi-nurse?
- Is the development of advanced nurse practitioners merely a response to the reduction in junior doctors' hours (Department of Health 1991)?
- Will the blurring of professional boundaries lead to better patient care or fragmentation of the nursing role?
- Will the public, nurses and other health professionals accept advanced nurse practitioners and support them?
- Will the advancing role of advanced nurse practitioners lead to confusion of accountability with medical staff (Dowling et al 1996)?

Jester (1997) believes that specialist/advanced nurses are in an ideal position to close the circle in the rehabilitation process (Johnson 1995), ensuring that interprofessional boundaries are not allowed to be detrimental to the patient's progress. She further suggests that their development encourages innovative practice development, and has a number of favourable aspects to commend it, as it:

- increases professional confidence and autonomy
- increases multidisciplinary collaboration
- minimises the divisions between professional boundaries
- increases the quality of holistic nurse-led care delivery
- enhances the specialist knowledge, skills and professional standing of nurses.

SCOPE OF PROFESSIONAL PRACTICE

Fundamental changes to the inherently diverse roles of the nurse have always occurred and will continue to do so. This provides opportunities, but is also a threat to those who feel they are struggling to keep up. This should be recognised, and support and education provided where necessary.

In the recent past nurses have given up many of their responsibilities. For example, when are we going to universally reclaim responsibility for prescribing simple medications and ensuring appropriate nutrition for patients and clients (Davis 1997)? The challenge is to ensure that we assume responsibility only for those areas of practice that we deem most appropriate for a nurse to undertake, and to be proactive and imaginative for the benefit of our patients/clients.

As it becomes more acceptable to the nursing, paramedical and medical fraternities that the traditional demarcation lines between the roles of professions can be safely crossed, there needs to be a translation of spoken acceptance into a usable written format. Nurses should also be continually aware of why they are taking on these roles. For example while the reduction in junior doctors' hours provides an opportunity for nurses to take on new roles, it should not be the reason for them to do so.

The ultimate responsibility for deciding competence is placed with the individual practitioner, who is expected to refuse to undertake tasks for which he feels he is not competent. Hunt & Wainwright (1994) explain that, as a result of the internal market and the creation of National Health Service (NHS) trusts, we are now seeing the production of protocols on the clinical responsibilities of nurses. These include many of the duties carried out by junior doctors. However, if they do not conflict with any statutory provision, and if the nurse is given the necessary training and support, then there is nothing illegal or undesirable about undertaking them.

The UKCC publication *Scope in Practice* (1997) describes 17 initiatives as examples of how *The Scope of Professional Practice* has enabled nurses, midwives and health visitors to improve the care they give to patients and clients. As recommended in the UKCC's *The Scope of Professional Practice* (1992), practice needs to be sensitive, relevant and responsive to the needs of individual patients and clients, with the capacity to adjust when and where appropriate to changing circumstances. The UKCC's position statement recommends six principles that should underpin a nurse's approach to taking on responsibility beyond the traditional boundaries of practice. The nurse should (UKCC 1997):

- be satisfied that patient and client needs are uppermost
- aim to keep up-to-date and develop knowledge, skills and competence
- recognise limits to personal knowledge and skill and remedy deficiencies
- ensure that new developments and responsibilities do not compromise existing nursing care
- acknowledge personal accountability
- avoid inappropriate delegation.

Many nurse practitioners are at the forefront of rehabilitation initiatives. Flasher (1997) describes an example of how rheumatology nursing practice was developed in one area of England utilising the UKCC's scope of practice. Box 9.2 illustrates the elements of a nurse practitioner's role in the speciality of rheumatology, but many of these elements can be applied to other specialties and are fundamental to rehabilitation nursing.

In these role developments, nursing autonomy through empowerment requires more than nurses acquainting themselves with biomedical knowledge. 'If nurse expansion is to be an expansion of nursing as opposed to an expansion of medicine into nursing, then nursing will need a new paradigm of what counts as health care knowledge' (Hunt & Wainwright 1994). Academic credit for any learning is desirable, as this may have an impact on issues of liability. The UKCC's 'Guidelines for Professional Practice' (1996b) is a helpful resource when addressing issues such as accountability, consent and working together.

■ **BOX 9.2 Scope of practice for the specialist nurse practitioner: Rheumatology**

Follow-up clinic
- Accurately record history and pre-senting features at each visit
- Prioritise problems in a treatment plan
- Manage the imple-mentation of a care package
- Monitor the effects of the treatment plan

Outreach clinics
- Drug management
- Follow-up care

Quality assurance and audit
- Initiate procedures to enhance quality and efficiency of practice*
- Develop protocols/guidelines/standards for care
- Recognise areas requiring protocols/guidelines/standards for care

Awareness of limitations

Professional and patient safety

Shared care
- Provide a link between primary and secondary care

Patient information
- Provide current information

- Provide access to information
- Recognise and bridge information gaps

Education (group and individual)
- Assess educational needs
- Assess access to resources
- General RA out-patient education programme
- Disease-specific out-patient programmes
- Practice nurse support information and education
- Registered nurse education
- Resource for health faculty

Competent patient assessment
- Administration of soft tissue injections, intra-articular aspiration and injection
- Carry out tests and procedures as specified within local protocols and guidelines
- Note disease features and assess their impact on the health of the individual
- Examination of the musculoskeletal system

Telephone helpline
- Information
- Advice/support
- Rapid access to treatment if required
- Progress reports

Drug management
- Gain informed con-sent for treatment
- Explore alternative medicine
- Issue prescription
- Increase dose

Following medical advice*
- Stop medication
- Reduce dose of medicine
- Interpret abnormalities
- Investigate abnormalities
- Order appropriate investigations
- Recognise unwanted effects
- Monitor efficacy

Resource management
- Understanding skills of multidisciplinary team
- Ordering and maintenance of equipment, supplies, educational supplies, etc.
- Awareness of issues surrounding income generation/loss

■ BOX 9.2 (contd)

Research
- Nursing
- Clinical
- Pharmaceutical

Counselling
- All aspects relating to rheumatological diseases and the effects thereof
- Referral and access to specialist agencies

Referral
- Rheumatologist
- Medical specialist*
- Surgical specialist*
- Radiographer*
- Special investigations*
- Occupational therapist
- Physiotherapist
- Surgical appliances

- General practitioner
- Practice nurse
- Phlebotomist
- Chiropodist
- Clinical psychologist
- Social support services
- Community services

*Components of role not yet confirmed.

HOW TO PROGRESS IN NURSING

It is recognised that many types of expertise exist within nursing. At the present time the profession of nursing has not developed sufficiently to be able to offer a definitive, or agreed, framework for determining the level at which a nurse is practising. The profession is unable to provide concise, valid and reliable descriptors, that are generally held and used by all nurses. For example, what is meant precisely by diploma level practice or advanced practice? Many present proposals are incomplete, as they fail to perceive theory and practice as equally important areas or to deal with them as interrelated. In addition, the personal development of the individual nurse has tended to be unrecognised as essential in any professional or academic development undertaken. The synthesis of elements of academic, professional and personal development should be included in any framework for levels of practice.

The concept of specialisation and specialist courses at different levels promotes the notion of a progressive hierarchy of development. Specialisation may be defined as 'a narrow focus on a part of the whole field of nursing. It entails the application of a broad range of theories to selected phenomena within the domain of nursing, in order to secure depth of understanding as a basis for advances in nursing' (American Nurses' Association 1984). The need for nurses who are specialists is proposed as essential (International Council of Nurses 1992). Specialisation enhances professionalism by enabling nurses to communicate and discuss with other disciplines on an equal level of knowledge and understanding. In addition, a developing body of specialist nursing knowledge and expertise clarifies, expands and develops nursing practice. It is therefore essential that post-registration courses are part of future quality assurance initiatives setting the benchmark for achievable criteria in standards of care (Davis 1994).

The growth in the number of specialist nurses is not necessarily to the exclusion of the generalist nurse, although some may argue this to be the case. Specialisation enables the nurturing of special nurses, who are then able to act as consultants to the generalist nurse. A generalist approach may require the acceptance of limited or restricted development in certain elements related to levels of practice.

There now exist, within nursing, many frameworks with which to gauge and recognise the level at which a nurse is practising. Some, such as clinical grading, have not provided the anticipated panacea. Others, such as the Credit Accumulation and Transfer Scheme (CATS) and the Open University's credit scheme from Higher Education, have been introduced from outside nursing. Even these academic frameworks have led to confusion due to their complexity and variety of types that bear no comparison to each other, and therefore are relatively incomparable for rating purposes. There is a need to identify the level at which a nurse is competent and capable.

LEVELS OF PRACTICE WITHIN NURSING

Davis (1994) proposed a way of linking levels of nursing practice to academic qualifications as simple guidance, to enable all nurses to be able to get a 'feel' for what different levels of practice actually mean and to promote discussion. A grid based on levels of academic qualifications was developed in order to produce a more holistic approach (Table 9.1). To bring meaning to the grid, Box 9.3 provides examples of nurses who may be considered as practising at a certain level. The grid could be useful in helping individual rehabilitation nurses to decide what is the most appropriate form and nature of the educational development they require in order to achieve their stated outcomes as part of their professional development.

RESEARCH AND REHABILITATION NURSING

Research continues to acquire an increasing importance in today's nursing. While research should not be ignored, it needs to be kept in perspective. Many nurses see research as a mystical undertaking for other nurses and not for themselves. There are several misconceptions about research and nursing, some of which are listed here.

- Research in nursing means you have to become a nurse researcher or acquire academic qualifications related to research processes.
- Research in nursing is the responsibility of a few elitist nurses and researchers.
- Most research is impossible to implement or utilise.
- Hard facts and figures are always better for developing and describing what nurses do than are personal reflections and intuition.
- If we ignore the issue of research it will go away, like many of the other fads that have been introduced and then disappeared.

As long ago as 1972, the Briggs Report (Department of Health and Social Security 1972) proclaimed that nursing should become a research-based

Table 9.1 Levels of practice

Element	Diploma	Bachelor's degree	Master's degree	Doctoral degree
Characteristics of knowledge	Broad-based overview	Broad and deep. Integration across categories	Focused and comprehensive. Specific	Very specific. New knowledge and theory generated, usually through research
Use of knowledge	Uses a framework to find the right answer	Begins to accept uncertainties	Fully accepts uncertainty	Able to deal with uncertainty
Understanding of ethics	Basic understanding	Recognises principles	Applies principles	Applies and develops principles in a balanced way
Nature of research studies	Critically reviews. Collects data for others. Uses others' evaluation of research. Assists with identification of research problems. Utilises research findings under supervision	Utilises research findings. Understands research process. Critically uses a range of literature to inform practice	Competent in research methods. Undertakes research. Implements research in practice. Collaborates in research studies	Possesses advanced research skills. Leads research-based practice. Postdoctoral: develops and coordinates funded research
Teacher/student relationships	Teacher/student contact high. Course structured by tutor	More able to work alone	Partnership negotiated within a structured curriculum	Tutor supervision, but locus of control with student
Self development and awareness	Perceives expertise as knowing everything about everything	Expects self to be proficient in a wide range of areas in order to be an expert	Begins to understand expertise can only be achieved in a limited number of areas and needs maintaining through continuous practice	Appreciates limited scope of area of expertise and functions within these limits

Table 9.1 (contd)

Element	Diploma	Bachelor's degree	Master's degree	Doctoral degree
Academic communication	Attends conferences	Presents own and others work at local level	Presents own work at national conferences and through journals and books	Presents own work at national and international inter-disciplinary conferences and publishes in peer-reviewed journals
Practice (Benner)	Novice/advanced beginner	Advanced beginner/competent	Proficient/expert	Expert
Professional development	Needs support in practice	Able to work autonomously with appropriate support	Works autonomously. Practice is creative/innovative and based on specialist knowledge	Develops support systems for self and others
PREP stages and CATS level	Initial practice. Period of support following registration. Level 2	Initial/specialist practice. Level 3	Advanced practice. Level M	Consultant practice
Promoting change	Limited understanding of the importance and nature of change	Beginning to understand the importance and nature of change	Supports and promotes change	Initiates and leads change
Management	Little appreciation of role of management and policy-making, although affected by it	Wider appreciation of management issues and policy but limited involvement	Appreciates role of management and policy-making process. May influence decision-making	Makes or directs policy decisions

CATS, Credit Accumulation and Transfer Scheme
PREP, Post-Registration Education and Practice.

■ BOX 9.3 Examples of nursing practice at each level

Diploma

A newly registered nurse, or one returning to nursing, who requires extensive support to determine and achieve her personal and professional developmental goals.

I've been in post now for one month and I know I need to develop my nursing but there is so much to learn and I'm not sure where to start. The staff nurse, who has been qualified for two years, has offered to help me identify priority areas for my development. For example, how to discuss with the new houseman the patient's prescription for analgesics that are inadequate to control the pain after surgery.

Bachelor's degree

An experienced nurse who requires guidance to further her personal and professional developmental goals.

My first formal appraisal is due as I've been in post now for 18 months. My manager and I feel that I've achieved most of the objectives we set a year ago. I'm interested in the lifting and handling of patients, and we both agree that the equipment, and its use, needs reviewing. One of my objectives for next year is to lead and coordinate a ward working group to carry out this review.

Master's degree

A nurse specialist who is seeking to increase the depth of his knowledge and skills in a specific area of nursing.

I've had several posts as a member of different primary healthcare teams. I now know that one of the areas of client care for which I'm responsible would benefit from an in-depth nursing study as I can find no suitable help from previous nursing research. The negotiations I've carried out with other professionals have gone well, but I will continue to work closely with them throughout the study.

Doctoral degree

An expert nurse who is contributing to the knowledge base and influencing the care within a highly specific aspect of nursing.

My expertise has become increasingly focused on a particular aspect of nursing care over the past several years. In collaboration with others I've devised a research programme and acquired the necessary funding. Although I'm supervising a small team of researchers, I realise the need to call on expert advice outside of my area of expertise when appropriate.

profession. But what does a research-based profession mean? It means that we have a professional responsibility to base our nursing on the current acceptable and accessible information (evidence-based practice). This means continually questioning our practice (reflective practice) and then doing something about it by implementing current findings (research utilisation). Both evidence-based practice and research utilisation mean that all nurses need to become research minded, but they do not mean that all nurses need to become researchers.

This approach to nursing and rehabilitation necessitates significant personal development. Basic computer skills are required to search the literature and communicate with colleagues. These skills are relatively easy to learn, but can be frightening when first confronted. A critical, questioning and balanced evaluation of current healthcare research needs to become part of one's working remit. A wide vision and tolerance of others' views needs to be developed. There are often several answers to the same question, many of which may be equally right or equally wrong. It is rare in health care to find a single answer to an issue or question, and many questions are still unanswerable.

THE REHABILITATION NURSING CURRICULUM

Rehabilitation nursing is broad and probably encompasses all aspects of nursing care across the age ranges. This presents a fundamental problem for educators. That is, what do you teach on programmes attended by rehabilitation nurses and how do you teach it? Decisions have to be made concerning the content of programmes (i.e. what should be included or left out). Material that is essential must not be omitted, and other material that is merely relevant or interesting often has to be put aside. These and many more examples of 'curriculum' issues need to be addressed by curriculum designers.

The curriculum for rehabilitation nursing education needs to be balanced. Beattie (1987) proposed a 'four-fold' framework for designing a curriculum to ensure this balance (Fig. 9.1). For example, a curriculum designed around 'key subjects' or 'basic skills' tends to be predetermined and lecturer

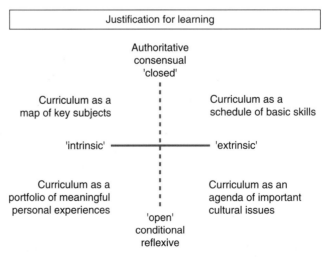

Figure 9.1 Beattie's four-fold curriculum (Beattie 1987).

prescribed, whereas one designed around 'meaningful personal experiences' and 'cultural issues' is based on experience or issues that students bring to the curriculum.

Education for rehabilitation nursing is not the sole responsibility of nurse educators. The nursing profession has traditionally been instrumental in the education of its own nurses. However, recent changes have widened the responsibility to include the corporate organisation, which consists of other healthcare professions and general managers, usually through consortia. In addition, the patient-centred nature of nurse education has been widened to include the participation of the student in shaping the curriculum. There has been a general move towards responding to market demands rather than professional regulation (Humphreys & Quinn 1994). Such rapid and radical changes in the provision of nursing education need to be recognised, confronted and utilised by rehabilitation nurses.

CONCLUSION

If rehabilitation nurses believe they can make a difference, for the better, to patient and client care then they need to grasp the opportunities presented. Rapid change can be threatening but it can also provide opportunities.

In the author's own area of nursing, orthopaedics, these opportunities exist but need to be taken. Santy (1998) describes the current care of elderly patients with fractured necks of femur as inappropriate. The surgery to repair the fracture is relatively straightforward and quick to perform and for the patient to recover from. However, the control of these patients' care is left with the orthopaedic surgeon and acute care orthopaedic nurses for too long. Care should be provided under the umbrella of an interdisciplinary team led by rehabilitation specialists. The significant problems these patients encounter are more chronic and long term in nature, and are not directly related to the initial fracture.

To change the organisation of healthcare provision, as in the example above, requires nurses with vision, confidence and competence. Through continuing education, at all levels, rehabilitation nurses can take the lead with their healthcare colleagues.

REFERENCES

American Nurses' Association 1984 Issues in professional nursing 2: specialisation in nursing practice. Kansas City, ANA
Bailey F C 1992 Some determinants that affect patient participation in decision-making about nursing care. Journal of Advanced Nursing 17:414–421
Beattie A 1987 Making a curriculum work. In: Allan A, Jolley M (eds) The curriculum in nursing education. Croom Helm, London
Benner P 1986 From novice to expert. Addison-Wesley, New York
Castledine G 1996 The role and criteria of an advanced nurse practitioner. British Journal of Nursing (5)5:288–289
Cohen S R 1997 Using a health belief model to promote increased well-being in obese patients with chronic low back pain. Journal of Orthopaedic Nursing 1(2):89–93
Davis P S 1994 How to define levels of practice. Nursing Standard 8(26):32–34
Davis P S 1997 Editorial – Scope of professional practice, opportunity or threat? Journal of Orthopaedic Nursing 1(3):109

Department of Health 1991 Junior doctors. The new deal. Making the best of the skills of nurses and midwives. DoH, London

Department of Health and Social Security 1972 Report of the committee on nursing – Briggs Report. DHSS, London

Dicks B 1996 Qualified success. Nursing Standard 10(48):14

Dowling S, Martin R, Skidmore P, Doyal L, Cameron A, Lloyd S 1996 Nurses takng on junior doctors' work: a confusion of accountability. British Medical Journal 312:1211–1214

Downie R S, Fyfe C, Tannahill A 1990 Health promotion models and values. Oxford University Press, Oxford

English National Board for Nursing, Midwifery and Health Visiting 1994 Creating lifelong learners: partnership for care. ENB, London

Fenton M, Hughes P 1989 Passivity to empowerment. Royal Association for Disability and Rehabilitation, London

Flasher N 1997 Developing the scope of practice for rheumatology nurse practitioners. Journal of Orthopaedic Nursing 1(3):123–126

Humphreys J, Quinn F M 1994 Health care education: towards a corporate paradigm. In: Humphreys J, Quinn F M (eds) Health care education. The challenge of the market. Chapman & Hall, London

Hunt G, Wainwright P 1994 Expanding the role of the nurse. Blackwell Scientific, Oxford

International Council of Nurses 1992 Guidelines on specialisation in nursing. ICN, Geneva

Jester R F 1997 The development and implementation of an orthopaedic pathway for a diploma/masters in health sciences leading to specialist/advanced practitioner status. Journal of Orthopaedic Nursing 1(2):85–88.

Johnson J 1995 Achieving effective rehabilitation outcomes- does the nurse have a role? British Journal of Therapy and Rehabilitation (2)3:113–118

Patterson C, Haddad B 1992 The advanced nurse practitioner: common attributes. Canadian Journal of Nursing Administration 18–22

Robertson A, Minkler M 1994 New health promotion movement: a critical examination. Health Education Quarterly 21(3):295–312

Rosenstock I M, Strecher V J, Becker M H 1998 Social learning theory and the health belief model. Health Education Quarterly 15(2):175–183

Rotter J B 1966 Generalised expectancies for internal versus external locus of control of reinforcement. Psychology Monograph 80:1–28

Santy J 1998 Rehabilitation of the patient with hip fracture – facing the challenge together. Journal of Orthopaedic Nursing 2(1):11–15

Smith R, Draper P 1994 Who is in control? An investigation of nurse and patient beliefs relating to control of their health care. Journal of Advanced Nursing 19:884–892

United Kingdom Central Council for Nurses, Midwives and Health Visitors 1992 The scope of professional practice. UKCC, London

United Kingdom Central Council for Nurses, Midwives and Health Visitors 1994 The future of professional practice – the Council's standards for education and practice following registration. UKKC, London

United Kingdom Central Council for Nurses, Midwives and Health Visitors 1995 PREP and you. UKCC, London

United Kingdom Central Council for Nurses, Midwives and Health Visitors 1996a PREP – the nature of advanced practice. An interim report. UKCC, London

United Kingdom Central Council for Nurses, Midwives and Health Visitors 1996b Guidelines for professional practice. UKCC, London

United Kingdom Central Council for Nurses, Midwives and Health Visitors 1997 Scope in practice. UKCC, London

A framework for developing an orientation programme

Part B

Paul Street

Adjusting to a new clinical area can be an overwhelming and demanding process for the newly appointed staff member (McKane & Schumacher 1997). Moreover, it is increasingly recognised that the provision of support during this process can allow the new member of staff to adjust better to their new clinical area and function more independently, than if they had no formal mechanism to help them achieve this (Kinley 1995). Hence, over the last decade there has been growing emphasis on the provision of orientation programmes to meet this end. However, it is noteworthy that there is much anecdotal activity in relation to the implementation of these programmes, but there is relatively little of this work published. In addition, there does not appear to be any evidence that describes the efficacy of such programmes, providing clear guidance as to development of programmes which are successful in achieving their aim.

Nevertheless, the issue of role adjustment has been highlighted further by the United Kingdom Central Council for Nursing, Midwifery and Health Visiting (UKCC) (Williams, 1997), within the standards for Post Registration Education and Practice (PREP). These state that newly qualified nurses, midwives and health visitors should be provided with a period of preceptor-ship to facilitate the transition from student to qualified practitioner (UKCC 1995). This requirement undoubtedly supports the development of effective orientation programmes that will not only take into account the needs of newly qualified staff, but also the needs of any newly appointed members of staff.

However, it is worth noting that the process of developing and implementing an orientation programme that achieves this is a challenge, and will undoubtedly place demands on the permanent staff within that clinical area (Wallace et al 1997). Therefore, identifying the available resources and planning their effective use is fundamental to ensure that the maximum benefit can be achieved from the programme. Moreover, it is crucial that any orientation programme does actually work in practice, rather than being just a paper exercise and not achieving its goals, otherwise the time and resources used for planning it will be wasted, and both the newly appointed staff member and the preceptor can be left feeling frustrated that the programme offered was not delivered.

The aim of this chapter is to guide the reader through the stages in the process of developing effective orientation programmes.

PLANNING THE DEVELOPMENT OF AN ORIENTATION PROGRAMME

Successful implementation of any initiative in practice is dependent on

■ **BOX 9.4 The aims of the orientation programme**

- Establishing the target group for the programme
- Identifying the resources to support the programme
- Identifying the structure of the programme
- Establishing the content of the programme
- Clarifying responsibilities of the new appointee and the ward staff during the programme
- Teaching and learning strategies
- Documenting the programme
- Preparation and evaluation of the programme

many factors, careful and thorough planning being one (Shaffer & Ward 1990). Implementing a programme too quickly can lead to either you, or the newly appointed person, not being able to meet the demands of the programme, or the programme failing because of a lack of organisation (Kidd & Sturt 1995).

The factors listed in Box 9.4 may help focus your thoughts in planning your programme, as they outline the major areas within development of an orientation programme. It is these issues that form the basis for this chapter, and each is examined in greater detail below.

THE AIMS OF THE ORIENTATION PROGRAMME

It is imperative that the first stage in the process should be the identification of the aims of the programme. This will provide the necessary base on which to structure your programme content, as well as offer outcomes through which evaluation can occur (Wallace et al 1997). As an

■ **BOX 9.5 Example of an orientation programme's aims**

The newly appointed member of staff is able to:

- be welcomed as a valued member of the ward and trust
- settle into the ward and perform his role to the optimum level within a specified period of time
- gain a focus for developing competencies and skills in relation to his practice area
- have a record of clinical time spent with his mentor or preceptor
- identify personal learning needs for the duration of the programme
- gain clinical and peer support from a named preceptor or mentor
- identify his starting point for individual performance review (IPR) beyond the orientation period.

(Reproduced with the kind permission of Colin Way, Lecturer/Practitioner, Paediatric Intensive Care Unit, Guy's Hospital London.)

example, Box 9.5 gives a list of aims adapted from an existing orientation programme in a Paediatric Intensive Care Unit at Guys Hospital which lasts for a period of 4–6 months. Although obviously not from a speciality perceived as having a rehabilitation focus, the aims regarding orientation of new staff are clearly transferable to any situation, despite the differences in content that will be required.

ESTABLISHING THE TARGET GROUP FOR THE PROGRAMME

Resolving this question is quite significant in devising an effective orientation programme, and such decisions need to be made in the early stages of planning (Shaffer & Ward 1990). Consideration needs to be given to the fact that potentially any grade of staff coming to work in a rehabilitation unit, from students to newly qualified nurses and from healthcare assistants to ward managers, will need an orientation programme. The major decision here is whether or not to have several programmes for different grades or have one programme with core and individualised elements. Whichever approach is chosen, you will need to consider what experience, knowledge and competencies are common to all grades, and what is specific to each grade. This will be discussed more fully below, in the section on establishing the content. The approach recommended and followed in the rest of this chapter focuses on a single programme with a core element for all staff and specific parts for individual staff.

ESTABLISHING THE DURATION OF THE PROGRAMME

When planning your orientation programme, you need to be realistic about the length of time over which you could effectively support the programme. There is little point in planning an elaborate 6-month programme if as a team in practice you cannot support one of that length. If an orientation programme is to work it has to be implemented fully and not left half done, as this will not fulfil the aims identified. Lack of completion of the programme will obviously be to the detriment of the new appointee, and the frustration of the persons designing and implementing the programme. Therefore, be realistic about the scope of the programme. Nevertheless, as the UKCC (1995) have stated that preceptorship should be for a period of 3–6 months, it may be worth designing your programme to run over at least 3 months. Then, no matter what grade the newly appointed person is, you will only have to develop one programme, providing the requirements of preceptorship and orientation together.

IDENTIFYING THE RESOURCES TO SUPPORT THE PROGRAMME

One of the first steps in planning an orientation programme is to identify what strategies and resources the ward already has that could help staff settle into their role (Shaffer & Ward 1990). There may be information booklets, you may already offer a mentor, or have a trust induction day. Gathering these together to see what is already available will prevent you from re-inventing the wheel and also give you some content and potential time frames to fit into your programme. Another consideration is the preparation needed by staff currently on the ward in order to implement the programme. For example, if an approach is used where the new appointee is asked to identify his own learning needs and write them as objectives as part of his programme, the staff in the ward will also need to be familiar with:

- setting objectives
- the content of the orientation programme
- the resources available that the new appointee may be directed to use.

Some of these issues will be resolved if the ward staff are involved in the development of the programme, as they will be familiar with its content. The ownership which this should create may encourage the ward staff to be more able and willing to ensure that the new appointee receives the help and guidance he needs during the implementation of the programme.

Furthermore, it is of importance to establish what staff time is available to support the development and implementation of the programme, as this will affect the duration of the programme and how the content is structured. If it is not possible to release the time of a current member of staff to act as a mentor, then the content of the programme may need to be highly structured and informative to facilitate the newly appointed staff finding out for themselves. In addition, the content would have to reflect how the supernumerary status of the newly appointed person will be managed (if it is going to be offered in the programme). The resources required to produce the programme also need to be considered (Messmer et al 1995). For example, if you intend to have a printed document or booklet, establishing who will produce it and what form of presentation it will take have to be considered, because both these factors have cost implications. This is discussed later when exploring documenting the programme.

IDENTIFYING THE STRUCTURE OF THE PROGRAMME

The essence of the programme needs a structure for the new appointee and existing staff to work around (Staab et al 1996). Structuring the content into the core and individual elements, and assigning priorities for these elements to be met, will give a basic framework. Possible approaches would be to list everything you consider essential for any new member of staff to know, and through the use of a staff questionnaire, to validate these. The areas of content thus identified can then be prioritised, and placed into the time frame you have decided for the programme. For example, you could identify what should be completed by the end of the first day, first week, etc., considering these priorities both from your own and the newly appointed person's perspective. The resources needed to support each of the elements of the programme can then be identified. Alternatively, you could use an existing appropriate framework to form the basis of the structure of your programme. The list of activities could then be formulated, placing and prioritising them under the headings in the framework. There may be some advantages in using a predetermined framework to structure your programme because it may also have other uses (e.g. demonstrating that you are implementing your trust's nursing strategy from the trust objectives). Another alternative could be to underpin an orientation programme with the ten key characteristics proposed by the English National Board of Nursing, Midwifery and Health Visiting (ENB) within their Higher Award. This may allow the orientation programme to be transferred directly into a Higher Award portfolio. However, it is worth pointing out that any defined framework you use to structure your programme can perhaps be used as part of the newly appointed staff member's personal professional portfolio required for re-registration and PREP.

The following are examples which could be used as frameworks to underpin, or as documents to inform, an orientation programme.

- Local frameworks and documents:
  - ward philosophy
  - local strategies (quality, education and training)
  - trust objectives
  - PERM (practice, education, research and management).

- National and professional documents:
  - *Vision for the Future* (National Health Service Management Executive 1993)
  - *ENB 10 Key Characteristics* (ENB 1991)
  - *From Novice to Expert* (Benner 1984).

For example, the PERM framework could be used, including some of the following under each of the framework elements as part of the programme.

- Practice:
  - emergency procedures
  - competency in aspects of care
  - explaining the model of care used.

- Education:
  - the new appointee to identify their own learning needs
  - familiarisation with the education and development available within the trust
  - strategies demonstrating education development (e.g. if the ward/unit supports the appointee on courses he has to perform at least one teaching session on the ward per semester).

- Research:
  - awareness of when the local research group meets, or when the wards hold their journal club.

- Management:
  - the management and organisation of self
  - reporting sickness
  - the appraisal or individual performance review (IPR) system.

ESTABLISHING THE CONTENT OF THE PROGRAMME

The aim of an orientation programme is to allow new staff to function at their optimal level within a set period of time following their appointment (McKane & Schumacher 1997). Therefore, any programme will require a balance of ward-set and individually defined learning objectives or competencies (Staab et al 1996). This balance will ensure not only that new members of staff have the required knowledge and skills to function safely, but also that they have the opportunity to develop the areas of knowledge or practice of interest or importance to them as individuals (Lockhart & Bryce 1996). Although each grade of nurse will have different needs to some degree, there will be many shared elements. Therefore, devising a programme with core and individualised elements should ensure that fundamental competencies and individual issues are covered in the programme.

These fundamental competencies will form part of the content directed by the ward and should include all the elements of care/management that you require of your staff, for them to be able to perform their role (Staab et al 1996). This core content will also include statutory and compulsory training (e.g. fire and resuscitation), as well as the basic nursing skills required in the particular rehabilitation speciality. To aid the identification of this type of content, a review of the job descriptions, ward philosophy, standards and policies can all inform the process. As well as these core elements required by all staff, in addition the knowledge and competencies specific to the new appointee's grade must be defined. Devising a simple survey questionnaire or obtaining views at a ward meeting or multigrade working group on the ward could all achieve this end. This itself does, of course, require time and resources, but can be very beneficial to the programme and its implementation, again by providing a sense of ownership and realism. Further information may be gained if this consultation is interprofessional and not exclusive to nursing. This is obviously the case within rehabilitation environments, as the emphasis is so much on the importance of an interdisciplinary approach.

The second aspect in the content for the programme is derived from the individual needs of the newly appointed staff member. This element will provide the necessary individualisation of the programme to meet the specific needs of each newly appointed member of staff. As the newly appointed staff member must be able to identify what it is he wants to know and experience in order to function well in his role, some degree of experience of the new situation may be necessary. Therefore, the setting of individual learning objectives may be planned to take place after a period of time (e.g. 2 weeks after commencing the new post). This flexibility in the programme is required because a newly registered nurse may have concerns about the administration of drugs alone or the management of the ward, whereas a newly appointed ward manager may be more concerned with familiarising himself with managing the ward budget or the mechanisms for devising new policies. Not only must this element of the programme include time for the newly appointed person to reflect and think about his own learning needs, but it must also aid in identifying his future learning needs once the programme has been completed.

RESPONSIBILITIES OF THE NEW APPOINTEE AND THE WARD STAFF DURING THE PROGRAMME

There is a strong influence in contemporary nursing and education of self-directed study, with individuals being responsible for their own learning (Hinchliff 1992). However, this needs to be put in the context of orientating someone to a new organisation; if left to find everything out for themselves, the time spent doing this may not only be expensive (Messmer et al 1995), but also may not be entirely successful. Therefore, the ward staff and the new appointee share the responsibility to some degree. Within the structure of the programme it must be stated who is responsible for each element of the programme. For example:

- identifying learning needs in week 2 of the programme would be the responsibility of the new appointee
- showing the new nurse around the hospital may be the responsibility of any member of staff
- explaining the IPR system may be the responsibility of a senior member of staff.

Box 9.6 provides more examples, but it is worth noting that many aspects may be shared by the new appointee and his mentor, including that of shared responsibility for operationalising the elements of the programme.

The UKCC (1995) standards for re-registration clearly state that each nurse, midwife and health visitor must maintain a record of their development within a portfolio. This portfolio is, of course, confidential to each nurse. However, through encouraging the process of reflection, the planning required in developing a portfolio will facilitate each nurse to some degree in identifying personal areas of development. The same applies to the individual performance review and personal development plan, as these also require the individual to identify areas of strength and areas for development.

TEACHING AND LEARNING STRATEGIES

Some educational theorists suggest that adopting a variety of teaching and learning styles within an individual teaching session and programme of study help the learner understand the subject more quickly than if just one method is used (Ogier 1989, Reece & Walker 1997). Approaches may include:

- departmental visits or exchanges
- shadowing or supervised practice
- reflection
- action planing
- allocated library time

■ **BOX 9.6 Example format for an orientation programme**

Elements to be completed on day 1 of your orientation programme	Resource person responsible	Date and signature when completed
1. Introduction to ward team	Any staff member	
2. Tour of the ward	Any staff member	
3. Explanation of orientation programme	Mentor	
4. Book CPR and fire training. Resuscitation officer Ms A. Heart, ext. 9090; fire officer Mr Ve Ryhot, ext. 2323	New appointee	
5. Identify individual learning needs for week 1	New appointee	
6. Negotiate individual learning needs with mentor, and identify time, resources and people to fulfil the needs	New appointee and mentor	
7. Time to address the individual learning need of: (state a topic/area specific to the individual needs)	New appointee and mentor. Appropriate other person	

- self-directed study
- guided study packs
- informal teaching sessions
- formal lectures.

Getting the balance right here will affect the use of resources, while making the programme more varied and enjoyable, but this does require additional planning and negotiation with the relevant people you want to involve. Once again these strategies should be identified within the programme.

DOCUMENTING THE PROGRAMME

The simplest way to do this is to have a formal document stating the elements of the orientation (Box 9.7), as this makes it quite explicit what is to be covered and by whom. This would have the advantage of providing clear expectations, as well as a clear record of the orientation. This record can then be used within the newly appointed staff member's portfolio. In addition, it allows simple auditing of whether the programme is being

■ BOX 9.7 Sample content of an orientation programme based on the PERM model

Month 1	Month 2	Month 3
Practice		
Emergency telephone numbers and procedures	Visit practice development team	Visit the nurse executive
Local guidelines for practice		
Care planning and computerised nurse information systems		
Philosophy of care, nursing model and care delivery system		
Observing multi-professional meetings	Participating in multi-professional meetings	Leading multi-professional meetings
Providing care to level of competency (supernumerary)	Providing care to level of competency	Providing care to level of competency
Liaison with other departments		
Identify individual competencies as practice learning needs	Identify individual competencies as practice learning needs	Identify individual competencies as practice learning needs for month 3 and the next year within IPR
Time to develop the above competencies	Time to develop the above competencies	Time to develop the above competencies
Education		
Identification of individual learning needs	Visit university	Contribute to the ward teaching programme
Aware of link lecturer	Identify trust learning resources (libraries, CD ROMS, etc.)	
Study-leave request		

■ BOX 9.7 (contd)

Month 1	Month 2	Month 3
Identifying individual competencies as educational learning needs	Identifying individual competencies as educational learning needs	Identifying individual competencies as educational learning needs for month 3, and the next year within IPR
Time to develop the above competencies	Time to develop the above competencies	Time to develop the above competencies
Research Ward audit programme	Clinical audit department Attend ward journal club	Attend hospital/ university research seminars Identify future audit/ research project
Identify individual competencies as research learning needs	Identify individual competencies as research learning needs	Identify individual competencies as research learning needs for month 3, and the next year within IPR
Time to develop the above competencies	Time to develop the above competencies	Time to develop the above competencies
Management Supernumerary status Sign human resources starting details Identity badge and uniforms Tour of the ward, directorate and trust	Supervised practice	Independent practice
Organisation of the ward Duty rostering and requests, annual leave entitlement		

■ BOX 9.7 (contd)

Month 1	Month 2	Month 3
Polices and procedures Complaints and compliments Identifying specific competencies as management learning needs	Identifying specific competencies as management learning needs	Identifying specific competencies as management learning needs for month 3 and for the next year within IPR
Time to develop the above competencies	Time to develop the above competencies	Time to develop the above competencies
Evaluation of month 1	Evaluation of month 2	Evaluation of total programme and initial IPR

completed and areas that may need to be re-examined. The documentation also provides evidence for the ward manager to command resources, as it demonstrates both the time and resources required for the training that is being provided by the staff on the ward. It also provides a record for the ward manager of the training that each individual has within their orientation. Documenting the individualised elements could easily be done by devising a learning contract to be included in the package, this stating what the individual needs to learn, when they will achieve this by, how they will go about doing this, and how they will know when they have successfully completed it.

Some hospitals produce the orientation programme in paperback book form, while others produce an A4 booklet, which can be easily photocopied. If there is an information technology department or reprographics department, they may be able to help make the format attractive, but may make a charge for this. If so, identifying money from your budget is important beforehand. However, if you have access to a personal computer, either on the ward, in a library or at home, this may provide the easiest way to produce the document. Remember though that you and your time are resources, so how long it will take you to produce the programme and where the computer is located must be taken into account (e.g. do you have to leave the ward to use the computer?). This option is probably the easiest one, as it allows you to update and change the programme to reflect changes in the ward and environment from staff completing the programme.

PREPARATION AND EVALUATION OF THE PROGRAMME

The time to start planning an orientation programme is not the night before your newly appointed member of staff is about to start. You will need to review the current situation, pull together resources, plan your content, produce the document, and ensure that your staff are aware of their involvement in the programme. Give yourself at least 3 months to plan and formulate your programme. During that time, regularly gain feedback from other members of the ward team and those who may be involved in the implementation or resourcing of your programme. Seek the help of other members in the trust (e.g. practice development nurses, link lecturers, quality department, human resources advisors, and other discipline team members). These staff will be able to help you prepare both the content of the programme and your staff for its implementation.

Evaluation needs to be planned for before the programme starts (Kidd & Sturt 1995). It is worth considering including a pre- and post-programme questionnaire in the orientation package; this will demonstrate the newly appointed person's expectations and then whether they have been fulfilled or not. Gaining advice from your research nurse or clinical audit department may provide you with some sound advice concerning the evaluation. However, it is worth contacting them at the beginning of the planning so that the method chosen for evaluation is built into the programme, rather than trying to evaluate something after the event and then realising you have not included something vital. As previously stated returning to the aims of the programme can provide a simple evaluation. Remember, hindsight is useful, but foresight is even better, so plan now for all stages of the orientation process and the development of the programme.

SUMMARY

The orientation of new staff to a clinical area is a vital component in the education of nurses. Clearly this has relevance to any nursing situation. However, it is especially pertinent in a rehabilitation environment, where the client often presents with complex problems and needs, and there is often a large team of professionals involved in delivering the service.

This chapter has aimed to provide the reader with a framework through which effectively to develop and implement an orientation programme. Not only will this result in a happier, more prepared workforce, but of course most importantly it will assist in the provision of high-quality nursing to the individuals we serve.

REFERENCES

Benner P 1984 From novice to expert: excellence and power in clinical nursing practice. Addison-Wesley, Menlo Park

English National Board of Nursing, Midwifery and Health Visiting 1991 ENB framework for continuing professional education for nurses, midwives and health visitors: guide to implementation (Summary card 1: 10 key characteristics). ENB, London

Hinchliff S 1992 The practitioner as teacher. Scutari, London

Kidd P, Sturt P 1995 Developing and evaluating an emergency nursing orientation pathway. Journal of Emergency Nursing 21(6):521–530

Kinley H 1995 Defining role models for staff orientation. Nursing Standard 10(8):27–29

Lockhart J S, Bryce J B 1996 A comprehensive plan to meet the unit based educational needs of nurses from several speciality units. Journal of Staff Development 12(3):135–138

McKane C L, Schumacher L 1997 Professional advancement model for critical care orientation. Journal of Nursing Staff Development 13(2):88–92

Messmer P R, Abelleria A, Erb P 1995 Code 50: an orientation matrix to track orientation cost. Journal of Staff Development 11(5):261–264

National Health Service Management Executive 1993 A vision for the future: the nursing, midwifery and health visiting contribution to health and health care. Department of Health, London

Ogier M E 1989 Working and learning: the learning environment in clinical nursing. Scutari, London

Reece I, Walker S 1997 A practical guide to teaching, training and learning, 2nd edn. Business Education, Sunderland

Shaffer A, Ward C 1990 Designing an orientation preceptorship: development, delivery and evaluation. Journal of Emergency Nursing 16(6):408–411

Staab S, Granneman S, Page-Reachr T 1996 Examining competency based orientation implementation. Journal of Staff Development 12(3):139–143

United Kingdom Central Council for Nursing, Midwifery and Health Visiting 1995 PREP and you: maintaining your registration and standards for education following registration. UKCC, London

Wallace K G, Graham K M, Venture M R, Burke R 1997 Lessons learnt in implementing a staff education programme in the acute care setting. Journal of Nursing Staff Development 13(1):24–31

Williams D 1997 Precpetorship for RGN's in a small community hospital. Nursing Times 1(6):2–3

Directions for rehabilitation in adult nursing practice

10

Mike Smith

INTRODUCTION

The focus of this chapter is the potential future changes in health care and nursing globally, and how these relate to rehabilitation in general nursing. The aim is to prepare the nurse for actual and potential future changes.

No one could fail to recognise the ever-changing nature of the provision of health care. Influences are many, including:

- changes in nursing
- government policy
- improving technology
- increasing expectations from clients and, potentially, professionals
- changing emphasis from acute to community services.

Add to these the desire for change in rehabilitation and in nursing within a rehabilitation setting, and it can be seen that an environment and culture has developed in which change is constant. All the authors in this book, through their suggestions on improving rehabilitation in adult nursing practice, have, in essence, prescribed the way forward, and therefore the desired future for rehabilitation. Overall it is clear that nursing must state and strengthen its position as the provider of rehabilitation. Nursing is an important, and indeed in most cases an essential, discipline within the provision of rehabilitation services. Not only does nursing bring many skills to the rehabilitation environment, but its unique way of working and, more implicitly, the skills which it can bring are vital.

THE NATURE OF CHANGE – AN OVERVIEW

Before reiterating the specific points raised by the contributors to this book, it is worth briefly revisiting some general issues about change itself.

The primary impact of change on a team and its individuals results in a change in behaviour. Change challenges, and requires adjustment from, familiar and traditional ways of approaching working practice and thinking. People facing change may experience a series of negative emotions (anger, denial, frustration and resignation) (Herzberg et al 1959). It is hardly suprising that the rapid change to which the National Health Service (NHS) has been subjected has resulted in a demotivation to change rehabilitation nursing practice. It has been suggested that people must be allowed to let go of the old way of doing things in a manner that maintains their self-esteem (Chaudhry Lawton & Lawton 1992). However this is surely increasingly difficult as one change is followed by another in quick succession. As morale and motivation are negatively influenced by the threat to self-esteem, the desire to participate in and embrace further change must logically diminish. This view was reinforced by Buchholz & Roth (1982), who stated: 'Past experiences and present beliefs can negatively affect group members' willingness to change.' It has also been suggested that resistance to change may have more to do with having the change imposed than the change itself, a situation most readers will be able to identify with within the NHS.

However, as change is a fact of life (Peters 1994), we must accept and even embrace it, and be proactive in our approaches, exploring new and innovative ways of working for the client's good and for the good of the profession. Promoting understanding and acceptance of this principle, both on an individual nurse and a team basis, is fundamental to managing change.

There is an apparent consensus among the authors mentioned above that a key factor in the successful implementation of change is the involvement of the people actually affected by the change (Buchholz & Roth 1982, Peters 1994). This should include an understanding of the need for change, as well as participating in and defining the nature of the change. This understanding is wholly dependent on the provision of accurate and comprehensive information as change is a learning experience for individuals. The fact that individuals learn at different rates may necessitate reinforcement and clarification, both at the commencement of and at regular intervals throughout the implementation of any change.

Such theories of change are applicable to most working environments and the need to develop rehabilitation nursing practice through some of the changes suggested within this text make them equally applicable to our situation.

CHANGES IN REHABILITATION NURSING

Based on the tradition of caring, which by its nature brings us close to the client, providing a continuous supply of this 'care', all nursing is fundamentally about rehabilitation if one looks at the premise on which this book is based. Even in the areas perceived as 'acute', the rehabilitation process actually begins as soon as an injury occurs or an illness is diagnosed.

Clearly there are specialties in which rehabilitation is more complex and requires the aggregation of expertise of specialist centres (e.g. neurorehabilitation and spinal cord injury). The role of these areas should be one of leading development and research and creating benchmarks of good rehabilitation practice, to enable other areas to develop tools that are applicable to their own clinical environment.

In Chapter 2, six key roles involved in nursing the patient undergoing rehabilitation were identified. Although some roles are already established to some degree, even these need to be reinforced and highlighted, not only to other professionals working within health care but also within nursing itself.

There are three overall issues that need to be addressed as a starting point.

1. The general belief that nursing has a lesser importance than other disciplines within rehabilitation needs to be quashed.

2. Greater guidance and direction from specialist rehabilitation centres is required, internally through effective dissemination (i.e. practising what is preached), and externally through the provision of expertise to other areas.

3. The focus of research should be moved from the apparent preoccupation with who we are, to what we do and could actually achieve as nurses within rehabilitation. I would suggest that this book and other similar texts offer sufficient guidance to actually start putting things into practice. Clearly, we need the relevant knowledge to underpin and rationalise nursing practice. However, in addition to this knowledge, practical advice is required to make the difference. This again was one of the primary aims of this book.

There are clear messages in each of the chapters in this book, many of which may involve a move away from traditional ways of working. Such moves will surely directly and positively influence the meeting of client needs, and strengthen rather than weaken nursing. This fact may help the reader through difficult times of change.

In Chapter 1 the principles underpinning rehabilitation were discussed. A definition of the key aims, expectations and characteristics of rehabilitation comprises the vital first stage in developing effective and meaningful rehabilitation services. Key characteristics were proposed, and include empowerment, independence, reduction of disability and handicap, and a client-centred approach. It is these factors on which rehabilitation nursing should be based.

In Chapter 2 the need to recognise the expertise that is inherent in nursing and to use this to its full potential was highlighted. Claiming different roles for nursing may upset some colleagues from other disciplines. However, if the process is managed properly, emphasising that some aspects of rehabilitation are nurse-led and that in others the nurse is involved in implementing interventions prescribed by others, may appease those struggling with the concept of nursing having a strong voice and clear direction. These issues were further explored in the discussion of the rehabilitation nurse as a technical expert and provider of care in Chapter 5.

Chapter 3 focused on the role of educator within rehabilitation. Although many areas have recognised and implemented programmes of patient and carer education, it is clear that some have not. Education is a fundamental component of rehabilitation, as it is congruous with the concepts of empowerment and gaining independence, and so needs to be formalised. Therefore, the evaluation of existing programmes and the development of new ones to meet current deficits in provision is vital.

Chapter 4 promoted the vital role of the nurse in providing psychological support for the client following illness or injury. Nursing will continue to fail in its desire to provide meaningful psychological care, until the lip-service given to this need is transformed into positive action. Educational institutions involved in the provision of nursing education have let nursing down in the lack of effective training for this role. Not only must psychological care be provided, but we must also develop ways to document this care. This is often the only means by which we can demonstrate that we are providing a service, and so we need such documentation in order to justify our working practices. In addition, the development of specialist nursing roles can not only contribute to the provision of improved client outcome, but can also benefit the profession as a whole.

The focus of Chapter 6 was our role as team workers, not only within a team of nurses but also within the wider team of rehabilitation professionals who are involved in the provision of rehabilitation services.

The need for the recognition of the value of the healthcare assistant was explored in Chapter 8. The need for appropriate and structured use (rather than abuse) of such assistants was emphasised. This will ensure that standards of care continue to be met, and will enable nursing to develop to its full potential. A great deal of the problem has been created by lack of direction from the professional bodies in nursing, and this has contributed to the situation of the nursing profession often perceiving the health care assistant as a threat rather than an opportunity. This view *must* change.

Chapter 9 focused on the education of rehabilitation nurses from two perspectives. First, the opportunities available for education and the principles underpinning the development of both the individual and the profession were outlined. Second, practically orientated guidelines were given, through which the clinical area can provide meaningful orientation and development of newer nurses to rehabilitation, not only facilitating their development but also having a direct relationship to quality nursing. Education for rehabilitation nursing is vital, and indeed is pivotal in facilitating the development of both individual nurses and nursing specialities.

Finally, for senior nursing colleagues, rehabilitation nursing itself must be empowered through creative and supportive leadership. Nurse managers must enable nursing to develop and promote such a service as being to the benefit of the population it serves. Nursing managers are, after all fundamentally responsible for fighting the nursing corner in allowing developments to happen.

WHERE DO WE START IN DEVELOPING REHABILITATION NURSING?

On a national basis:

- recognise what we are achieving (give a national pat on the back for what nursing has achieved and continues to achieve)
- benchmark optimum practice through specialist groups (e.g. the Royal College of Nursing rehabilitation nurses forum)
- disseminate information to all nurses by creating a national

network that encompasses more than just specialist rehabilitation units

- continue with the development of standards and research which will positively impact on rehabilitation nursing.

Within your clinical area:

- recognise what you are achieving (provide a pat on the back for what you have achieved as a ward team)
- identify deficits in current practices
- prioritise action areas
- create meaningful alliances, so spreading the load (work with clinical areas both within the organisation in which you work and those local to your area); delegate different areas of practice development, openly sharing results and experiences
- be realistic in the pace of the change you desire, but hold firm to your vision for rehabilitation nursing even in the tougher times (and there will be some).

Finally the author would encourage all nurses to shout from the rooftops that nursing is valuable and should be valued within rehabilitation. No one should convince us otherwise. While doing this we need to demonstrate to those who may doubt the value of nursing that we are as good as we know we are through evidence of effectiveness. Happy rehabilitating.

REFERENCES

Buchholz S, Roth T 1982 Focused on the future – is change really a change? In: Creating the high-performance team. Wilson Learning Corporation/Wiley, New York, ch 6, pp 91–109
Chaudhry Lawton R, Lawton R 1992. There has to be a better way. In: Ignition – sparking organisational change. BCA, London, ch 3, pp 71–101
Herzberg F, Maisner B, Snyderman B 1959 The motivation to work. Wiley, New York
Peters T 1994 Beyond decentralisation. In: The Tom Peters seminar – crazy times call for crazy organisations. Macmillan, London, ch 2, pp 25–63

Index

About the
PROFESSIONAL DEVELOPMENT RECORD

The United Kingdom Central Council (UKCC) PREP regulations require you to maintain a personal professional portfolio, in which you record evidence of your professional development.

This book provides you with excellent educational material to assist your study and develop your practice. Reading all or parts of it can contribute to your professional development.

The *Professional Development Record* (overleaf) is designed to help you record your study activity in your portfolio and show how it has enhanced your practice. To use the Record, you can do either of the following:

- photocopy the Record and place it directly into your portfolio, or

- use it as a basis for your own individual entry.

The aim of the Record is to help you plan how this book assists your professional development, to the benefit of yourself, your colleagues and your patients/clients.

Further information:

- If you do not have a portfolio and would like to purchase one, please contact your local bookseller or, in case of difficulty, phone our Customer Services Department on 0181 308 5710.

- If you need further information about PREP, you should contact the UKCC on: 0171 333 6550.

PROFESSIONAL DEVELOPMENT RECORD

Book (fill in author, title, year of publication, publisher):

Date of completion of book (or selections from book):

Duration of study time:

Reason for reading the book:

Intended learning outcomes:

Evaluation of material read:

Planned influence on practice:

Evaluation of influence on practice:

Learning outcomes achieved: